Gastroparesis

Editors

HENRY P. PARKMAN
PANKAJ JAY PASRICHA

GASTROENTEROLOGY
CLINICS OF NORTH AMERICA

www.gastro.theclinics.com

Consulting Editor
GARY W. FALK

March 2015 • Volume 44 • Number 1

ELSEVIER

1600 John F. Kennedy Boulevard • Suite 1800 • Philadelphia, Pennsylvania, 19103-2899
http://www.theclinics.com

GASTROENTEROLOGY CLINICS OF NORTH AMERICA Volume 44, Number 1
March 2015 ISSN 0889-8553, ISBN-13: 978-0-323-35656-5

Editor: Kerry Holland
Developmental Editor: Susan Showalter

Gastroenterology Clinics of North America (ISSN 0889-8553) is published quarterly by Elsevier Inc., 360 Park Avenue South, New York, NY 10010-1710. Months of issue are March, June, September, and December. Business and Editorial Offices: 1600 John F. Kennedy Blvd., Suite 1800, Philadelphia, PA 19103-2899. Customer Service Office: 6277 Sea Harbor Drive, Orlando, FL 32887-4800. Periodicals postage paid at New York, NY and additional mailing offices. Subscription prices are $320.00 per year (US individuals), $160.00 per year (US students), $530.00 per year (US institutions), $350.00 per year (Canadian individuals), $651.00 per year (Canadian institutions), $445.00 per year (international individuals), $220.00 per year (international students), and $651.00 per year (international institutions). Foreign air speed delivery is included in all *Clinics* subscription prices. All prices are subject to change without notice. **POSTMASTER**: Send address changes to *Gastroenterology Clinics of North America*, Elsevier Health Sciences Division, Subscription Customer Service, 3251 Riverport Lane, Maryland Heights, MO 63043. Telephone: 1-800-654-2452 (U.S. and Canada); 314-447-8871 (outside U.S. and Canada). Fax: 314-447-8029. E-mail: journalscustomerservice-usa@elsevier.com (for print support); journalsonlinesupport-usa@elsevier.com (for online support).

Reprints. For copies of 100 or more, of articles in this publication, please contact the Commercial Reprints Department, Elsevier Inc., 360 Part Avenue South, New York, New York 10010-1710. Tel. 212-633-3874, Fax: 212-633-3820, E-mail: reprints@elsevier.com.

Gastroenterology Clinics of North America is also published in Italian by Il Pensiero Scientifico Editore, Rome, Italy; and in Portuguese by Interlivros Edicoes Ltda., Rua Commandante Coelho 1085, 21250 Cordovil, Rio de Janeiro, Brazil.

Gastroenterology Clinics of North America is covered in *MEDLINE/PubMed (Index Medicus), Excerpta Medica, Current Contents/Clinical Medicine, Science Citation Index, ISI/BIOMED*, and *BIOSIS*.

Contributors

CONSULTING EDITOR

GARY W. FALK, MD, MS
Professor of Medicine, Division of Gastroenterology, Hospital of the University of Pennsylvania, University of Pennsylvania Perelman School of Medicine, Philadelphia, Pennsylvania

EDITORS

HENRY P. PARKMAN, MD
Professor of Medicine, and Director, GI Motility Laboratory, School of Medicine, Temple University, Temple University Hospital, Philadelphia, Pennsylvania

PANKAJ JAY PASRICHA, MD
Director, Department of Medicine, Johns Hopkins Center for Neurogastroenterology; Professor of Medicine and Neurosciences, Johns Hopkins School of Medicine; Professor of Innovation Management, Johns Hopkins Carey School of Business, Baltimore, Maryland

AUTHORS

THOMAS L. ABELL, MD, FACP
Division of Gastroenterology, GI Motility Clinic, University of Louisville, Louisville, Kentucky

ANDRES ACOSTA, MD, PhD
Clinical Enteric Neuroscience Translational and Epidemiological Research (C.E.N.T.E.R.); Fellow, Division of Gastroenterology and Hepatology, Mayo Clinic, Rochester, Minnesota

ADIL E. BHARUCHA, MBBS, MD
Professor of Medicine, Clinical Enteric Neuroscience Translational and Epidemiological Research Program, Division of Gastroenterology and Hepatology, Mayo Clinic, Rochester, Minnesota

JORGE CALLES-ESCANDÓN, MD
Professor of Internal Medicine, Chief, Section on Endocrinology, MetroHealth Regional, Case Western Reserve University School of Medicine, Cleveland, Ohio

MICHAEL CAMILLERI, MD
Clinical Enteric Neuroscience Translational and Epidemiological Research (C.E.N.T.E.R.); Professor of Medicine, Pharmacology and Physiology, Mayo Clinic, Rochester, Minnesota

JIANDE CHEN, PhD
Director, Clinical Motility Lab, Professor of Medicine, Division of Gastroenterology and Hepatology, Johns Hopkins University School of Medicine, Baltimore, Maryland

JOHN O. CLARKE, MD
Associate Professor of Medicine, Division of Gastroenterology & Hepatology, Johns Hopkins University, Baltimore, Maryland

BRIAN DAVIS, MD
Department of Surgery, Paul L. Foster School of Medicine, Texas Tech University Health Sciences Center, El Paso, Texas

EVELIN EICHLER, MS, RD, LD
Division of Gastroenterology, Founding Chair, Department of Internal Medicine, Paul L. Foster School of Medicine, Texas Tech University Health Sciences Center, El Paso, Texas

GIANRICO FARRUGIA, MD
Enteric NeuroScience Program, Mayo Clinic, Rochester, Minnesota

WILLIAM L. HASLER, MD
Professor, Division of Gastroenterology, University of Michigan Health System, Ann Arbor, Michigan

KENNETH L. KOCH, MD
Professor of Internal Medicine, Chief, Section on Gastroenterology, Wake Forest School of Medicine, Winston-Salem, North Carolina

LINDA A. LEE, MD
Associate Professor of Medicine, Division of Gastroenterology and Hepatology, Director, Johns Hopkins Integrative Medicine & Digestive Center, Johns Hopkins University School of Medicine, Lutherville, Maryland

RICHARD W. McCALLUM, MD
Division of Gastroenterology, Department of Internal Medicine, Paul L. Foster School of Medicine, Texas Tech University Health Sciences Center, El Paso, Texas

LINDA ANH NGUYEN, MD
Division of Gastroenterology, Department of Medicine, Stanford University, Palo Alto, California

GREGORY O'GRADY, MBChB, PhD, FRACS
Department of Surgery, University of Auckland, Auckland, New Zealand

HENRY P. PARKMAN, MD
Professor of Medicine, and Director, GI Motility Laboratory, School of Medicine, Temple University, Temple University Hospital, Philadelphia, Pennsylvania

CAROL REES PARRISH, MS, RD
Nutrition Support Specialist, Digestive Health Center, University of Virginia Health System, Charlottesville, Virginia

PANKAJ JAY PASRICHA, MD
Director, Department of Medicine, Johns Hopkins Center for Neurogastroenterology; Professor of Medicine and Neurosciences, Johns Hopkins School of Medicine; Professor of Innovation Management, Johns Hopkins Carey School of Business, Baltimore, Maryland

EAMONN M.M. QUIGLEY, MD, FRCP, FACP, FACG, FRCPI
David M Underwood Chair of Medicine in Digestive Disorders; Professor of Medicine, Weill Cornell Medical College; Chief, Division of Gastroenterology and Hepatology, Houston Methodist Hospital, Weill Cornell Medical College, Houston, Texas

IRENE SAROSIEK, MD
Division of Gastroenterology, Department of Internal Medicine, Paul L. Foster School of Medicine, Texas Tech University Health Sciences Center, El Paso, Texas

WILLIAM J. SNAPE Jr, MD
Division of Gastroenterology, Department of Medicine, California Pacific Medical Center, San Francisco, California

JIEYUN YIN, MD
Research Investigator, Veterans Research and Education Foundation, VA Medical Center, Oklahoma City, Oklahoma

Contents

Gastroparesis is a chronic symptomatic disorder of the stomach characterized by delayed emptying without evidence of mechanical obstruction.
Symptoms of gastroparesis include nausea, vomiting, early satiety,
postprandial fullness, and upper abdominal pain. The 3 main causes are
diabetic, postsurgical, and idiopathic. Diagnosis is confirmed by demonstrating delayed gastric emptying. Gastric emptying rates measured by
gastric motor testing generally correlate poorly with symptoms and quality
of life in patients with gastroparesis. It may be appropriate to reconsider the
definition of gastroparesis, recognizing it as a broader spectrum of gastric
neuromuscular dysfunction.

Gastroparesis is characterized by delayed gastric emptying and symptoms
thereof in the absence of gastric outlet obstruction. Most studies on the
epidemiology of gastroparesis have been conducted in selected case series rather than in the population at large. In the only community-based
study of gastroparesis in diabetes mellitus (DM), the average cumulative
incidence of symptoms and delayed gastric emptying over 10 years was
higher in type 1 DM (5%) than in type 2 DM (1%) and controls (1%). In
the United States, the incidence of hospitalizations related to gastroparesis
increased substantially between 1995 and 2004, and particularly after
2000.

Gastroparesis is a heterogeneous disorder defined by delay in gastric
emptying. Symptoms of gastroparesis are nonspecific, including nausea,
vomiting, early satiety, bloating, and/or abdominal pain. Normal gastric motor function and sensory function depend on a complex coordination between the enteric and central nervous system. This article discusses the
pathophysiology of delayed gastric emptying and the symptoms of gastroparesis, including antropyloroduodenal dysmotility, impaired gastric accommodation, visceral hypersensitivity, and autonomic dysfunction. The
underlying pathophysiology of gastroparesis is complex and multifactorial.

The article discusses how a combination of these factors leads to symptoms of gastroparesis.

The cellular abnormalities that lead to diabetic gastroparesis are increasingly being understood. Several key cell types are affected by diabetes, leading to gastroparesis. These changes include abnormalities in the extrinsic innervation to the stomach, loss of key neurotransmitters at the level of the enteric nervous system, smooth muscle abnormalities, loss of interstitial cells of Cajal, and changes in the macrophage population resident in the muscle wall. This article reviews the current understanding with a focus on data from human studies when available.

Gastroparesis is a complication of long-standing type 1 and type 2 diabetes mellitus. Symptoms associated with gastroparesis include early satiety, prolonged postprandial fullness, bloating, nausea and vomiting, and abdominal pain. Mortality is increased in patients with diabetic gastroparesis. A subset of patients with diabetic gastroparesis have pylorospasm that results in obstructive gastroparesis. Current treatment approaches include improving glucose control with insulin and prescribing antinauseant drugs, prokinetic agents, and gastric electric stimulation. Future directions include improved diet counseling based on gastric emptying rate, continuous insulin delivery systems with glucose sensor-augmented monitoring, and drugs for correcting gastric neural and electric abnormalities.

Gastroparesis is a chronic symptomatic disorder of the stomach characterized by delayed emptying without evidence of mechanical obstruction. Idiopathic gastroparesis refers to gastroparesis of unknown cause not from diabetes; not from prior gastric surgery; not related to other endocrine, neurologic, rheumatologic causes of gastroparesis; and not related to medications that can delay gastric emptying. There is overlap in the symptoms of idiopathic gastroparesis and functional dyspepsia. Patients with idiopathic gastroparesis often have a constellation of symptoms including nausea, vomiting, early satiety, postprandial fullness, and upper abdominal pain. Current treatment options of dietary management, prokinetics agents, antiemetic agents, and symptom modulators do not adequately address clinical need for idiopathic gastroparesis.

Although many surgical procedures originally associated with gastroparesis are less commonly performed nowadays, several more recently developed upper abdominal procedures may be complicated by the development of gastroparesis. Gastroparesis has been described in association with neurologic disorders ranging from Parkinson disease to muscular dystrophy, and its presence may have important implications for patient management and prognosis. Although scleroderma is most frequently linked with gastrointestinal motility disorder, gastroparesis has been linked to several other connective tissue disorders. The management of these patients presents several challenges, and is best conducted in the context of a dedicated and skilled multidisciplinary team.

Gastroparesis, or delayed gastric emptying, has many origins and can wax and wane depending on the underlying cause. Not only do the symptoms significantly alter quality of life, but the clinical consequences can also be life threatening. Once a patient develops protracted nausea and vomiting, providing adequate nutrition, hydration, and access to therapeutics such as prokinetics and antiemetics can present an exceptional challenge to clinicians. This article reviews the limited evidence available for oral nutrition, as well as enteral and parenteral nutritional support therapies. Practical strategies are provided to improve the nutritional depletion that often accompanies this debilitating condition.

Prokinetic agents are medications that enhance coordinated gastrointestinal motility and transit of content in the gastrointestinal tract, mainly by amplifying and coordinating the gastrointestinal muscular contractions. In addition to dietary therapy, prokinetic therapy should be considered as a means to improve gastric emptying and symptoms of gastroparesis, balancing benefits and risks of treatment. In the United States, metoclopramide remains the first-line prokinetic therapy, because it is the only approved medication for gastroparesis. Newer agents are being developed for the management of gastroparesis. This article provides detailed information about prokinetic agents for the treatment of gastroparesis.

Although prokinetic agents typically are used for gastroparesis, antiemetic, analgesic, and neuromodulatory medications may help manage nausea, vomiting, pain, or discomfort. Antiemetic benefits are supported by few case reports. An open series reported symptom reductions with transdermal granisetron in gastroparesis. Opiates are not advocated in gastroparesis because they worsen nausea and delay emptying. Neuromodulators have theoretical utility, but the tricyclic agent nortriptyline showed no benefits over placebo in an idiopathic gastroparesis study raising doubts about this strategy. Neurologic and cardiac toxicities of these medications are recognized. Additional controlled study is warranted to define antiemetic, analgesic, and neuromodulator usefulness in gastroparesis.

Gastroparesis is a syndrome characterized by delayed gastric emptying with associated symptoms. Gastric emptying is a complex process and pyloric dysfunction may play a key role in select subsets of patients with gastroparesis. Diagnostic tests to measure pyloric physiology are now available and have the potential to be more widely used in clinical practice. Targeted therapies including botulinum toxin, transpyloric stent placement, surgical pyloroplasty and endoscopic pyloromyotomy have been developed. Data are emerging regarding efficacy and durability, but these therapies may play a prominent role in select patients with gastroparesis and pyloric dysfunction.

Complementary and alternative medicine is of great interest to patients with gastrointestinal disorders and some will choose to ask their health care providers about those therapies for which some scientific evidence exists. This review focuses on those therapies most commonly used by patients, namely acupuncture/electroacupuncture and various herbal formulations that have been the focus of clinical and laboratory investigation. A discussion of their possible mechanisms of action and the results of clinical studies are summarized.

Gastric electrical stimulation (GES) is neurostimulation; its mechanism of action is affecting central control of nausea and vomiting and enhancing vagal function. GES is a powerful antiemetic available for patients with refractory symptoms of nausea and vomiting from gastroparesis of idiopathic and diabetic causes. GES is not indicated as a way of reducing abdominal pain in gastroparetic patients. The need for introducing a jejunal feeding tube means intensive medical therapies are failing, and is an indication for the implantation of the GES system, which should always be accompanied by a pyloroplasty to guarantee accelerated gastric emptying.

Gastric arrhythmias occur in gastroparesis but their significance is debated. An improved understanding is currently emerging, including newly-defined histopathologic abnormalities in gastroparesis. In particular, the observation that interstitial cells of Cajal are depleted and injured provides mechanisms for arrhythmogenesis in gastroparesis. Electrogastrography has been the dominant clinical method of arrhythmia analysis, but is limited by summative nature, low signal quality, and incomplete sensitivity and specificity. Recently, high-resolution (HR; multi-electrode) mapping has emerged, providing superior spatial data on arrhythmic patterns and mechanisms. However, HR mapping is invasive, and low-resolution approaches are being assessed as bridging techniques until endoscopic mapping is achieved.

Understanding of gastroparesis is evolving, in part because of systematic studies on the pathology, pathophysiology, and outcomes. It is clear that simply accelerating gastric emptying may not effectively control symptoms in this syndrome and more creative approaches are required that address aberrant sensation (vagal and spinal) as well as regional disturbances in motility. Further, with the growing recognition of a possible inflammatory basis, the prospects of disease modifying now seem realistic.

GASTROENTEROLOGY
CLINICS OF NORTH AMERICA

NOW AVAILABLE FOR YOUR iPhone and iPad

Foreword

Gastroparesis

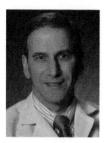

Gary W. Falk, MD, MS
Consulting Editor

Gastroparesis is undoubtedly one of the most frustrating disorders in gastroenterology for both patients and clinicians. The disease may be profoundly debilitating and, unfortunately, treatment options remain limited and have not progressed dramatically over the years. Furthermore, little has changed in the diagnostic approach to this disease, which continues to be based on radionuclide gastric-emptying studies. In this issue of *Gastroenterology Clinics of North America*, Drs Henry Parkman and Pankaj Jay Pasricha have assembled a group of leaders in the field of gastroparesis to provide an update on many of the relevant issues of this vexing disorder. In addition to the entire spectrum of diagnosis and treatment, exciting new information is presented on underlying mechanisms of disease as well as urgently needed new therapies. Taken together, this issue of *Gastroenterology Clinics of North America* provides the reader with the perspective of experts in the field to allow for optimal management of these very challenging patients.

Gary W. Falk, MD, MS
Division of Gastroenterology
University of Pennsylvania
Perelman School of Medicine
9th Floor Penn Tower
1 Convention Avenue
Philadelphia, PA 19104-4311, USA

E-mail address:
gary.falk@uphs.upenn.edu

Gastroenterol Clin N Am 44 (2015) xiii
http://dx.doi.org/10.1016/j.gtc.2014.12.002
0889-8553/15/$ – see front matter © 2015 Published by Elsevier Inc.

Preface

Improving Our Understanding of Gastroparesis

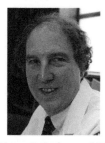 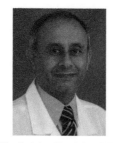

Henry P. Parkman, MD   Pankaj Jay Pasricha, MD
Editors

This issue of *Gastroenterology Clinics of North America* was written to help provide physicians and clinical investigators a better understanding of gastroparesis, a symptomatic chronic disorder of the stomach characterized by delayed gastric emptying. Gastroparesis is an increasingly recognized and diagnosed disorder. Symptoms of gastroparesis can be variable and include early satiety, nausea, vomiting, postprandial fullness, and upper abdominal pain. These symptoms can range from mild to severe, leading to such complications as malnutrition, functional disability, and multiple hospitalizations. The three most common etiologies are diabetes, postsurgical complications, and idiopathic causes. Treatment consists of dietary manipulation, medical treatment, and surgical therapy and can be extremely challenging. New and effective therapies for symptomatic control and, ultimately, disease control, are needed; these will come through better understanding of the pathophysiology of gastroparesis and the biological basis of the disease. This issue provides a comprehensive and in-depth review that captures new and emerging information on this syndrome. Each article is written by an expert in the area, enabling the reader with a better appreciation of the

Gastroenterol Clin N Am 44 (2015) xv–xvi
http://dx.doi.org/10.1016/j.gtc.2014.12.001
0889-8553/15/$ – see front matter © 2015 Published by Elsevier Inc.

gastro.theclinics.com

clinical spectrum of gastroparesis, its pathogenesis, symptomatic treatment, and the unmet clinical and research needs.

Henry P. Parkman, MD
GI Section–Parkinson Pavilion 8th Floor
Temple University School of Medicine
3401 North Broad Street
Philadelphia, PA 19140, USA

Pankaj Jay Pasricha, MD
Johns Hopkins Center
for Neurogastroenterology
Johns Hopkins School of Medicine
Johns Hopkins Carey School of Business
720 Rutland Street, Ross 958
Baltimore, MD 21205, USA

E-mail addresses:
henry.parkman@temple.edu (H.P. Parkman)
ppasric1@jhmi.edu (P.J. Pasricha)

Gastroparesis

Definitions and Diagnosis

Pankaj Jay Pasricha, MD[a,b], Henry P. Parkman, MD[c],*

KEYWORDS

- Gastroparesis • Gastric emptying • Nausea • Vomiting • Diabetes

KEY POINTS

- Gastroparesis is a chronic symptomatic disorder of the stomach characterized by delayed emptying without evidence of mechanical obstruction.
- Symptoms of gastroparesis include nausea, vomiting, early satiety, postprandial fullness, and, in some patients, upper abdominal pain.
- Diagnosis is confirmed by demonstrating delayed gastric emptying: scintigraphy has been the standard for diagnosis; breath testing and wireless motility capsule can also be used.
- Gastric emptying rates generally correlate poorly with symptoms and quality of life in patients with gastroparesis.
- Perhaps gastroparesis should be considered as a broader spectrum of gastric neuromuscular dysfunction, marked by nausea, vomiting, early satiety, postprandial fullness, and epigastric discomfort.

The longer I live, the more I am convinced that…half the unhappiness in the world proceeds from little stoppages, from a duct choked up, from food pressing in the wrong place, from a vexed duodenum or an agitated pylorus.
        —*Sydney Smith, English clergyman, wit and essayist, 1771–1845*

INTRODUCTION

Gastroparesis is often defined as a chronic symptomatic disorder of the stomach manifested by delayed emptying without evidence of mechanical obstruction.[1,2] This classic motility disorder of the stomach can lead to symptoms in patients that reduce the quality of life. Although in many patients symptoms can be controlled with dietary and medical therapy, some patients remain markedly symptomatic with

Dr P.J. Pasricha is supported by a grant from the NIH (NIDDK 073983).
a Johns Hopkins Center for Neurogastroenterology, Johns Hopkins School of Medicine, 720 Rutland Street, Ross 958, Baltimore, MD 21205, USA; b Johns Hopkins Carey School of Business, Baltimore, MD, USA; c GI Section, Temple University School of Medicine, Parkinson Pavilion 8th Floor, 3401 North Broad Street, Philadelphia, PA 19140, USA
* Corresponding author.
E-mail address: henry.parkman@temple.edu

Gastroenterol Clin N Am 44 (2015) 1–7
http://dx.doi.org/10.1016/j.gtc.2014.11.001

progressive weight loss. This article provides an overview of the definitions and diagnosis of gastroparesis and updates the present status of the understanding of this disorder.

SYMPTOMS

Common symptoms of gastroparesis include nausea (>90% of patients), vomiting (84% of patients), and early satiety (60% of patients).[3] Other symptoms include postprandial fullness and abdominal pain.[4,5] Symptoms can be persistent or can manifest as episodic flares. Weight loss, malnutrition, and dehydration may be prominent in severe cases. In diabetic patients, gastroparesis may adversely affect glycemic control. In addition, poor glycemic control can worsen the delayed gastric emptying and symptoms.

Symptom profile is established and symptom severity assessed with the Gastroparesis Cardinal Symptom Index (GCSI), a subset of the Patient Assessment of Upper Gastrointestinal Symptoms.[6,7] The GCSI comprises 3 subscales (nausea and vomiting, postprandial fullness and early satiety, and bloating) that the patient scores from no symptom to very severe symptoms with reference to the preceding 2 weeks.[6] The GCSI daily diary, assessing nausea, vomiting, early satiety, postprandial fullness, and upper abdominal pain, is used to record symptoms on a daily basis and may be more accurate in recording symptoms.[8]

Although it has been a common assumption that the gastrointestinal symptoms can be attributed to delay in gastric emptying, most investigations have observed only weak correlations between symptom severity and the degree of gastric stasis. In general, the symptoms that seem to be best correlated with a delay in gastric emptying include nausea, vomiting, early satiety, and postprandial fullness.[9,10] Some symptoms that have been present in patients with gastroparesis, such as bloating and upper abdominal pain, are not correlated with delayed gastric emptying and might be related to sensory alterations that might also be present in patients with gastroparesis.[5,11] There is an overlap of symptoms of gastroparesis and functional dyspepsia. Abdominal pain or discomfort may be present to varying degrees in patients with gastroparesis, but it is not usually the predominant symptom, as it can be in functional dyspepsia.[12]

ETIOLOGY

Major causes of gastroparesis are diabetic, postsurgical, and idiopathic.[1,2,13] Less common causes of gastroparesis include connective tissue disease, neurologic disease such as Parkinson disease, eating disorders, metabolic or endocrine conditions (hypothyroidism), critical illness, and medications such as opiate narcotic analgesics and anticholinergic agents.[11] In addition, glucagon-like peptide-1 analogues, such as exenatide, used for treatment of type 2 diabetes mellitus can delay gastric empting.[1]

Gastroparesis is a common complication of diabetes; delayed gastric emptying has been found to occur in approximately 40% of patients with longstanding type 1 diabetes and approximately 20% of patients with type 2 diabetes.[11] These estimates are from academic medical centers, and true estimates may be lower in the general population in patients seeing primary care physicians. Diabetic gastroparesis is often attributed to chronic hyperglycemia-induced damage to the vagus nerve and is frequently observed in association with other diabetic complications such as neuropathy, retinopathy, and nephropathy. Glucose can modify gastric emptying tests and symptoms; hyperglycemia can delay gastric emptying and worsen symptoms of gastroparesis, whereas hypoglycemia may accelerate gastric emptying.

Postsurgical gastroparesis can occur with many types of operations but is most often observed after upper abdominal procedures because of injury to or sectioning of the vagus nerve.[1] In the past, surgery for peptic ulcer disease, such as antrectomy with vagotomy, was associated with the development of gastroparesis. However, this type of surgery is being performed less often because of the use of proton pump inhibitor treatments of ulcers and treatment of Helicobacter pylori. Nisson fundoplication is probably the more common surgical procedure associated with gastroparesis. Bariatric surgeries and pancreatic surgery have also been associated with gastroparesis.

Idiopathic gastroparesis, with no obvious cause for the gastroparesis, is a common classification for gastroparesis. Characteristics of 243 patients with idiopathic gastroparesis enrolled in the National Institute of Diabetes and Digestive and Kidney Diseases Gastroparesis Clinical Research Consortium Registry were reported.[14] Patients' mean age was 41 years, and most (88%) were women. The most common presenting symptoms were nausea (34%), vomiting (19%), and abdominal pain (23%). Severe delay in gastric emptying (>35% retention at 4 hours) was present in 28% of patients. Severe delay in gastric emptying was associated with more severe symptoms of nausea and vomiting and loss of appetite compared with patients with mild or moderate delay. About 86% met criteria for functional dyspepsia, predominately postprandial distress syndrome. Thus, idiopathic gastroparesis is a heterogeneous syndrome that primarily affects young women and can occur even in overweight or obese individuals. Half of the patients had acute onset of symptoms, with a minority of patients with idiopathic gastroparesis (19%) reporting an initial infectious prodrome such as gastroenteritis or respiratory infection.[14] It has been suggested that idiopathic gastroparesis of acute onset with infectious prodrome could constitute postviral or viral injury to the neural innervation of the stomach or the interstitial cells of Cajal in the stomach. In some series, patients with postviral gastroparesis improve over time, generally several years.

PATHOPHYSIOLOGY

Gastric emptying is mediated by the vagus nerve, which helps regulate fundic accommodation, antral contraction, and pyloric relaxation.[1] These regional gastric motility changes with food ingestion are then mediated through smooth muscle cells, which control stomach contractions; interstitial cells of Cajal, which regulate gastric pacemaker activity; and enteric neurons, which initiate smooth muscle cell activity.[1] The pathophysiology of gastroparesis has not been fully elucidated but seems to involve abnormalities in functioning of several elements, including autonomic nervous system, smooth muscle cells, enteric neurons, and interstitial cells of Cajal. Histologic studies demonstrate defects in the morphology of enteric neurons, smooth muscle cells, and interstitial cells of Cajal and increased concentrations of inflammatory cells in gastric tissue.[15,16]

DIAGNOSIS

Differential diagnosis of gastroparesis entails excluding other possible causes, including peptic ulcer disease, gastric outlet obstruction, neoplasm, and small-bowel obstruction.[9] For evaluation of these, an upper gastrointestinal endoscopy is performed.

For evaluating gastric emptying, the standard test is gastric emptying scintigraphy, which uses a labeled isotope bound to solid food to image gastric emptying.[17] There is variable methodology used at different centers. Standardization of gastric emptying among different centers has been suggested using the 4-hour imaging protocol with scans taken at 0, 1, 2, and 4 hours after ingestion of a radioactive technetium Tc

99m–labeled low-fat egg white with jam and 2 pieces of toast.[18,19] Delayed gastric emptying is defined as greater than 60% retention at 2 hours postprandially and/or greater than 10% retention at 4 hours. Imaging for gastric emptying out to 4 hours increases the detection of delayed gastric emptying and is now recommended as the standard for gastric emptying scintigraphy to obtain reliable results for the detection of gastroparesis. When gastric scintigraphy is performed for shorter durations, the test is less reliable possibly because of large variations in normal gastric emptying. Because there is not a close correlation between a delay in gastric emptying and symptoms, the gastric emptying test alone should probably not be used for grading the severity of the clinical disorder of gastroparesis. Grading the severity of the delay in gastric emptying has been performed in clinical research studies and might be used clinically.[17,18] Grading for severity of delayed gastric emptying based on the 4-hour value has been proposed: mild delay, 11% to 20% retention at 4 hours; moderate delay, 21% to 35% retention at 4 hours; severe delay, 36% to 50% retention at 4 hours; and very severe delay, greater than 50% retention at 4 hours.

Use of the wireless motility capsule to quantify luminal pH and pressure is an alternative to gastric emptying scintigraphy.[17] The gastric emptying of the wireless motility capsule is identified by a sharp increase in pH, representing the capsule passing from the acidic stomach to the alkaline small intestine. This gastric emptying of the wireless motility capsule represents the emptying of an undigested solid material, which generally occurs with the return of the fasting phase III motility complex after eating, suggesting that the gastric residence time of the wireless motility capsule represents a time near the end of the emptying of a solid meal.[20] A wireless motility capsule gastric residence cutoff time of 5 hours was best in distinguishing between subjects with delayed emptying and those with normal gastric emptying based on scintigraphy on the day of the test (83% sensitivity, 83% specificity).[21] The wireless motility capsule also measures whole-gut transit, that is, gastric emptying, small-bowel transit, and colonic transit.

Breath tests for gastric emptying, another alternative to gastric emptying scintigraphy, measure labeled nonradioactive $^{13}CO_2$ in exhaled breath samples after ingestion of a $^{13}CO_2$-labeled meal.[17] The nonradioactive isotope carbon 13 is used to label octanoate, a medium-chain triglyceride, which can be bound into a solid meal. Studies have also been carried out using ^{13}C-labeled proteinaceous algae (Spirulina). After ingestion and emptying from the stomach, octanoate is absorbed by the small intestine. The octanoate is metabolized to carbon dioxide in the liver and the ^{13}C is excreted from the lungs during respiration. The rate-limiting step for excretion of ^{13}C is gastric emptying. By measuring ^{13}C in breath samples, gastric emptying can be indirectly determined. Breath samples are obtained periodically over several hours. The exhaled $^{13}CO_2$ represents the gastric emptying, duodenal absorption, hepatic metabolism, and pulmonary excretion, whereby gastric emptying is the rate limiting step.[17] Gastric emptying using breath testing correlates well with results of gastric emptying scintigraphy.[22] This test is used clinically in Europe, whereas in the United States, breath tests are most often used in research studies and rarely used in the clinic.

Gastric emptying testing is useful in diagnosing gastroparesis. However, there are several drawbacks. First, gastric emptying rates measured by gastric motor testing generally correlate poorly with symptoms and quality of life in patients with gastroparesis.[23,24] This finding suggests that factors in addition to slow gastric emptying contribute to symptoms. High interindividual and intraindividual variability in gastric emptying rates measured with gastric motor testing constitutes another limitation of gastric motor testing.[13] The relative contributions to these variabilities of gastric motor testing methodology and biologic inconsistency in gastric emptying are not currently known.

GASTROPARESIS—TIME FOR A CHANGE

Despite such historic recognition of the importance of gastrointestinal motility in the maintenance of health and well-being, physicians have made surprisingly little progress in developing effective methods of treatment. This fact applies particularly to the syndrome known as gastroparesis, a disorder of gastric neuromuscular function characterized by delayed gastric emptying with symptoms including chronic nausea that affects patients, most of whom are women, in the prime of their life.[14,25] Inadequate understanding about the pathogenesis of this condition, coupled with a general lack of awareness of the disease among most clinicians, has led to a haphazard and often ineffective approach to treatment.

The traditional concept of gastroparesis being defined as a disorder of delayed gastric emptying has dominated physician thinking for decades, with considerable implications for the field. First, the relationship between gastric emptying and symptoms is a loose one and a rigid adherence to this definition may result in the patient being labeled as either suffering from a less severe illness (functional dyspepsia, or other) or sometimes even outright dismissal. Second, it follows that prokinetic agents by themselves are unlikely to provide global relief. Finally, preoccupation with gastric emptying has distracted attention from symptoms such as nausea and pain and diverted resources that could have led to the development of effective therapies for them.

For all these reasons, it is perhaps appropriate to reconsider the definition of gastroparesis, recognizing it as a broader spectrum of gastric neuromuscular dysfunction, marked by nausea, vomiting, early satiety and postprandial fullness, and epigastric discomfort. By this definition, many patients who have been labeled with "nonulcer dyspepsia" or "chronic unexplained nausea and vomiting" will be included.[24] However, the authors believe this is not necessarily inappropriate, as there seems to be much overlap between the 2 groups symptomatically and pathophysiologically.[26]

By this definition, gastroparesis may be thought of as having at least 2 broad types: one with delayed emptying and one without. However, closer reflection suggests that such a classification may be premature, in part because of the limitations and gaps in the knowledge about gastric motility and how it is measured clinically. To begin with, it is not confidently known that gastric emptying, even as measured by standardized testing, varies with time in the same patient. So labeling a patient as having gastroparesis (or not) based on a single point in time may not be accurate. Second, it is not known whether measuring gastric emptying of a standardized meal truly reflects what happens chronically in patients in real life, depending on the nature and quantity of what they eat. Most of us are familiar with the occasional patient with a food bezoar in the stomach seen endoscopically but with normal gastric emptying. On a related subject, there is also a discrepancy between liquid and solid phase gastric emptying, and if only the latter were measured, a significant number of patients with "gastroparesis" may be missed. Finally, gastric emptying is only one (and perhaps most extreme) manifestation of disordered gastric motility; it is possible that subtler forms of dysmotility within different regions of the stomach are more responsible for the pathogenesis of symptoms rather than overall delayed emptying. This fact may account for the lack of correlation between improvement in symptoms and change in gastric emptying in response to therapeutic agents.

Going beyond gastric emptying, there may be other subtypes of gastroparesis that may be of pathophysiologic and clinical importance. Thus, some patients may have predominant fundic dysfunction, whereas in others the pathophysiology may be dominated by pyloric dysfunction. It is clear that symptoms do not necessarily distinguish between these groups, yet the therapeutic implications are rather different. Similarly, it is possible that pathologic differences exist among patients with varying degrees of damage to nerves, interstitial cells of Cajal, and muscle. There is therefore a need for better and clinically practical ways to phenotype gastroparesis physiologically and pathologically to truly tailor treatment to individual patients.

The aforementioned and many other questions are addressed in various articles in this issue, authored by well-known experts in the field. Although the answers may not be forthcoming in all instances, it is clear that many advances have been made in this field and that the future is exciting and full of possibility.

REFERENCES

1. Camilleri M, Parkman HP, Shafi MA, et al. Clinical guideline: management of gastroparesis. Am J Gastroenterol 2013;108:18–37.
2. Parkman HP, Hasler WL, Fisher RS. American Gastroenterological Association technical review on the diagnosis and treatment of gastroparesis. Gastroenterology 2004;127:1592–622.
3. Soykan I, Sivri B, Sarosiek I, et al. Demography, clinical characteristics, psychological and abuse profiles, treatment, and long-term follow-up of patients with gastroparesis. Dig Dis Sci 1998;43:2398–404.
4. Cherian D, Sachdeva P, Fisher RS, et al. Abdominal pain is a frequent symptom of gastroparesis. Clin Gastroenterol Hepatol 2010;8:676–81.
5. Hasler WL, Wilson LA, Parkman HP, et al. Factors related to abdominal pain in gastroparesis: contrast to patients with predominant nausea and vomiting. Neurogastroenterol Motil 2013;25:427–38.
6. Rentz AM, Kahrilas P, Stanghellini V, et al. Development and psychometric evaluation of the patient assessment of upper gastrointestinal symptom severity index (PAGI-SYM) in patients with upper gastrointestinal disorders. Qual Life Res 2004; 13:1737–49.
7. Revicki DA, Rentz AM, Dubois D, et al. Development and validation of a patient-assessed gastroparesis symptom severity measure: the Gastroparesis Cardinal Symptom Index. Aliment Pharmacol Ther 2003;18:141–50.
8. Revicki DA, Camilleri M, Kuo B, et al. Development and content validity of a gastroparesis cardinal symptom index daily diary. Aliment Pharmacol Ther 2009;30: 670–80.
9. Pathikonda M, Sachdeva P, Malhotra N, et al. Gastric emptying scintigraphy: is four hours necessary? J Clin Gastroenterol 2012;46:209–15.
10. Cassilly DW, Wang YR, Friedenberg FK, et al. Symptoms of gastroparesis: use of the gastroparesis cardinal symptom index in symptomatic patients referred for gastric emptying scintigraphy. Digestion 2008;78:144–51.
11. Hasler WL, Wilson LA, Parkman HP, et al. Bloating in gastroparesis: severity, impact, and associated factors. Am J Gastroenterol 2011;106:1492–502.
12. Tack J, Talley NJ, Camilleri M, et al. Functional gastroduodenal disorders. Gastroenterology 2006;130:1466–79.
13. Hasler WL. Gastroparesis: pathogenesis, diagnosis, and management. Nat Rev Gastroenterol Hepatol 2011;8:438–53.
14. Parkman HP, Yates K, Hasler WL, et al. Clinical features of idiopathic gastroparesis vary with sex, body mass, symptom onset, delay in gastric emptying, and gastroparesis severity. Gastroenterology 2011;140:101–15.

15. Harberson J, Thomas R, Harbison S, et al. Gastric neuromuscluar pathology of gastroparesis: analysis of full-thickness antral biopsies. Dig Dis Sci 2010;55: 359–70.
16. Grover M, Farrugia G, Lurken MS, et al, NIDDK Gastroparesis Clinical Research Consortium. Cellular changes in diabetic and idiopathic gastroparesis. Gastroenterology 2011;140(5):1575–85.
17. Parkman HP. Assessment of gastric emptying and small-bowel motility: scintigraphy, breath tests, manometry, and SmartPill. Gastrointest Endosc Clin N Am 2009;19:49–55.
18. Abell TL, Camilleri M, Donohoe K, et al, American Neurogastroenterology and Motility Society. Consensus recommendations for gastric emptying scintigraphy. A joint report of the Society Of Nuclear Medicine. Am J Gastroenterol 2008;103: 753–63.
19. Guo JP, Maurer AH, Urbain JL, et al. Extending gastric emptying scintigraphy from two to four hours detects more patients with gastroparesis. Dig Dis Sci 2001;46:24–9.
20. Cassilly D, Kantor S, Knight L, et al. Gastric emptying of a nondigestible solid: assessment with simultaneous SmartPill pH and pressure capsule, antroduodenal manometry, gastric emptying scintigraphy. Neurogastroenterol Motil 2008; 20(4):311–9.
21. Kuo B, McCallum RW, Koch K, et al. Comparison of gastric emptying of a nondigestible capsule to a radiolabeled meal in healthy and gastroparetic subjects. Aliment Pharmacol Ther 2008;27(2):186–96.
22. Szarka LA, Camilleri M, Vella A, et al. A stable isotope breath test with a standard meal for abnormal gastric emptying of solids in the clinic and in research. Clin Gastroenterol Hepatol 2008;6(6):635–43.
23. Horowitz M, Maddox AF, Wishart JM, et al. Relationships between oesophageal transit and solid and liquid gastric emptying in diabetes mellitus. Eur J Nucl Med 1991;18:229–34.
24. Pasricha PJ, Colvin R, Yates K, et al. Characteristics of patients with chronic unexplained nausea and vomiting and normal gastric emptying. Clin Gastroenterol Hepatol 2011;9:567–76.e1–4.
25. Parkman HP, Yates K, Hasler WL, et al. Similarities and differences between diabetic and idiopathic gastroparesis. Clin Gastroenterol Hepatol 2011;9:1056–64.
26. Tack J, Bisschops R, Sarnelli G. Pathophysiology and treatment of functional dyspepsia. Gastroenterology 2004;127:1239–55.

Epidemiology and Natural History of Gastroparesis

Adil E. Bharucha, MBBS, MD

KEYWORDS

- Gastroparesis • Epidemiology • Quality of life • Natural history
- Diabetic gastroparesis • Idiopathic gastroparesis

KEY POINTS

- Gastroparesis is a syndrome characterized by delayed gastric emptying and symptoms thereof in the absence of gastric outlet obstruction.
- Most studies on the epidemiology of gastroparesis have been conducted in selected case series rather than in the population at large.
- In the only community-based study, the age-adjusted prevalence of idiopathic gastroparesis per 100,000 persons was higher in women (37.8; 95% CI, 23.3–52.4) than men (9.6; 95% CI, 1.8–17.4).
- In the only community-based study of gastroparesis in diabetes mellitus (DM), the average cumulative incidence of symptoms and delayed gastric emptying over 10 years was higher in type 1 DM (5%) than in type 2 DM (1%) and controls (1%).
- In the United States, the incidence of hospitalizations related to gastroparesis increased substantially between 1995 and 2004, and particularly after 2000.

INTRODUCTION

Gastroparesis is a syndrome characterized by delayed gastric emptying (GE) and symptoms thereof in the absence of gastric outlet obstruction. In diabetes mellitus (DM), delayed GE is often asymptomatic.[1] This term should be reserved for patients with delayed GE and upper gastrointestinal symptoms. DM and idiopathic disease are the 2 primary causes associated with gastroparesis. Only 2 studies have evaluated the epidemiology of gastroparesis in the population.[2,3] Even these studies are based on data collected from patients who presented for medical attention rather from than a

Disclosures: Dr A.E. Bharucha has received consulting fees from Asubio Pharmaceuticals, Ironwood Pharmaceuticals, GICare Pharmaceuticals, and Medspira Inc, and has licensed a patent to Medspira Inc.

This work was supported in part by United States Public Health Service, National Institutes of Health grant P01 DK68055.

Clinical Enteric Neuroscience Translational and Epidemiological Research Program, Division of Gastroenterology and Hepatology, Mayo Clinic, 200 1st Street Southwest, Rochester, MN 55905, USA

E-mail address: bharucha.adil@mayo.edu

random sample of people in the community. Currently, GE can only be assessed with scintigraphy, which requires specialized laboratories and radiation exposure, limiting population-based studies of the epidemiology of gastroparesis. Hence, understanding of many facets of the epidemiology of gastroparesis is primarily based on case series or hospital-based databases rather than on the population. These studies suggest that gastroparesis is not uncommon and can impair quality of life. The incidence of hospitalizations associated with a diagnosis of gastroparesis has increased considerably since 2000.[4]

Several organic diseases affect gastric neuromuscular functions through causing an extrinsic or enteric neuropathy or a myopathy. Among patients who do not have an underlying disorder that is known to be associated with gastroparesis, the pathogenesis of gastroparesis is poorly understood.

PREVALENCE AND INCIDENCE

Only 1 study on the epidemiology of idiopathic gastroparesis in the population has been published.[2] That study, which was conducted in the Rochester Epidemiology Project, defined gastroparesis as definite (ie, delayed GE according to standard scintigraphy and typical symptoms for >3 months), probable (ie, typical symptoms and food retention on endoscopy or upper gastrointestinal study), and possible (ie, typical symptoms alone or delayed GE according to scintigraphy without gastrointestinal symptoms). A total of 83 patients had definite gastroparesis, 127 had definite or probable, and 222 had any of the 3 definitions. On January 1, 2007, the age-adjusted prevalence of definite gastroparesis per 100,000 persons was approximately 4-fold higher in women (37.8; 95% CI, 23.3–52.4) than in men (9.6; 95% CI, 1.8–17.4). Likewise, the age-adjusted incidence per 100,000 person-years of definite gastroparesis for 1996 through 2006 was approximately 4-fold higher in women (9.8; 95% CI, 7.5–12.1) than in men (2.4; 95% CI, 1.2–3.8).

Earlier reports from tertiary referral centers observed that up to 60% of patients with long-standing type 1 DM (T1DM) and gastrointestinal symptoms had diabetic gastroparesis.[5,6] However, these studies predated the routine use of intensive insulin therapy for T1DM.

More recently, population-based studies of gastrointestinal symptoms in DM have been based on symptoms alone or symptoms and delayed GE. Compared with the studies in selected populations mentioned previously, the cumulative incidence of diabetic gastroparesis among patients with DM in the community is lower. In the only community-based study from Olmsted County, MN, the cumulative incidence of symptoms and delayed GE over 10 years was 5% in T1DM (hazard ratio [HR], 33; 95% CI, 4.0, 274; adjusted for age and gender vs controls), 1% in type 2 DM (T2DM) (HR, 7.5; 95% CI, 0.8, 68; adjusted for age and gender vs controls) and 1% in controls (**Table 1**).[3] The risk of gastroparesis in T1DM was significantly greater than in T2DM (HR, 4.4; 95% CI, 1.1, 17). Gastroparesis was documented by physician diagnosis, evaluating GE with scintigraphy, or symptoms and retained food at endoscopy. Because gastroparesis was identified only in people who presented for care, people in whom GE was not evaluated may not have been identified. Hence, this study assessed the cumulative incidence of diabetic gastroparesis (over 10 years) rather than the prevalence of diabetic gastroparesis.

Several studies have evaluated the epidemiology of upper gastrointestinal symptoms but not GE among people with diabetes in the community. In most community-based studies, the prevalence of gastrointestinal symptoms was not significantly higher in people with diabetes than in asymptomatic controls. In the

Table 1
Community-based epidemiologic studies of gastrointestinal symptoms in diabetes mellitus

	Respondents	Response Rate (Number of Respondents)	Key Findings
Dyck et al,[7] 1993	Residents of Rochester, MN with DM	44% (T1DM: n = 102; T2DM: n = 278)	Gastroparesis: 0% T1DM, 1% T2DM
Janatuinen et al,[55] 1993	All residents in a hospital district with DM and a randomly selected control group	92%–100% (T1DM: n = 89; T2DM: n = 481; controls: n = 635)	Symptoms of nausea and vomiting were not different between cases with DM and controls without
Maleki et al,[8] 2000	Samples of Olmsted County residents with T1DM, T2DM, and corresponding age- and sex-stratified controls	59% (T1DM: n = 138; T2DM: n = 217; controls: n = 388)	No difference in proportions with stomach symptoms between DM and controls; less heartburn reported by patients with T1DM
Bytzer et al,[9] 2001; Hammer et al,[56] 2003	Gender-stratified sample of 15,000 people in Sydney, Australia	60% for entire sample (423 of 8555 respondents had DM; 95% had T2DM)	Small differences were detected with the highest adjusted OR for vomiting 1.7% vs 1.1% (mean OR, 2.51) When upper gut dysmotility symptoms were evaluated, the results were 18.2% vs 15.3% (OR, 1.75)
Talley et al,[10] 2002	Two surveys of subjects with T2DM on mailing list of Diabetes Australia at 3-y interval	64% returned second survey (892 with T2DM in first survey)	NA
Choung et al,[3] 2012	Follow-up of 1374 subjects (T1DM: n = 269; T2DM: n = 409) and controls matched for age and gender (n = 735) in Olmsted County, MN	89% (1226 subjects) authorized review of medical records; questionnaires at interviews were not performed	Over 10 y, gastroparesis developed in 5.2% (T1DM), 1.0% (T2DM), and 0.2% (controls) Higher risk (HR, 4.4; CI, 1.1, 17) in T1DM than T2DM

All surveys used a mailed questionnaire.
Abbreviations: T1DM, type 1 diabetes mellitus; T2DM, type 2 diabetes mellitus; HR, hazard ratio; NA, not available; OR, odds ratio.
Data from Refs.[3,7–10,55]

Rochester Diabetic Neuropathy Study from Olmsted County, MN, only 1% of patients had symptoms of gastroparesis (**Table 2**).[7] Another study from Olmsted County observed that the prevalence for nausea and/or vomiting or dyspepsia was not significantly different in people with T1DM or T2DM relative to controls.[8] That study did not assess GE. However, in an Australian community-based study of 423 patients with

Table 2
Pathogenesis and cause of gastroparesis

Mechanism	Common Causes	Uncommon Causes
Extrinsic neuropathy	Iatrogenic vagotomy (eg, surgery for peptic ulcer disease, fundoplication), DM neuropathy	Other central nervous system diseases (eg, stroke, other causes of autonomic neuropathy, Parkinson disease, spinal cord injury)
Intrinsic or enteric neuropathy	Postinfectious gastroparesis,[1] DM	Paraneoplastic syndrome
Myopathy		Polymyositis, scleroderma[2]
Drugs and metabolic disorders		Opiates, anticholinergic drugs, hypothyroidism, hyperparathyroidism, Addison disease
Miscellaneous		After lung transplantation, anorexia nervosa, pregnancy

predominantly (95%) T2DM, the prevalence of several upper gastrointestinal symptoms, including abdominal pain or discomfort, early satiety, postprandial fullness, bloating, heartburn, nausea, vomiting, and dysphagia, was higher in a sample of people predominantly with T2DM than in controls.[9] Taken together, these data suggest that gastrointestinal symptoms are not uncommon among people with DM. The risk of gastroparesis is higher in T1DM than in T2DM.

Longitudinal studies from Australia suggest that, similar to functional gastrointestinal disorders, gastrointestinal symptom turnover also occurs in DM. Turnover refers to appearance and disappearance of symptoms over time. In the first study, considerable turnover in gastrointestinal symptoms was seen 3 years after the initial assessment in patients with T2DM.[10] However, appearance and resolution were balanced; hence, overall prevalence was comparable at follow-up. Several factors, but not glycemic control, predicted symptom change; these factors varied among symptoms. In another cohort of 139 subjects with diabetes, of whom approximately 50% had T1DM and 5% had severe autonomic dysfunction, symptom turnover varied between 15% and 25% in the group with diabetes and was not significantly different from that of controls.[11] Symptom turnover was not associated with glycemic control or autonomic neuropathy, but rather with depression (ie, appearance and disappearance of depression were associated with gain and loss of gastrointestinal symptoms, respectively).

No studies that have assessed symptoms and GE among randomly selected people in a community, perhaps because scintigraphy is cumbersome and involves radiation exposure. GE breath tests (GEBTs) use ^{13}C, which is a stable isotope, and offer an alternative approach for measuring solid-phase GE without elaborate detection equipment or radiation exposure in the office or bedside.[12,13] The U.S. Food and Drug Administration (FDA) is currently reviewing a ^{13}C-spirulina GEBT for use in the United States. GE can also be measured with a nondigestible capsule, SmartPill (Given Imaging, Ltd., Yoqneam, Israel), which records luminal pH, temperature, and pressure during gastrointestinal transit, providing a measure of GE time.[14]

Although most attention has focused on delayed GE, DM is also associated with rapid GE. In a Mayo Clinic tertiary referral study of 129 patients with diabetes and upper gastrointestinal symptoms undergoing scintigraphy, 42% had normal, 36% delayed, and 22% rapid GE.[15] Each category had an approximately equal number of patients with T1DM and T2DM. However, the prevalence of rapid GE among people with diabetes in the community is unknown.

HOSPITALIZATION

Although the incidence of gastroparesis did not change significantly between the periods 1996 to 2000 and 2001 to 2006,[2] data from the Nationwide Inpatient Sample (NIS), which comprises a nationally representative sample of 5 to 8 million hospitalizations, demonstrate a 138% increase in the hospitalizations related to gastroparesis between 1995 and 2004.[4] DM was listed as a comorbidity in 21.0% of these patients in 1995 and 26.7% in 2004. Gastroparesis was the primary or secondary diagnosis for these hospitalizations. The former increased by 158% between 1995 and 2004, and most of this change (138%) occurred between 2000 and 2004. In comparison, changes were smaller over that period in diabetes-related hospitalizations (53% increase), all hospitalizations (13% increase), and hospitalizations with 4 other gastrointestinal conditions, such as gastroesophageal reflux disease (GERD), gastric ulcer, gastritis, or nonspecific nausea/vomiting as the primary diagnosis (ranging from a 3% decrease to 76% increase). Conceivably, this increase in hospitalizations for gastroparesis may reflect an increased prevalence of DM or gastroparesis; changes in diagnostic criteria, severity, and treatment of gastroparesis; or better recognition and/or diagnosis of this disorder. Several possible explanations exist for the striking increase after 2000. The withdrawal of the prokinetic agent cisapride from the market might have increased the number of symptomatic patients. The FDA provided humanitarian device exemption to gastric electric stimulation around 2000. This device often entails hospitalization for surgical placement of the stimulator.[16] Increased recognition of the disorder gastroparesis and a change in hospital coding practices may also contribute.

Compared with the 4 gastrointestinal conditions as the primary diagnosis (GERD, gastric ulcer, gastritis, and nonspecific nausea/vomiting), the length of stay was also longer for gastroparesis listed as the primary diagnosis (increase of 15.4%–66.2%; all P<.001). The total charges for hospitalization in patients with gastroparesis listed as the primary ($20,573) or secondary ($24,965) diagnosis in 2004 were also higher than these other diagnoses except for gastric ulcer, for which the total charge was $23,259. Similar trends for gastroparesis versus other diagnoses were observed in 1995.

The Nationwide Inpatient Sample study[4] did not clearly discriminate between hospitalization for idiopathic versus diabetic gastroparesis. In the National Institute of Diabetes, Digestive and Kidney Diseases (NIDDK) consortium, patients with gastroparesis from T1DM reported more hospitalizations (ie, 5.1 ± 6.4 per year, mean ± SD), mostly for vomiting and dehydration, than those with idiopathic gastroparesis (1.6 ± 3.0) or T2DM (2.7 ± 5.7).[17] In a study from the Beth Israel Deaconess Medical Center and the Joslin Diabetes Center, patients with diabetic gastroparesis also had more hospital days than those with DM and gastrointestinal symptoms but normal GE (ie, 25.5 vs 5.1 per 1000 patient days).[18]

RISK FACTORS AND ASSOCIATED CONDITIONS

Table 2 identifies the mechanisms of and diseases associated with gastroparesis. Among patients who do not have these underlying disorders, the pathogenesis of gastroparesis is poorly understood. A tertiary referral series of patients with idiopathic gastroparesis observed that the onset of symptoms was consistent with a viral origin in 23% and began after a cholecystectomy in 8%.[19] In the NIDDK Gastroparesis Clinical Research Consortium, approximately 19% of patients with idiopathic gastroparesis and 14% each with T1DM and T2DM had features of an infectious prodrome; 36% of patients with idiopathic or diabetic gastroparesis had a cholecystectomy.[17,20]

Patients with cholecystectomy had more comorbidities, particularly chronic fatigue syndrome, fibromyalgia, depression, and anxiety. Whether cholecystectomy is an independent risk for gastroparesis is unclear.

Acute hyperglycemia delays GE.[21] However, the relationship between long-term control of glycemia and GE is unclear. Increased glycated hemoglobin (HbA1c) levels were associated with gastrointestinal symptoms in people with T2DM.[22] However, HbA1c levels were not significantly different among participants with DM with gastrointestinal symptoms and delayed GE, DM with gastrointestinal symptoms and normal GE, and DM without gastrointestinal symptoms.[18] Also, improved glycemic control did not accelerate GE in participants with T1DM or T2DM and delayed GE.[23] This finding is in contrast to the those of the Diabetes Control and Complications Trial (DCCT), wherein 6.5 years of intensive insulin therapy reduced the risk of diabetic retinopathy, nephropathy, and peripheral and cardiac autonomic neuropathy by 40% to 60% compared with conventional insulin therapy.[24] Moreover, these differences between the former intensive and conventional treatment groups have persisted for as long as 14 years despite the loss of glycemic separation.[25–27]

Other than an association with autonomic neuropathy,[28] the relationship between diabetic gastroparesis and other complications of longstanding DM is incompletely understood. In the only community-based study, symptoms of peripheral or autonomic neuropathy were not associated with diabetic gastroparesis.[3]

NATURAL HISTORY AND OUTCOMES

In the Olmsted County epidemiology study, one-third of all incident cases of gastroparesis died and another one-third required hospitalization, medications, or tube feeding related to gastroparesis.[2] Overall survival in patients with gastroparesis was significantly lower than that of the Minnesota white population.

Minimal data are available on the natural history of diabetic gastroparesis. From a group of 86 patients assessed at a tertiary referral center, 20 patients, of whom 16 had T1DM, were reevaluated 12 years later and only 13 patients (12 had T1DM) were reevaluated approximately 25 years after the first study.[23,29] Although GE was not significantly different 25 years after the baseline assessment, correlation between initial and subsequent assessments was limited, as evidenced by a correlation coefficient of 0.56.[23]

IMPACT ON QUALITY OF LIFE

Although nausea and vomiting are the cardinal symptoms of gastroparesis, data from the NIDDK Gastroparesis Clinical Research Consortium suggest that upper abdominal pain or discomfort is not uncommon and is often severe.[30] Moderate to severe pain was associated with more severely delayed GE, worse quality of life, depression, and anxiety.[30] Moreover, among patients with moderate to severe pain, 48% were taking opiates. The 36-Item Short Form Health Survey (SF-36) physical and mental component scores indicate a severe impact on quality of life. To what extent this impact is related to gastrointestinal symptoms per se versus comorbid conditions (eg, depression) and/or medications (eg, opiates) is unclear.

Data on the impact of gastrointestinal symptoms on quality of life among patients with gastroparesis in the community are limited. Among a cohort of people with predominantly T2DM in the community, the physical and mental quality of life as assessed by the SF-36 were lower in patients with diabetes with gastrointestinal symptoms compared with population norms.[31] The quality of life scores in all subscales decreased markedly with increasing numbers of distinct gastrointestinal symptom groups. The association between gastrointestinal symptoms and poorer quality of life in DM was independent of age, gender, smoking, alcohol use, and type of diabetes. However, the absolute SF-36 scores in this study were approximately 2-fold higher than those seen in the data from the NIDDK consortium.[30,31]

Race has also been shown to be associated with the impact of gastrointestinal symptoms on quality of life in patients with DM. One study reported that nonwhite patients with gastroparesis had more severe symptoms, poorer quality of life, and used more health care resources than white patients.[32] The 2 groups differed in health care use, with 49% of nonwhite patients reporting more than 4 gastroparesis-related emergency department visits and 42% reporting more than 4 gastroparesis-related hospitalizations, compared with 20% and 14% of white patients, respectively. In this study, nonwhite race, sex, age, and age of onset were independently associated with symptom scores, whereas cause of gastroparesis and GE times were not. High unemployment rates, lower household income, and work absenteeism are also variably associated with gastroparesis.[17,33]

MORTALITY RATES

Overall survival in patients with idiopathic gastroparesis was significantly lower than the age- and sex-specific expected survival computed from the Minnesota white population.[2] A review of several case series observed that the mortality rates in patients with gastroparesis range from 4% and 38%.[34] The best outcomes were observed in a largely outpatient-based group of patients followed for approximately 2 years, and the highest death rates were reported in patients with diabetes with gastroparesis requiring nutritional support.[2,19,23,35–38] In a study of 86 patients with diabetes, approximately 25% had died by follow-up at least 9 years later, but gastroparesis was not associated with mortality after adjustment for other disorders.[39] However, this study did not ascertain the relationship between diabetic gastroparesis and other medical conditions. Whether this increased mortality is driven by gastroparesis is unknown. Data on long-term natural history in the community are lacking.

CLINICAL IMPLICATIONS

The clinical features of gastroparesis are detailed in other articles elsewhere in this issue. This section focuses on selected aspects that pertain to the epidemiology of gastroparesis.

During GE scintigraphy, postprandial scans at 1 hour can identify accelerated GE, whereas scans at 2 and 4 hours distinguish normal function from delayed GE with a sensitivity of 90% and a specificity of 70%.[40] For solid-phase testing, most centers use a technetium 99m sulfur colloid-labeled egg sandwich as the test meal, with imaging performed at 0, 1, 2, and 4 hours. The Society of Nuclear Medicine and the American Neurogastroenterology and Motility Society recommend a 4-hour test using a radiolabeled Egg Beaters meal with jam, toast, and water.[41]

The cardinal upper gastrointestinal symptoms of dyspepsia and gastroparesis are similar. Although dyspepsia is not defined by delayed GE, approximately one-third of patients with functional dyspepsia have delayed GE.[42] Hence, the distinction between dyspepsia with delayed GE and gastroparesis, either functional or diabetic, is blurred,[42] Because the term *gastroparesis* implies a paralyzed stomach, its use should be restricted to patients with severe symptoms and markedly delayed GE. No accepted GE value exists to discriminate between delayed GE and gastroparesis. When the delay in GE is not severe, the term *dyspepsia* is perhaps more appropriate.

Up to 40% of patients with diabetic gastroparesis are asymptomatic.[1] Likewise, a limited correlation exists between symptoms and delayed GE in idiopathic gastroparesis.[42] During therapeutic trials for gastroparesis, improvements in GE and symptoms were not correlated.[43] Hence, the utility of using GE as an end point in therapeutic trials for gastroparesis has been questioned.[43] Perhaps this limited correlation between symptoms and delayed GE is explained by other features, such vagal dysfunction[44] or increased sensitivity to gastric distention,[45] that influence the expression of GE disturbance (ie, as symptoms). Similar discrepancies between symptoms and objective findings exist in other diseases (eg, Crohn disease). For example, in one study, the correlation between symptoms evaluated by the Crohn's Disease Activity Index and endoscopic findings in Crohn disease was not significant.[46] In addition to gastrointestinal symptoms, delayed GE may also predispose patients with T1DM to hypoglycemia.[47] Hence, consideration should be given to evaluating GE in patients with unexplained hypoglycemia without gastrointestinal symptoms.

By convention, delayed GE is defined by scintigraphy. However, delayed GE may also manifest with retained food in the stomach after an overnight fast. Clinical observations suggest that some patients with retained food in the stomach at endoscopy have normal GE by scintigraphy. This discrepancy may be explained by day-to-day variations in GE, the use of medications (eg, opioids) that can delay GE before either study, ingestion of food before an endoscopy, or differences between the gastric motor mechanisms responsible for antral motility and emptying of smaller particles during scintigraphy (ie, type 2 antral motor activity) and indigestible larger particles (ie, $\geq$3 mm) ingested with meals, which are emptied by the antral component of the migrating motor complex during fasting or sleeping.

Among patients with an idiopathic disorder, DM, an autonomic neuropathy, or postural orthostatic tachycardia syndrome, dyspeptic symptoms may also be associated with rapid GE.[48–54] Because symptoms are of limited utility for discriminating between delayed and rapid GE, this function must be measured to ascertain whether it is normal, delayed, or rapid.

SUMMARY

Diabetic and idiopathic gastroparesis are not uncommon conditions that can substantially impair quality of life. Most studies on the epidemiology of gastroparesis have been conducted in selected case series rather than in the population. More studies are needed to better understand the incidence and prevalence, risk factors, and natural history of gastroparesis.

REFERENCES

1. Camilleri M, Bharucha AE, Farrugia G. Epidemiology, mechanisms, and management of diabetic gastroparesis. Clin Gastroenterol Hepatol 2011;9:5–12 [quiz: e7].
2. Jung HK, Choung RS, Locke GR 3rd, et al. The incidence, prevalence, and outcomes of patients with gastroparesis in Olmsted County, Minnesota, from 1996 to 2006. Gastroenterology 2009;136:1225–33.
3. Choung RS, Locke GR 3rd, Schleck CD, et al. Risk of gastroparesis in subjects with type 1 and 2 diabetes in the general population. Am J Gastroenterol 2012; 107:82–8.
4. Wang YR, Fisher RS, Parkman HP. Gastroparesis-related hospitalizations in the United States: trends, characteristics, and outcomes, 1995-2004. Am J Gastroenterol 2008;103:313–22.

5. Feldman M, Schiller LR. Disorders of gastrointestinal motility associated with diabetes mellitus. Ann Intern Med 1983;98:378–84.

6. Jones KL, Russo A, Stevens JE, et al. Predictors of delayed gastric emptying in diabetes. Diabetes Care 2001;24:1264–9.

7. Dyck PJ, Kratz KM, Karnes JL, et al. The prevalence by staged severity of various types of diabetic neuropathy, retinopathy, and nephropathy in a population-based cohort: the Rochester Diabetic Neuropathy Study. Neurology 1993;43:817–24 [Erratum appears in Neurology 1993;43(11):2345].

8. Maleki D, Locke GR 3rd, Camilleri M, et al. Gastrointestinal tract symptoms among persons with diabetes mellitus in the community. Arch Intern Med 2000;160:2808–16.

9. Bytzer P, Talley NJ, Leemon M, et al. Prevalence of gastrointestinal symptoms associated with diabetes mellitus: a population-based survey of 15,000 adults. Arch Intern Med 2001;161:1989–96.

10. Talley NJ, Howell S, Jones MP, et al. Predictors of turnover of lower gastrointestinal symptoms in diabetes mellitus [comment]. Am J Gastroenterol 2002;97:3087–94.

11. Quan C, Talley NJ, Jones MP, et al. Gain and loss of gastrointestinal symptoms in diabetes mellitus: associations with psychiatric disease, glycemic control, and autonomic neuropathy over 2 years of follow-up. Am J Gastroenterol 2008;103:2023–30.

12. Szarka LA, Camilleri M, Vella A, et al. A stable isotope breath test with a standard meal for abnormal gastric emptying solids in the clinic and in research. Clin Gastroenterol Hepatol 2008;6:635–43.

13. Bharucha AE, Camilleri M, Veil E, et al. Comprehensive assessment of gastric emptying with a stable isotope breath test. Neurogastroenterol Motil 2013;25:e60–9.

14. Kuo B, McCallum RW, Koch KL, et al. Comparison of gastric emptying of a non-digestible capsule to a radio-labelled meal in healthy and gastroparetic subjects. Aliment Pharmacol Ther 2008;27:186–96.

15. Bharucha AE, Camilleri M, Forstrom LA, et al. Relationship between clinical features and gastric emptying disturbances in diabetes mellitus. Clin Endocrinol (Oxf) 2008;70:415–20.

16. Cutts TF, Luo J, Starkebaum W, et al. Is gastric electrical stimulation superior to standard pharmacologic therapy in improving GI symptoms, healthcare resources, and long-term health care benefits? Neurogastroenterol Motil 2005;17:35–43.

17. Parkman HP, Yates K, Hasler WL, et al, National Institute of Diabetes Digestive Kidney Diseases Gastroparesis Clinical Research Consortium. Similarities and differences between diabetic and idiopathic gastroparesis. Clin Gastroenterol Hepatol 2011;9:1056–64 [quiz: e133–4].

18. Hyett B, Martinez FJ, Gill BM, et al. Delayed radionucleotide gastric emptying studies predict morbidity in diabetics with symptoms of gastroparesis. Gastroenterology 2009;137:445–52.

19. Soykan I, Sivri B, Sarosiek I, et al. Demography, clinical characteristics, psychological and abuse profiles, treatment, and long-term follow-up of patients with gastroparesis. Dig Dis Sci 1998;43:2398–404.

20. Parkman HP, Yates K, Hasler WL, et al. Cholecystectomy and clinical presentations of gastroparesis. Dig Dis Sci 2013;58:1062–73.

21. Fraser RJ, Horowitz M, Maddox AF, et al. Hyperglycaemia slows gastric emptying in type 1 (insulin-dependent) diabetes mellitus. Diabetologia 1990;33:675–80.

22. Bytzer P, Talley NJ, Hammer J, et al. GI symptoms in diabetes mellitus are associated with both poor glycemic control and diabetic complications. Am J Gastroenterol 2002;97:604–11.
23. Jones KL, Russo A, Berry MK, et al. A longitudinal study of gastric emptying and upper gastrointestinal symptoms in patients with diabetes mellitus [see comment]. Am J Med 2002;113:449–55.
24. Kilpatrick ES, Rigby AS, Atkin SL. The diabetes control and complications trial: the gift that keeps giving. Nat Rev Endocrinol 2009;5:537–45.
25. Writing Team for the Diabetes Control and Complications Trial/Epidemiology of Diabetes Interventions and Complications Research Group. Effect of intensive therapy on the microvascular complications of type 1 diabetes mellitus. JAMA 2002;287:2563–9.
26. Writing Team for the Diabetes Control and Complications Trial/Epidemiology of Diabetes Interventions and Complications Research Group. Sustained effect of intensive treatment of type 1 diabetes mellitus on development and progression of diabetic nephropathy: the Epidemiology of Diabetes Interventions and Complications (EDIC) study. JAMA 2003;290:2159–67.
27. Martin CL, Albers JW, Pop-Busui R, DCCT/EDIC Research Group. Neuropathy and related findings in the diabetes control and complications trial/epidemiology of diabetes interventions and complications study. Diabetes Care 2014;37:31–8.
28. Bharucha AE, Camilleri M, Low PA, et al. Autonomic dysfunction in gastrointestinal motility disorders. Gut 1993;34:397–401.
29. Chang J, Russo A, Bound M, et al. A 25-year longitudinal evaluation of gastric emptying in diabetes. Diabetes Care 2012;35:2594–6.
30. Hasler WL, Wilson LA, Parkman HP, et al. Factors related to abdominal pain in gastroparesis: contrast to patients with predominant nausea and vomiting. Neurogastroenterol Motil 2013;25:427–38 e300–1.
31. Talley NJ, Young L, Bytzer P, et al. Impact of chronic gastrointestinal symptoms in diabetes mellitus on health-related quality of life. Am J Gastroenterol 2001;96: 71–6.
32. Friedenberg FK, Kowalczyk M, Parkman HP. The influence of race on symptom severity and quality of life in gastroparesis. J Clin Gastroenterol 2013;47:757–61.
33. Bielefeldt K, Raza N, Zickmund SL. Different faces of gastroparesis. World J Gastroenterol 2009;15:6052–60.
34. Bielefeldt K. Gastroparesis: concepts, controversies, and challenges. Scientifica 2012;2012:424802.
35. Chaudhuri TK, Fink S. Prognostic implication of gastroparesis in patients with diabetes mellitus. Clin Auton Res 1992;2:221–4.
36. Fontana RJ, Barnett JL. Jejunostomy tube placement in refractory diabetic gastroparesis: a retrospective review. Am J Gastroenterol 1996;91:2174–8.
37. Dudekula A, O'Connell M, Bielefeldt K. Hospitalizations and testing in gastroparesis. J Gastroenterol Hepatol 2011;26:1275–82.
38. McCallum RW, Lin Z, Forster J, et al. Gastric electrical stimulation improves outcomes of patients with gastroparesis for up to 10 years. Clin Gastroenterol Hepatol 2011;9:314–9.e1.
39. Kong MF, Horowitz M, Jones KL, et al. Natural history of diabetic gastroparesis. Diabetes Care 1999;22:503–7.
40. Camilleri M, Zinsmeister AR, Greydanus MP, et al. Towards a less costly but accurate test of gastric emptying and small bowel transit. Dig Dis Sci 1991;36:609–15.
41. Abell TL, Camilleri M, Donohoe K, et al, American Neurogastroenterology and Motility Society and the Society of Nuclear Medicine. Consensus

recommendations for gastric emptying scintigraphy: a joint report of the American Neurogastroenterology and Motility Society and the Society of Nuclear Medicine. Am J Gastroenterol 2008;103:753–63 [Reprint in J Nucl Med Technol 2008;36(1):44–54].

42. Lacy BE. Functional dyspepsia and gastroparesis: one disease or two? Am J Gastroenterol 2012;107:1615–20.

43. Janssen P, Harris MS, Jones M, et al. The relation between symptom improvement and gastric emptying in the treatment of diabetic and idiopathic gastroparesis. Am J Gastroenterol 2013;108:1382–91.

44. Rathmann W, Enck P, Frieling T, et al. Visceral afferent neuropathy in diabetic gastroparesis. Diabetes Care 1991;14:1086–9.

45. Farre R, Vanheel H, Vanuytsel T, et al. In functional dyspepsia, hypersensitivity to postprandial distention correlates with meal-related symptom severity. Gastroenterology 2013;145:566–73.

46. Jones J, Loftus EV Jr, Panaccione R, et al. Relationships between disease activity and serum and fecal biomarkers in patients with Crohn's disease. Clin Gastroenterol Hepatol 2008;6:1218–24.

47. Chang J, Rayner CK, Jones KL, et al. Diabetic gastroparesis and its impact on glycemia. Endocrinol Metab Clin North Am 2010;39:745–62.

48. Phillips WT, Schwartz JG, McMahan CA. Rapid gastric emptying of an oral glucose solution in type 2 diabetic patients. J Nucl Med 1992;33:1496–500.

49. Frank JW, Saslow SB, Camilleri M, et al. Mechanism of accelerated gastric emptying of liquids and hyperglycemia in patients with type II diabetes mellitus. Gastroenterology 1995;109:755–65.

50. Schwartz JG, Green GM, Guan D, et al. Rapid gastric emptying of a solid pancake meal in type II diabetic patients [see comment]. Diabetes Care 1996;19: 468–71.

51. Charles F, Phillips SF, Camilleri M, et al. Rapid gastric emptying in patients with functional diarrhea. Mayo Clin Proc 1997;72:323–8.

52. Weytjens C, Keymeulen B, Van Haleweyn C, et al. Rapid gastric emptying of a liquid meal in long-term type 2 diabetes mellitus. Diabet Med 1998;15:1022–7.

53. Bertin E, Schneider N, Abdelli N, et al. Gastric emptying is accelerated in obese type 2 diabetic patients without autonomic neuropathy. Diabete Metab 2001;27: 357–64.

54. Lawal A, Barboi A, Krasnow A, et al. Rapid gastric emptying is more common than gastroparesis in patients with autonomic dysfunction. Am J Gastroenterol 2007;102:618–23.

55. Janatuinen E, Pikkarainen P, Laakso M, et al. Gastrointestinal symptoms in middle-aged diabetic patients. Scand J Gastroenterol 1993;28:427–32.

56. Hammer J, Howell S, Bytzer P, et al. Symptom clustering in subjects with and without diabetes mellitus: a population-based study of 15,000 Australian adults. Am J Gastroenterol 2003;98:391–8.

Clinical Presentation and Pathophysiology of Gastroparesis

 CrossMark

Linda Anh Nguyen, MD[a],*, William J. Snape Jr, MD[b],*

KEYWORDS

- Gastroparesis • Pathophysiology • Gastric motor function • Gastric emptying
- Visceral hypersensitivity • Gastric accommodation

KEY POINTS

- Symptoms of gastroparesis go beyond delay in gastric emptying.
- There is significant overlap between idiopathic gastroparesis and functional dyspepsia in terms of symptoms and pathophysiology.
- Abdominal pain is an under-recognized symptom of gastroparesis that is associated with decreased quality of life.

Gastroparesis is a heterogeneous disorder defined as delayed gastric emptying in the absence of a mechanical obstruction. Symptoms of gastroparesis include nausea, vomiting, bloating, early satiety, and/or abdominal pain.[1]

ETIOLOGIES OF GASTROPARESIS

The most common forms of gastroparesis are idiopathic, diabetic, and postsurgical.[2] In earlier studies, idiopathic gastroparesis comprised approximately 35% of all gastroparetic patients. However, a larger multicenter study found that 67% of patients had idiopathic gastroparesis.[3] Additionally, other conditions can lead to gastroparesis (Table 1). Independent of etiology, gastroparesis affects women more commonly than men.

CLINICAL MANIFESTATIONS

Symptoms of gastroparesis are variable and include nausea, vomiting, early satiety, bloating, postprandial fullness, abdominal pain/discomfort, and anorexia (Table 2).[1–4] However, despite its prevalence in gastroparesis, consensus publications have traditionally not considered pain as a predominant factor.[1] Additionally, there is significant

Disclosures: None.
[a] Division of Gastroenterology, Department of Medicine, Stanford University, 900 Blake Wilbur Drive, 2nd Floor, Palo Alto, CA 94305, USA; [b] Division of Gastroenterology, Department of Medicine, California Pacific Medical Center, 2340 Clay Street, Suite 210, San Francisco, CA 94115, USA
* Corresponding authors.
E-mail addresses: nguyenLB@stanford.edu; snapew@sutterhealth.org

Table 1
Etiologies of gastroparesis

Etiology	N = 146	%	Female (%)
Idiopathic Postviral	52 (12)	35.6 (8.2)	90.4
Diabetes	42	28.8	76.2
Postsurgical	19	13.0	73.7
Parkinson disease	11	7.5	81.8

Collagen vascular disease
  Scleroderma
  Systemic lupus erythematosus
  Raynaud
	7	4.8	85.7

Intestinal pseudo-obstruction	6	4.1	66.7

Miscellaneous
  Stiffman syndrome
  Charcot-Marie-Tooth syndrome
  Wardenburg syndrome
  Superior mesenteric artery syndrome
  Median arcuate ligament syndrome
  Paraneoplastic syndrome
  Systemic mastocytosis
	9	6.2	55.6

Data from Soykan I, Sivri B, Saroseik I, et al. Demography, clinical characteristics, psychological and abuse profiles, treatment, and long-term follow-up of patients with gastroparesis. Dig Dis Sci 1998;43(11):2398–404.

overlap between symptoms of gastroparesis and functional dyspepsia. In a recent multicenter study, 86% of patients with idiopathic gastroparesis met Rome III criteria for functional dyspepsia.[5] Likewise, delayed gastric emptying has been found to present in 23% to 33% of patients with functional dyspepsia.[6,7] Many of the patients had a previous cholecystectomy prior to the diagnosis of gastroparesis.[8] Cholecystectomy was more common in patients with type 2 diabetes and idiopathic gastroparesis than in patients with type 1 diabetes. Patients who had a cholecystectomy had a higher prevalence of comorbidities including chronic fatigue, fibromyalgia, depression, and anxiety. These symptoms led to a worse quality of life.

Patients with type 1 diabetes mellitus had increased vomiting and retching, whereas the idiopathic gastroparesis group had increased prevalence of early satiety, postprandial fullness, and abdominal pain (**Table 3**).

Table 2
Gastroparesis symptom prevalence

Symptom	%
Nausea	80–92
Vomiting	66–84
Bloating	55–75
Early satiety	54–60
Abdominal pain	46–68

Data from Soykan I, Sivri B, Saroseik I, et al. Demography, clinical characteristics, psychological and abuse profiles, treatment, and long-term follow-up of patients with gastroparesis. Dig Dis Sci 1998;43(11):2398–404; and Parkman H, Yates K, Hasler WL, et al. Similarities and differences between diabetic and idiopathic gastroparesis. Clin Gastroenterol Hepatol 2011;9(12):1056–64.

Table 3
Symptom pattern—idiopathic versus diabetic gastroparesis

Symptom	Idiopathic (%)	Type 1 DM (%)	Type 2 DM (%)
Nausea	84.3	84.6	94.9[a]
Vomiting	59.8	88.5[a]	91.5[a]
Bloating	57.5	56.4	62.7
Early satiety	57.5	47.4	74.6[a]
Abdominal pain	76.0	60.3[a]	69.5
Weight loss	46.5	52.6	52.5

[a] $P<.05$ when compared with idiopathic gastroparesis.
Data from Parkman H, Yates K, Hasler WL, et al. Similarities and differences between diabetic and idiopathic gastroparesis. Clin Gastroenterol Hepatol 2011;9(12):1056–64.

Not all patients with chronic nausea and vomiting have a delay in gastric emptying.[9] The Gastroparesis Registry enrolled 106 patients (25%) with normal emptying and chronic nausea and vomiting. The symptoms in patients with normal gastric emptying, including nausea, vomiting and abdominal pain, had a similar severity as in patients with delayed gastric emptying. The majority of patients in either the normal or delayed gastric emptying group satisfied Rome III criteria for functional dyspepsia. Both groups remained equally symptomatic at 48-week follow-up.

In addition to nausea and vomiting, abdominal pain is a major symptom in patients with gastroparesis.[10] Abdominal pain often has been an overlooked symptom in patients with gastroparesis. Classical teaching dictates that patients with pain predominance should undergo additional evaluation for other causes. This in part may be due to the overlap between idiopathic gastroparesis and functional dyspepsia and the broad differential diagnoses for abdominal pain. However, in a large multicenter cohort study, the prevalence of moderate-to-severe abdominal pain (approximately 60%) was similar between patients with idiopathic and diabetic gastroparesis.[10] In this study, 20% of patients with gastroparesis reported pain predominance compared with 44% reporting nausea/vomiting predominance. The presence of pain predominance was associated with decreased quality of life and increased depression and anxiety. The delay in gastric emptying was similar in patients with predominant pain and predominant nausea and vomiting. Moderate-to-severe abdominal pain was more prevalent in idiopathic gastroparesis and in those patients who did not have an infectious prodrome. Compared with patients with predominant nausea/vomiting, the patients with pain had greater use of opiates and less use of antiemetics.

MEASURES OF SYMPTOM SEVERITY

The Patient Assessment of Upper Gastrointestinal Disorders Symptoms (PAGI-SYM) was developed to assess symptom severity of upper gastrointestinal (GI) symptoms in patients with gastroesophageal reflux disease (GERD), dyspepsia, and gastroparesis.[11] The PAGI-SYM consists of 20 questions and 6 subscales: heartburn/regurgitation, nausea/vomiting, postprandial fullness/early satiety, bloating, upper abdominal pain, and lower abdominal pain. The subscale scores are calculated by taking the mean of the items in each of the subscales.

The Gastroparesis Cardinal Symptom Index (GCSI) is derived from the PAGI-SYM and validated as a tool to assess patient-derived symptom severity in patients with upper gut symptoms.[12] Based on review of the literature, physician interviews, and patient focus groups, the GCSI was constructed with 9 items that categorized gastroparesis into 3 subscales: nausea/vomiting, postprandial fullness/early satiety, and bloating. The purpose of the GCSI is to provide a patient-reported tool that can be used in clinical trials to assess patient responses to therapy. However, the GCSI does not address the impact of pain on treatment outcomes.

Psychological dysfunction is associated with increased severity of symptoms as measured with the Beck Depression Inventory and the State–Trait Anxiety Inventory.[13] All 3 indexes were greater for GCSI scores greater than 3.1. The measures of psychological dysfunction were not different for diabetic or idiopathic gastroparesis and were not related to the severity of gastric retention. Nausea, vomiting, bloating, and postprandial fullness were increased in patients with higher depression or anxiety inventories.

NORMAL GASTRIC MOTOR FUNCTION

Normal GI function depends on a complex coordination between smooth muscles of the gastric fundus, antrum, pylorus, and duodenum under the control of the enteric (intrinsic) and central (extrinsic) nervous systems. Central nervous system control of digestion is mediated through the autonomic nervous system. Parasympathetic control is mediated through the vagus, while sympathetic control is mediated through the spinal cord at T5 to T10 via the celiac ganglia.[14] Vagal efferents arise from the dorsal motor nucleus and terminate in the myenteric plexus. The vagus effects gastric motility indirectly via the enteric nervous system rather than direct innervation of gastric smooth muscles.

Distention of the antrum by a solid meal triggers the fundus to relax to store food as the rest of the meal enters the stomach.[15] This accommodation response effectively increases the gastric volume without raising the intragastric pressure. Tonic contractions of the proximal stomach transfer food to the gastric antrum, where high amplitude contractions break down the food into particles 1 to 2 mm in size through trituration.[16] These particles are able to pass through the pylorus into the duodenum. Particles greater than 2 mm that cannot pass the pylorus during the postprandial phase are cleared during the interdigestive period by phase 3 of the migrating motor complexes (MMCs), which are cyclical contractions of the antrum and small bowel that propel undigestable solids distally.[17]

Motor dysfunction anywhere in the stomach may delay gastric emptying.

PATHOPHYSIOLOGY OF DELAYED GASTRIC EMPTYING
Impaired Gastric Accommodation

Regulation of proximal gastric tone and accommodation is vagally mediated through activation of nonadrenergic, noncholinergic myenteric neurons that release nitric oxide (NO).[18,19] NO produced by neuronal NO synthase in nitrergic neurons diffuses to the smooth muscle cells and inhibits gastric tone via guanosine 3',5'-cyclic monophosphate (cGMP).[15] Inhibition of cholinergic pathways can also increase gastric accommodation. There are presynaptic inhibitory α2-adrenoceptors and 5-HT1A receptors on cholinergic neurons in the stomach.[20] Disruption of these can lead to impaired gastric accommodation. The impaired accommodation may increase sensory afferent input into the chemoreceptor's trigger zone, causing nausea and vomiting.

Antral Hypomotility

The antrum is responsible for the trituration and emptying of solid foods from the stomach.[16] Postprandial antral hypomotility occurs in 70% of patients with unexplained nausea and vomiting[21] and 46% of patients with delayed gastric emptying.[22]

The presence of acute hyperglycemia is associated with antral hypomotility, especially at glucose levels of at least 250 mg/dL, but it can occur at levels as low as 140 mg/dL.[23]

Pylorospasm

In a preliminary study, 58% of DM patients had elevated pyloric tone,[24] which correlates with the number of patients who had improvement in symptoms and gastric emptying at 2 and 6 weeks after injection of botulinum toxin.[24–26] These studies suggest that pyloric pressure, including both tonic and phasic contractions, can be elevated in patients with gastroparesis. However, double-blind trials, which may have been underpowered, did not demonstrate improvement in symptoms in patients with gastroparesis.[27,28]

Duodenal Dysmotility

Coordination of antral and duodenal contractions is important in gastric emptying.[29] In this study of 12 patients with gastroparesis, simultaneous gastric emptying scintigraphy and antropyloroduodenal manometry found that postprandial coordination of antroduodenal contractions was impaired. Cisapride stimulated increased frequency of coordinated antroduodenal contractions that was associated with faster gastric emptying.

Autonomic Dysfunction

Dysfunction of the autonomic nervous system, including the parasympathetic and sympathetic systems, may contribute to gastroparesis. Vagal afferents convey sensory signals from the upper GI tract to the central nervous system (CNS). Vagal efferents mediate smooth muscle contraction and motility. Patients with orthostatic intolerance frequently have chronic GI complaints, most commonly abdominal pain, nausea, and vomiting.[30] However, the nausea often resolves with treatment of the orthostasis. Autonomic dysfunction can cause symptoms by altering either afferent or efferent pathways.

Visceral Hypersensitivity

Gastric sensation is mediated by mechano- and chemoreceptors in the stomach that transmit signals to the CNS.[31] Mechanosensitivity can be studied using the gastric barostat, which can deliver isobaric or isovolumetric distentions of the stomach during fasting or postprandially. Visceral hypersensitivity or a lowered gastric sensory threshold can be measured using the gastric barostat. The presence of visceral hypersensitivity has been described in functional dyspepsia.[19] Similarly, in a small study of patients with diabetic gastroparesis, 55% demonstrated hypersensitivity to pressure distention during fasting, while all patients exhibited hypersensitivity to distention in the postprandial state.[32]

PATHOPHYSIOLOGY OF SYMPTOMS

There is poor correlation between severity of gastroparesis symptoms and the degree of delayed gastric emptying.[33–35] Additionally, changes in gastric emptying correlated poorly with symptom response in treatment trials.[36–38] It is postulated that the presence of visceral hypersensitivity and/or impaired gastric accommodation may explain part of this disparity.

Because of the vague and heterogeneous nature of symptoms, classifying patients based on symptom predominance was proposed, in hopes of providing a framework for treating gastroparesis symptoms and gaining a better understanding of the pathophysiology. A study validating the classification of gastroparesis subgroups (**Table 4**)

Table 4	
Definition of symptom subtypes	
Symptom Subtype	**Definition of Most Bothersome Symptom(s)**
Nausea/vomiting predominant	Nausea, vomiting and/or retching
Pain/dyspepsia predominant	Upper abdominal pain/discomfort or fullness
Regurgitation predominant	Effortless regurgitation of food or heartburn

Data from Harrell S, Studts JL, Dryden GW, et al. A novel classification scheme for gastroparesis based on predominant-symptom presentation. J Clin Gastroenterol 2008;42(5):455–9; and Hasler W, Wilson LA, Parkman HP, et al. Factors related to abdominal pain in gastroparesis: contrast to patients with predominant nausea and vomiting. Neurogastroenterol Motil 2013;25(5):427–38.

found that there was concordance between patient and physician classifications. Additionally, when comparing symptom predominance with a validated 20-item symptom severity questionnaire (PAGI-SYM), there was good correlation between vomiting predominance with the nausea/vomiting subscale and regurgitation predominance with the heartburn/regurgitation subscale. However, the dyspepsia predominant group did not correlate well with any of the PAGI-SYM subscales.[39] This study also found that regurgitation predominant patients were heavier than the other 2 groups, while vomiting predominant patients were younger.

Nausea and Vomiting

Nausea and vomiting are the most common symptoms in patients with gastroparesis, with over 40% of patients reporting that these are the most bothersome symptoms.[10] However, the pathogenesis of these symptoms is heterogeneous and often multifactorial.

Centrally, the receptor site for vomiting is located in the area postrema at the base of the fourth ventricle (chemoreceptor trigger zone). Peripheral receptor sites include the vagus and vestibular apparatus. Stimulation of vagal afferents triggers emesis.[40]

Early Satiety/Fullness

Early satiety and fullness are common symptoms among patients with idiopathic and diabetic gastroparesis, especially those with type 2 diabetes.[3] Impaired gastric accommodation has been found in 43% of patients with idiopathic gastroparesis, and it contributes to patients' inability to complete eating a normal meal.[35] In this group of patients, symptoms of early satiety and weight loss were more prevalent. Similarly, impaired gastric accommodation was found in 40% of patients with functional dyspepsia.[41] A smaller study of 10 diabetic gastroparesis patients who were refractory to prokinetic therapy found that 90% of patients had impaired gastric accommodation.[32]

Several medications have been shown to increase gastric accommodation in healthy subjects as well as patients with functional dyspepsia (see **Table 5**). Moreover,

Table 5	
Medications that stimulate gastric accommodation	
Medication	**Mechanism of Action**
Sildenafil[43]	Phosphodiesterase inhibitor
Paroxetine[44]	Selective serotonin reuptake inhibitor
Cisapride[45]	5-HT4 agonist, 5-HT3 antagonist
Tegaserod[46]	Partial 5-HT4 agonist
Clonidine[20]	α2-adrenoceptor agonist
Buspirone[47]	5-HT1A agonist

Table 6 Mechanisms of bloating	
Functional Gastrointestinal Disorder	**Pathophysiology**
Functional dyspepsia[51]	Abnormal intragastric distribution of food to the distal half of the stomach
IBS with visible distention[52]	Lower sensory threshold
IBS-C[53]	Delayed colonic and/or orocecal transit

buspirone also resulted in improvement in functional dyspepsia symptoms, notably postprandial fullness, bloating, and early satiety.[42]

Bloating

Bloating is a common symptom among functional GI disorders (**Table 6**) including gastroparesis, irritable bowel syndrome (IBS), and functional dyspepsia.[48] There is no association between rate of gastric emptying and severity of bloating.[49] The presence of bloating is associated with a poor response to medical therapy.[50] A large multicenter study including 335 patients found bloating was present in 76% of patients with gastroparesis, with 41% suffering severe symptoms.[49] This study also found an association between use of norepinephrine reuptake inhibitors (predominantly tricyclic antidepressants) and minimal symptoms of bloating.

Abdominal Pain

Although a common feature of gastroparesis, abdominal pain studies have consistently shown that the severity of pain does not correlate with the severity of the delay in gastric emptying.[10,35] Patient defined pain predominance was found in approximately 20% of patients referred to the NIDDK (National Institute of Diabetes and Digestive and Kidney Diseases) Gastroparesis Clinical Research Consortium.[10]

Visceral hypersensitivity, defined as lowered threshold for eliciting visceral pain, is common among functional GI disorders, including functional dyspepsia and IBS. The presence of visceral hypersensitivity was found in 29% of patients with idiopathic gastroparesis[35] and 55% of patients with diabetic gastroparesis.[32] The presence of hypersensitivity to intragastric balloon distention was associated with a higher prevalence of abdominal pain, early satiety, and weight loss. Among these patients, the presence of hypersensitivity was also associated with greater symptom severity.

SUMMARY

There is significant overlap between idiopathic gastroparesis and functional dyspepsia in terms of symptoms and pathophysiology. This suggests that idiopathic gastroparesis and functional dyspepsia are on a spectrum a single disorder. Once thought to be a minor aspect of gastroparesis, abdominal pain is common and associated with decreased quality of life. Approximately 20% of patients describe pain as their predominant symptom. Patients with a severe delay in gastric emptying have a greater correlation between emptying and symptoms. Patients with less severe delays in emptying may benefit in classification by symptom to direct therapy.

REFERENCES

1. Parkman HP, Hasler WL, Fisher RS. American Gastroenterological Association medical position statement: diagnosis and treatment of gastroparesis. Gastroenterology 2004;127(5):1589–91.

2. Soykan I, Sivri B, Sarosiek I, et al. Demography, clinical characteristics, psychological and abuse profiles, treatment, and long-term follow-up of patients with gastroparesis. Dig Dis Sci 1998;43(11):2398–404.
3. Parkman HP, Yates K, Hasler WL, et al. Similarities and differences between diabetic and idiopathic gastroparesis. Clin Gastroenterol Hepatol 2011;9(12): 1056–64 [quiz: e133–4].
4. Hoogerwerf WA, Pasricha PJ, Kalloo AN, et al. Pain: the overlooked symptom in gastroparesis. Am J Gastroenterol 1999;94(4):1029–33.
5. Parkman HP, Yates K, Hasler WL, et al. Clinical features of idiopathic gastroparesis vary with sex, body mass, symptom onset, delay in gastric emptying, and gastroparesis severity. Gastroenterology 2011;140(1):101–15.
6. Sarnelli G, Caenepeel P, Geypens B, et al. Symptoms associated with impaired gastric emptying of solids and liquids in functional dyspepsia. Am J Gastroenterol 2003;98(4):783–8.
7. Stanghellini V, Tosetti C, Paternico A, et al. Risk indicators of delayed gastric emptying of solids in patients with functional dyspepsia. Gastroenterology 1996;110(4):1036–42.
8. Parkman HP, Yates K, Hasler WL, et al. Cholecystectomy and clinical presentations of gastroparesis. Dig Dis Sci 2013;58(4):1062–73.
9. Pasricha PJ, Colvin R, Yates K, et al. Characteristics of patients with chronic unexplained nausea and vomiting and normal gastric emptying. Clin Gastroenterol Hepatol 2011;9(7):567–76.e1-4.
10. Hasler WL, Wilson LA, Parkman HP, et al. Factors related to abdominal pain in gastroparesis: contrast to patients with predominant nausea and vomiting. Neurogastroenterol Motil 2013;25(5):427–38.
11. Rentz AM, Kahrilas P, Stanghellini V, et al. Development and psychometric evaluation of the patient assessment of upper gastrointestinal symptom severity index (PAGI-SYM) in patients with upper gastrointestinal disorders. Qual Life Res 2004; 13(10):1737–49.
12. Revicki DA, Rentz AM, Dubois D, et al. Development and validation of a patient-assessed gastroparesis symptom severity measure: the gastroparesis cardinal symptom index. Aliment Pharmacol Ther 2003;18(1):141–50.
13. Hasler WL, Parkman HP, Wilson LA, et al. Psychological dysfunction is associated with symptom severity but not disease etiology or degree of gastric retention in patients with gastroparesis. Am J Gastroenterol 2010;105(11):2357–67.
14. Wood JD, Alpers DH, Andrews PL. Fundamentals of neurogastroenterology. Gut 1999;45(Suppl 2):II6–16.
15. Kindt S, Tack J. Impaired gastric accommodation and its role in dyspepsia. Gut 2006;55(12):1685–91.
16. Camilleri M, Malagelada JR, Brown ML, et al. Relation between antral motility and gastric emptying of solids and liquids in humans. Am J Physiol 1985;249(5 Pt 1): G580–5.
17. Takahashi T. Interdigestive migrating motor complex -its mechanism and clinical importance. J Smooth Muscle Res 2013;49:99–111.
18. Azpiroz F. Control of gastric emptying by gastric tone. Dig Dis Sci 1994;39(Suppl 12):18S–9S.
19. Carbone F, Tack J. Gastroduodenal mechanisms underlying functional gastric disorders. Dig Dis 2014;32(3):222–9.
20. Thumshirn M, Camilleri M, Choi MG, et al. Modulation of gastric sensory and motor functions by nitrergic and alpha2-adrenergic agents in humans. Gastroenterology 1999;116(3):573–85.

21. Kerlin P. Postprandial antral hypomotility in patients with idiopathic nausea and vomiting. Gut 1989;30(1):54–9.
22. Camilleri M, Brown ML, Malagelada JR. Relationship between impaired gastric emptying and abnormal gastrointestinal motility. Gastroenterology 1986;91(1): 94–9.
23. Barnett JL, Owyang C. Serum glucose concentration as a modulator of interdigestive gastric motility. Gastroenterology 1988;94(3):739–44.
24. Mearin F, Camilleri M, Malagelada JR. Pyloric dysfunction in diabetics with recurrent nausea and vomiting. Gastroenterology 1986;90(6):1919–25.
25. Ezzeddine D, Jit R, Katz N, et al. Pyloric injection of botulinum toxin for treatment of diabetic gastroparesis. Gastrointest Endosc 2002;55(7):920–3.
26. Miller LS, Szych GA, Kantor SB, et al. Treatment of idiopathic gastroparesis with injection of botulinum toxin into the pyloric sphincter muscle. Am J Gastroenterol 2002;97(7):1653–60.
27. Arts J, Holvoet L, Caenepeel P, et al. Clinical trial: a randomized-controlled crossover study of intrapyloric injection of botulinum toxin in gastroparesis. Aliment Pharmacol Ther 2007;26(9):1251–8.
28. Friedenberg FK, Palit A, Parkman HP, et al. Botulinum toxin A for the treatment of delayed gastric emptying. Am J Gastroenterol 2008;103(2):416–23.
29. Fraser RJ, Horowitz M, Maddox AF, et al. Postprandial antropyloroduodenal motility and gastric emptying in gastroparesis–effects of cisapride. Gut 1994; 35(2):172–8.
30. Sullivan SD, Hanauer J, Rowe PC, et al. Gastrointestinal symptoms associated with orthostatic intolerance. J Pediatr Gastroenterol Nutr 2005;40(4):425–8.
31. Camilleri M, Coulie B, Tack JF. Visceral hypersensitivity: facts, speculations, and challenges. Gut 2001;48(1):125–31.
32. Kumar A, Attaluri A, Hashmi S, et al. Visceral hypersensitivity and impaired accommodation in refractory diabetic gastroparesis. Neurogastroenterol Motil 2008;20(6):635–42.
33. Horowitz M, Su YC, Rayner CK, et al. Gastroparesis: prevalence, clinical significance and treatment. Can J Gastroenterol 2001;15(12):805–13.
34. Talley NJ, Verlinden M, Jones M. Can symptoms discriminate among those with delayed or normal gastric emptying in dysmotility-like dyspepsia? Am J Gastroenterol 2001;96(5):1422–8.
35. Karamanolis G, Caenepeel P, Arts J, et al. Determinants of symptom pattern in idiopathic severely delayed gastric emptying: gastric emptying rate or proximal stomach dysfunction? Gut 2007;56(1):29–36.
36. Talley NJ, Verlinden M, Snape W, et al. Failure of a motilin receptor agonist (ABT-229) to relieve the symptoms of functional dyspepsia in patients with and without delayed gastric emptying: a randomized double-blind placebo-controlled trial. Aliment Pharmacol Ther 2000;14(12):1653–61.
37. Silvers D, Kipnes M, Broadstone V, et al. Domperidone in the management of symptoms of diabetic gastroparesis: efficacy, tolerability, and quality-of-life outcomes in a multicenter controlled trial. DOM-USA-5 Study Group. Clin Ther 1998;20(3):438–53.
38. Arts J, Caenepeel P, Verbeke K, et al. Influence of erythromycin on gastric emptying and meal related symptoms in functional dyspepsia with delayed gastric emptying. Gut 2005;54(4):455–60.
39. Harrell SP, Studts JL, Dryden GW, et al. A novel classification scheme for gastroparesis based on predominant-symptom presentation. J Clin Gastroenterol 2008; 42(5):455–9.

40. Urayama Y, Yamada Y, Nakamura E, et al. Electrical and chemical stimulation of the nucleus raphe magnus inhibits induction of retching by afferent vagal fibers. Auton Neurosci 2010;152(1–2):35–40.
41. Tack J, Piessevaux H, Coulie B, et al. Role of impaired gastric accommodation to a meal in functional dyspepsia. Gastroenterology 1998;115(6):1346–52.
42. Tack J, Janssen P, Masaoka T, et al. Efficacy of buspirone, a fundus-relaxing drug, in patients with functional dyspepsia. Clin Gastroenterol Hepatol 2012; 10(11):1239–45.
43. Sarnelli G, Sifrim D, Janssens J, et al. Influence of sildenafil on gastric sensorimotor function in humans. Am J Physiol Gastrointest Liver Physiol 2004;287(5): G988–92.
44. Tack J, Broekaert D, Coulie B, et al. Influence of the selective serotonin re-uptake inhibitor, paroxetine, on gastric sensorimotor function in humans. Aliment Pharmacol Ther 2003;17(4):603–8.
45. Tack J, Broekaert D, Coulie B, et al. The influence of cisapride on gastric tone and the perception of gastric distension. Aliment Pharmacol Ther 1998;12(8):761–6.
46. Tack J, Janssen P, Bisschops R, et al. Influence of tegaserod on proximal gastric tone and on the perception of gastric distention in functional dyspepsia. Neurogastroenterol Motil 2011;23(2):e32–9.
47. Van Oudenhove L, Kindt S, Vos R, et al. Influence of buspirone on gastric sensorimotor function in man. Aliment Pharmacol Ther 2008;28(11–12):1326–33.
48. Jiang X, Locke GR 3rd, Choung RS, et al. Prevalence and risk factors for abdominal bloating and visible distention: a population-based study. Gut 2008;57(6): 756–63.
49. Hasler WL, Wilson LA, Parkman HP, et al. Bloating in gastroparesis: severity, impact, and associated factors. Am J Gastroenterol 2011;106(8):1492–502.
50. Anaparthy R, Pehlivanov N, Grady J, et al. Gastroparesis and gastroparesis-like syndrome: response to therapy and its predictors. Dig Dis Sci 2009;54(5): 1003–10.
51. Troncon LE, Bennett RJ, Ahluwalia NK, et al. Abnormal intragastric distribution of food during gastric emptying in functional dyspepsia patients. Gut 1994;35(3): 327–32.
52. Agrawal A, Houghton LA, Lea R, et al. Bloating and distention in irritable bowel syndrome: the role of visceral sensation. Gastroenterology 2008;134(7):1882–9.
53. Agrawal A, Houghton LA, Reilly B, et al. Bloating and distension in irritable bowel syndrome: the role of gastrointestinal transit. Am J Gastroenterol 2009;104(8): 1998–2004.

Histologic Changes in Diabetic Gastroparesis

Gianrico Farrugia, MD

KEYWORDS

- Interstitial cells of Cajal • Gastric emptying • Macrophages • Enteric nerves • Vagus
- Smooth muscle

KEY POINTS

- Several key cell types are affected by diabetes leading to gastroparesis.
- Diabetic gastroparesis is associated with damage to the extrinsic innervation to the stomach, loss of key neurotransmitters at the level of the enteric nervous system, smooth muscle abnormalities, loss of interstitial cells of Cajal (ICC) and changes in the macrophage population resident in the muscle wall.
- Macrophages seem to be a key cell type underlying injury to other cell types.
- Targeting macrophages may allow for the development of a disease-modifying strategy for treating diabetic gastroparesis with the potential to markedly change how diabetic gastroparesis is managed.

INTRODUCTION

The cellular abnormalities that lead to diabetic gastroparesis are increasingly being understood. Several key cell types are affected by diabetes, leading to gastroparesis. These changes include abnormalities in the extrinsic innervation to the stomach, loss of key neurotransmitters at the level of the enteric nervous system, smooth muscle abnormalities, loss of ICC, and changes in the macrophage population resident in the muscle wall. This article reviews the current understanding with a focus on data from human studies when available.

EXTRINSIC INNERVATION IN DIABETIC GASTROPARESIS

Diabetic gastroparesis was first described by Dr Kassander in 1958. After the initial description, investigations centered on the role of abnormalities in the extrinsic innervation to the stomach in the causation of diabetic gastroparesis. Both sympathetic

Disclosure statement: The author has nothing to disclose.
Supported by NIH grants DK74008, DK68055, DK57061.
Enteric NeuroScience Program, Mayo Clinic, 200 First Street Southwest, Rochester, MN 55905, USA
E-mail address: Farrugia.gianrico@mayo.edu

Gastroenterol Clin N Am 44 (2015) 31–38
http://dx.doi.org/10.1016/j.gtc.2014.11.004
0889-8553/15/$ – see front matter © 2015 Elsevier Inc. All rights reserved.

and parasympathetic abnormalities were described, with increasing evidence over the years for a defect in the vagal innervation to the stomach and indeed the upper gastro-intestinal tract.[1] Damage to the vagal innervation of the stomach was shown by a sham feeding test, which takes advantage of the innervation of the pancreas by the vagus. During the cephalic phase of food digestion, stimulation of the vagus results in release of pancreatic polypeptide. Patients with advanced diabetic gastroparesis have a blunted pancreatic polypeptide response as well as reduced gastric secretion in response to sham feeding suggesting vagus nerve dysfunction.[2,3] Abnormalities in vagal innervation of the stomach may contribute to the motor abnormalities seen, including abnormal relaxation of the pylorus. However, the initial histologic report in 1988[4] in 16 diabetic patients of whom 5 had gastroparesis failed to show any histolog-ic defects. In retrospect, this was likely due to the small n value and the limited tech-niques available at that time (hematoxylin and eosin, Gomori trichrome, Luxol fast blue, and Holmes silver stains). In subsequent animal and human studies abnormal-ities have been described, including abnormalities at a histologic level both in myelin-ated and unmyelinated nerve fibers of the vagus nerve,[1,5] which were also reported to be smaller in the biobreeding rat model of spontaneous diabetes. Sympathetic ner-vous system abnormalities have also been described, with changes in the axons and dendrites within the prevertebral sympathetic ganglia.

SMOOTH MUSCLE

In the past relatively, rarely, patients with severe symptoms of diabetic gastroparesis, often unremitting nausea and vomiting, had gastrectomies as a treatment of their symptoms with variable results. An examination of the resected tissue showed evi-dence of smooth muscle degeneration and fibrosis, with eosinophilic inclusion bodies.[6] In a study of 2 patients with severe diabetic gastroparesis, one had no fibrosis and the other showed fibrosis with the use of a trichrome stain.[7] A study of full-thickness biopsies at the time of gastric stimulation implantation did not show signif-icant fibrosis,[8] suggesting that the fibrosis seen in the earlier studies may represent a more end-stage aspect of the disease.

Nonobese diabetic (NOD) mice are an often used model of diabetic gastroparesis. NOD mice develop a leukocytic infiltrate of the pancreatic islets, resulting in a type 1 type of diabetes. Studies on organotypic cultures from the stomachs of these mice have shown a loss of smooth muscle–derived insulin-like growth factor 1,[9] suggesting that smooth muscle function may be impaired before the onset of overt fibrosis.

ENTERIC NERVES

After the initial discovery that extrinsic nervous system defects are present in diabetic gastroparesis, work on animal models found that the intrinsic nervous system was also affected. Initial work was carried out in rats. Rats made diabetic with streptozo-tocin[10] showed an increase in vasoactive intestinal peptide-like immunoreactivity in nerve cell bodies and nerve fibers, with no change in level of substance (SP). These changes were reversible with insulin administration.[11] The same rat model also showed evidence for altered enteric nerve ion transport.[12] A study[13] using spontane-ously non-insulin-dependent diabetic rats demonstrated depolarization of the smooth muscle membrane potential, an attenuation of nonadrenergic noncholinergic inhibi-tory neurotransmission, and a reduction in reactivity of adrenoceptors to noradrena-line. Work carried out using spontaneously diabetic biobreeding/Worcester (BB/W) rats showed that the number of neuronal nitric oxide synthase (nNOS)-containing neu-rons in the gastric myenteric plexus and NOS activity were significantly reduced in diabetic BB/W rats, suggesting a nitrergic defect.[14] Similar results were found in streptozotocin-induced diabetes in rats. Gastric relaxation correlates better with the dimerized form of nNOS rather than with absolute nNOS levels, suggesting that post-translational modification is important and in fact may be more relevant than overall quantification of nNOS.[15] Work in mice has similarly shown loss of nNOS expression in diabetes, both in the stomach[16] and in other regions of the gastrointestinal tract.[17]

Studies in humans have also highlighted the role of nNOS in diabetic gastroenteropathy. Work using human colon showed enteric nerves cells with enhanced apoptosis and loss of peripherin, nNOS, neuropeptide Y, and choline acetyl transferase neurons, with evidence for increased oxidative stress.[18] A study on male patients with gastric cancer, with and without type 2 diabetes, showed reduced number of ICC, nNOS, and substance P (SP) in the antrum of patients with diabetes.[4] In a study of 16 patients with diabetic gastroparesis, 6 had reduced myenteric nerve cell bodies.[19] The study from the Gastroparesis Clinical Research Consortium (GpCRC) funded by the National Institutes of Health examined tissue from the gastric body of 20 patients with diabetic gastroparesis. Overall, there was no statistical difference in the level of PGP9.5 (a marker of neurons) or nNOS-containing neurons between patients with diabetic gastroparesis and controls, although 4 patients did have a greater than 25% decrease in the number of nNOS-containing neurons. At the electron microscopic level, several patients had empty secretory vesicles in nerve terminals suggesting altered neurotransmission.[20] These data suggest that, given the relative sparing of enteric neurons, the enteric neuronal abnormalities seen, such as loss of nNOS expression, may be more reversible than initially thought. One needs to understand the regulation of the expression of nNOS and other key proteins to target their expression.

INTERSTITIAL CELLS OF CAJAL

In the early 1990s, several studies reported on the requirement for an intact ICC network for normal gastrointestinal motility. Loss of ICC has been associated with several diseases, including chronic intestinal pseudo-obstruction and slow transit constipation.[21] ICC generate an electric event known as the slow wave that sets the smooth muscle membrane potential, thereby regulating contractility. ICCs are also involved in cholinergic and nitrergic neurotransmission, with enteric nerves innervating both ICC and smooth muscle,[22] and in mechanotransduction. Loss of ICC is the most common abnormality seen in diabetic gastroparesis. Loss of ICC was first reported in mouse models of diabetic gastroparesis,[23] but it soon became apparent that loss of ICC is also seen in humans.[24] The GpCRC study that reported on enteric nerve changes also studied the numbers of ICC and found that 50% of patients with diabetic gastroparesis had a significant decrease in the number of ICC.[8] At an ultrastructural level, even when the number of ICC was not reduced there were significant changes to ICC and the surrounding stroma, with 95% (19/20) of patient tissue examined showing ICC abnormalities and a thick stroma separating ICC from smooth muscle cells[20] and nerves. A protein key to the electrical function of ICC is Ano-1, a calcium-activated chloride channel. Ano-1 expression is altered in diabetic gastroparesis,[25] and patients with diabetic gastroparesis have variants of Ano-1 different from those in diabetic patients without gastroparesis. These variants were associated with altered electrical activity of the ion channel, suggesting that even when structurally normal, the function of ICC may be impaired in diabetic gastroparesis.[26]

Loss of ICC impairs gastric function. Loss of ICCs in diabetic gastroparesis is associated with disruption of the generation and propagation of electrical slow waves, resulting in gastric dysrhythmias.[27] A decrease in frequency of the slow wave is referred to as bradygastria, with tachygastria referring to an increase in frequency. These changes are often transient, and both have been reported in diabetic gastroparesis with symptoms related to meals.[28,29] Refractory diabetic gastroparesis was found to correlate with both loss of ICC and abnormal results in electrogastrogram. Animal studies have shown that not only the absolute number of ICCs leads to electrical dysrhythmias but also a patchy disruption of ICC networks may result in reentrant tachyarrhythmias as well as loss of generation of the slow waves resulting in bradyarrhythmias. A recent study reported severe ICC loss in 12 of 34 patients with refractory diabetic gastroparesis and correlated loss of ICC with abnormal results in electrogastrogram showing tachygastria.[30] Loss of ICC is correlated with development of delayed gastric emptying, with a more severe loss of ICC associated with a more severe delay in gastric emptying.[31]

FIBROBLAST-LIKE CELLS

A recent addition to our understanding of the cell types required for normal gastric motor function is a type of interstitial cell with fibroblast-like ultrastructure that is referred to as fibroblast-like cells (FLCs).[32,33] These cells were shown to have gap junctions with smooth muscle cells and to be close to but distinct from ICC.[34,35] A distinct feature of this cell type is the high expression of SK3 (small conductance calcium-activated potassium channels type 3) channels and platelet-derived growth factor receptor α.[36–38] FLCs are involved in enteric neurotransmission, specifically purinergic neurotransmission.[39–41] Given that FLCs, like ICC, are involved in enteric neurotransmission and the number of ICCs is decreased in diabetic gastroparesis, the question was soon raised on whether FLCs are also altered in diabetic gastroparesis. The one study that addressed this question did not find any difference in the number or distribution of FLCs in diabetic gastroparesis,[42] suggesting that diabetic gastroparesis is not due to structural changes to this cell type.

IMMUNE CELLS

Type 1 diabetes is associated with an immune-related destruction of pancreatic islets. This has led to the suggestion that diabetic gastroparesis may have an inflammatory component. In a study on antral biopsies from 14 patients with diabetic gastroparesis, a mild lymphocytic infiltrate was found in the myenteric plexus in 6 of the 14 patients.[19] These findings were not borne out in a subsequent study comparing gastric body tissue from patients with diabetes and diabetic gastroparesis. Immune cells in the circular muscle layer were studied using antibodies to CD45, CD206, iNOS, and the putative human macrophage markers HAM56, CD68, and EMR1. Overall, no difference in CD45-positive cells was found between the 2 groups, but an association was found between CD206-positive cells and ICC numbers.[43] These data suggest that the type of infiltrate may be more relevant than the absolute number of immune cells (see later discussion).

MACROPHAGES

Mouse models of diabetes have strongly suggested a critical role for macrophages in the development of delayed gastric emptying. Diabetes is associated with increased oxidative stress. In NOD mice, development of diabetes was accompanied by upregulation of heme oxygenase 1 (HO1) in macrophages.[16] The muscle wall of the stomach is populated with resident macrophages that have been described to play a role in neuronally mediated regulation of contractility.[44] In response to various stimuli, mouse macrophages polarize to either the classically activated proinflammatory M1 macrophage or the anti-inflammatory alternatively activated M2 (CD206-positive) macrophage. Development of diabetes was associated with upregulation of HO1 in CD206-positive M2 macrophages. Onset of delayed gastric emptying did not alter the number of macrophages, but there was selective loss of CD206-positive/HO1-positive M2 macrophages and an increase in the number of M1 macrophages.[45] Treatment of diabetic mice with delayed gastric emptying with hemin or interleukin 10 to upregulate HO1 resulted in repopulation of the stomach wall with M2 macrophages and normalization of gastric emptying. These data suggest that HO1-positive M2 macrophages are required for the prevention of diabetes-induced delayed gastric emptying and that M1 macrophages are associated with the development of delayed gastric emptying. HO1 breaks down heme into iron, biliverdin, and carbon monoxide. Diabetic NOD mice with delayed gastric emptying treated with carbon monoxide inhalation at low levels (100 ppm) showed reduced oxidative stress, restored Kit (a marker of ICC) expression, and normalized delayed gastric emptying, suggesting that carbon monoxide mediates, at least in part, the effects of HO1.[46]

A role for macrophages in the development of diabetic macrophages seems to also hold true for humans. In a study from the GpCRC, full-thickness gastric body biopsies were studied from nondiabetic controls, diabetic controls, and patients with diabetic gastroparesis. The number of CD206-positive cells correlated with the number of ICC, suggesting that in humans, like mice, CD206-positive macrophages may play a cytoprotective role in diabetes.[43]

SUMMARY/DISCUSSION

A major issue with the current therapies for diabetic gastroparesis is that they are all symptom based, including use of prokinetics.[47–49] Although a prokinetic helps restore the synchronicity between delivery of food and hormone and peptide release, it does not target the underlying defects. To truly treat diabetic gastroparesis, disease-modifying agents must be developed, and to do so, the mechanisms of disease must be better understood. It is now known that several cell types are affected in diabetic gastroparesis. These cell types include extrinsic nerves, the enteric nervous system, and ICC, with ICC loss being the most common cellular defect seen. Advances in the understanding of the role macrophages play in the stomach wall and the role of activated macrophages in diabetic gastroparesis suggest that gastric macrophages may be central to the development of the diverse cellular damage that leads to gastroparesis. Sustained expression of HO1 by CD206-positive macrophages protects against the injurious effect of mediators released by M1 macrophages. Not every patient with diabetes develops gastroparesis, and the duration between the onset of diabetes and the onset of gastroparesis varies widely, with some patients developing the disease only after 3 to 4 years. This observation strongly suggests other factors, including genetics and epigenetics, may play a significant role in the polarization of macrophages and the increase in expression of HO1, and this is an area of high interest that needs further study. Understanding the role macrophages play in diabetic gastroparesis as the key cell type that underlies injury to other cell types would allow the development of a disease-modifying strategy for treating diabetic gastroparesis with potential to markedly change how diabetic gastroparesis is managed at present.

REFERENCES

1. Duchen LW, Anjorin A, Watkins PJ, et al. Pathology of autonomic neuropathy in diabetes mellitus. Ann Intern Med 1980;92:301–3.

2. Buysschaert M, Donckier J, Dive A, et al. Gastric acid and pancreatic polypeptide responses to sham feeding are impaired in diabetic subjects with autonomic neuropathy. Diabetes 1985;34:1181–5.

3. Schwartz TW. Pancreatic polypeptide: a hormone under vagal control. Gastroenterology 1983;85:1411–25.

4. Iwasaki H, Kajimura M, Osawa S, et al. A deficiency of gastric interstitial cells of Cajal accompanied by decreased expression of neuronal nitric oxide synthase and substance P in patients with type 2 diabetes mellitus. J Gastroenterol 2006;41:1076–87.

5. Guy RJ, Dawson JL, Garrett JR, et al. Diabetic gastroparesis from autonomic neuropathy: surgical considerations and changes in vagus nerve morphology. J Neurol Neurosurg Psychiatry 1984;47:686–91.

6. Ejskjaer NT, Bradley JL, Buxton-Thomas MS, et al. Novel surgical treatment and gastric pathology in diabetic gastroparesis. Diabet Med 1999;16:488–95.

7. Pasricha PJ, Pehlivanov ND, Gomez G, et al. Changes in the gastric enteric nervous system and muscle: a case report on two patients with diabetic gastroparesis. BMC Gastroenterol 2008;8:21.

8. Grover M, Farrugia G, Lurken MS, et al. Cellular changes in diabetic and idiopathic gastroparesis. Gastroenterology 2011;140:1575–85.e8.

9. Horvath VJ, Vittal H, Ordog T. Reduced insulin and IGF-I signaling, not hyperglycemia, underlies the diabetes-associated depletion of interstitial cells of Cajal in the murine stomach. Diabetes 2005;54:1528–33.

10. Belai A, Lincoln J, Milner P, et al. Enteric nerves in diabetic rats: increase in vasoactive intestinal polypeptide but not substance P. Gastroenterology 1985;89:967–76.

11. Burnstock G, Mirsky R, Belai A. Reversal of nerve damage in streptozotocin-diabetic rats by acute application of insulin in vitro. Clin Sci (Lond) 1988;75:629–35.

12. Perdue MH, Davison JS. Altered regulation of intestinal ion transport by enteric nerves in diabetic rats. Am J Physiol 1988;254:G444–9.

13. Imaeda K, Takano H, Koshita M, et al. Electrical properties of colonic smooth muscle in spontaneously non-insulin-dependent diabetic rats. J Smooth Muscle Res 1998;34:1–11.

14. Takahashi T, Nakamura K, Itoh H, et al. Impaired expression of nitric oxide synthase in the gastric myenteric plexus of spontaneously diabetic rats. Gastroenterology 1997;113:1535–44.

15. Gangula PR, Maner WL, Micci MA, et al. Diabetes induces sex-dependent changes in neuronal nitric oxide synthase dimerization and function in the rat gastric antrum. Am J Physiol Gastrointest Liver Physiol 2007;292:G725–33.

16. Choi KM, Gibbons SJ, Nguyen TV, et al. Heme oxygenase-1 protects interstitial cells of Cajal from oxidative stress and reverses diabetic gastroparesis. Gastroenterology 2008;135:2055–64, 2064.e1–2.

17. Yarandi SS, Srinivasan S. Diabetic gastrointestinal motility disorders and the role of enteric nervous system: current status and future directions. Neurogastroenterol Motil 2014;26:611–24.

18. Chandrasekharan B, Anitha M, Blatt R, et al. Colonic motor dysfunction in human diabetes is associated with enteric neuronal loss and increased oxidative stress. Neurogastroenterol Motil 2011;23:131–8 e26.

19. Harberson J, Thomas RM, Harbison SP, et al. Gastric neuromuscular pathology in gastroparesis: analysis of full-thickness antral biopsies. Dig Dis Sci 2010;55:359–70.

20. Faussone-Pellegrini MS, Grover M, Pasricha PJ, et al. Ultrastructural differences between diabetic and idiopathic gastroparesis. J Cell Mol Med 2012;16:1573–81.
21. Farrugia G. Interstitial cells of Cajal in health and disease. Neurogastroenterol Motil 2008;20(Suppl 1):54–63.
22. Lies B, Groneberg D, Friebe A. Toward a better understanding of gastrointestinal nitrergic neuromuscular transmission. Neurogastroenterol Motil 2014;26:901–12.
23. Ordog T, Takayama I, Cheung WK, et al. Remodeling of networks of interstitial cells of Cajal in a murine model of diabetic gastroparesis. Diabetes 2000;49: 1731–9.
24. He CL, Soffer EE, Ferris CD, et al. Loss of interstitial cells of Cajal and inhibitory innervation in insulin-dependent diabetes. Gastroenterology 2001;121:427–34.
25. Gomez-Pinilla PJ, Gibbons SJ, Bardsley MR, et al. Ano1 is a selective marker of interstitial cells of Cajal in the human and mouse gastrointestinal tract. Am J Physiol Gastrointest Liver Physiol 2009;296:G1370–81.
26. Mazzone A, Bernard CE, Strege PR, et al. Altered expression of Ano1 variants in human diabetic gastroparesis. J Biol Chem 2011;286:13393–403.
27. O'Grady G, Angeli TR, Du P, et al. Abnormal initiation and conduction of slow-wave activity in gastroparesis, defined by high-resolution electrical mapping. Gastroenterology 2012;143:589–98.e1–3.
28. Koch KL. Diabetic gastropathy: gastric neuromuscular dysfunction in diabetes mellitus: a review of symptoms, pathophysiology, and treatment. Dig Dis Sci 1999;44:1061–75.
29. Koch KL. Electrogastrography: physiological basis and clinical application in diabetic gastropathy. Diabetes Technol Ther 2001;3:51–62.
30. Forster J, Damjanov I, Lin Z, et al. Absence of the interstitial cells of Cajal in patients with gastroparesis and correlation with clinical findings. J Gastrointest Surg 2005;9:102–8.
31. Grover M, Bernard CE, Pasricha PJ, et al. Clinical-histological associations in gastroparesis: results from the Gastroparesis Clinical Research Consortium. Neurogastroenterol Motil 2012;24:531–9 e249.
32. Rumessen JJ, Thuneberg L. Interstitial cells of Cajal in human small intestine. Ultrastructural identification and organization between the main smooth muscle layers. Gastroenterology 1991;100:1417–31.
33. Rumessen JJ, Thuneberg L, Mikkelsen HB. Plexus muscularis profundus and associated interstitial cells. II. Ultrastructural studies of mouse small intestine. Anat Rec 1982;203:129–46.
34. Horiguchi K, Komuro T. Ultrastructural observations of fibroblast-like cells forming gap junctions in the W/W(nu) mouse small intestine. J Auton Nerv Syst 2000;80: 142–7.
35. Vanderwinden JM, Rumessen JJ, De Laet MH, et al. CD34+ cells in human intestine are fibroblasts adjacent to, but distinct from, interstitial cells of Cajal. Lab Invest 1999;79:59–65.
36. Fujita A, Takeuchi T, Jun H, et al. Localization of Ca2+-activated K+ channel, SK3, in fibroblast-like cells forming gap junctions with smooth muscle cells in the mouse small intestine. J Pharmacol Sci 2003;92:35–42.
37. Fujita A, Takeuchi T, Saitoh N, et al. Expression of Ca(2+)-activated K(+) channels, SK3, in the interstitial cells of Cajal in the gastrointestinal tract. Am J Physiol Cell Physiol 2001;281:C1727–33.
38. Vanderwinden JM, Rumessen JJ, de Kerchove d'Exaerde A Jr, et al. Kit-negative fibroblast-like cells expressing SK3, a Ca2+-activated K+ channel, in the gut musculature in health and disease. Cell Tissue Res 2002;310:349–58.

39. Blair PJ, Bayguinov Y, Sanders KM, et al. Relationship between enteric neurons and interstitial cells in the primate gastrointestinal tract. Neurogastroenterol Motil 2012;24:e437–49.
40. Kurahashi M, Mutafova-Yambolieva V, Koh SD, et al. Platelet-derived growth factor receptor-alpha-positive cells and not smooth muscle cells mediate purinergic hyperpolarization in murine colonic muscles. Am J Physiol Cell Physiol 2014;307: C561–70.
41. Kurahashi M, Zheng H, Dwyer L, et al. A functional role for the 'fibroblast-like cells' in gastrointestinal smooth muscles. J Physiol 2011;589:697–710.
42. Grover M, Bernard CE, Pasricha PJ, et al. Platelet-derived growth factor receptor alpha (PDGFRalpha)-expressing "fibroblast-like cells" in diabetic and idiopathic gastroparesis of humans. Neurogastroenterol Motil 2012;24:844–52.
43. Bernard CE, Gibbons SJ, Mann IS, et al. Association of low numbers of CD206-positive cells with loss of ICC in the gastric body of patients with diabetic gastroparesis. Neurogastroenterol Motil 2014;26:1275–84.
44. Muller PA, Koscso B, Rajani GM, et al. Crosstalk between muscularis macrophages and enteric neurons regulates gastrointestinal motility. Cell 2014;158: 300–13.
45. Choi KM, Kashyap PC, Dutta N, et al. CD206-positive M2 macrophages that express heme oxygenase-1 protect against diabetic gastroparesis in mice. Gastroenterology 2010;138:2399–409, 2409.e1.
46. Kashyap PC, Choi KM, Dutta N, et al. Carbon monoxide reverses diabetic gastroparesis in NOD mice. Am J Physiol Gastrointest Liver Physiol 2010;298:G1013–9.
47. Abell TL, Bernstein RK, Cutts T, et al. Treatment of gastroparesis: a multidisciplinary clinical review. Neurogastroenterol Motil 2006;18:263–83.
48. Rabine JC, Barnett JL. Management of the patient with gastroparesis. J Clin Gastroenterol 2001;32:11–8.
49. Stevens JE, Jones KL, Rayner CK, et al. Pathophysiology and pharmacotherapy of gastroparesis: current and future perspectives. Expert Opin Pharmacother 2013;14:1171–86.

Diabetic Gastroparesis

Kenneth L. Koch, MD[a],*, Jorge Calles-Escandón, MD[b]

KEYWORDS

- Type 1 and type 2 diabetes mellitus • Gastroparesis • Gastric dysrhythmias
- Prokinetic and antinauseant drugs • Gastric electric stimulation • Nausea • Vomiting

KEY POINTS

- Gastroparesis is delayed gastric emptying in the absence of obstruction, a complication that affects patients with type 2 as well as type 1 diabetes mellitus.
- Symptoms associated with gastroparesis are nonspecific, and the diagnoses should be confirmed with gastric emptying tests.
- Patients are often overweight and have nutritional deficiencies.
- Obstructive gastroparesis, a subset of gastroparesis, is caused by pyloric dysfunction, and botulinum toxin A injections may be helpful.
- Trending postprandial glucose excursions with continuous glucose monitoring aids in the dosing and timing of insulin administration in diabetic patients with gastroparesis.

INTRODUCTION

When gastroparesis afflicts patients with type 1 diabetes mellitus (T1DM) or type 2 diabetes mellitus (T2DM), the consequences are particularly severe. Symptoms associated with gastroparesis, such as early satiety, prolonged fullness, nausea, and vomiting of undigested food, not only reduce the quality of life but also compound difficulties in controlling blood glucose levels.

Gastroparesis is defined as a delay in the emptying of ingested food in the absence of mechanical obstruction of the stomach or duodenum.[1] Many patients with diabetes (as well as their physicians) do not appreciate that gastroparesis has developed. In diabetic patients with gastroparesis, ingested food is not emptied in a predictable period of time; thus, the anticipated nutrient absorption is not the reality. Consequently, the selected dose and timing of insulin therapy to control postprandial glucose may be inappropriate.

In many patients with gastroparesis, erratic postcibal glucose levels result in swings from hypoglycemia to severe hyperglycemia and even ketoacidosis.[2,3] Hyperglycemia

Disclosures: 3 CPM Company, Shareholder; GlaxoSmithKline, Consultant (K.L. Koch, MD); The author has nothing to disclose (J. Calles-Escandón, MD).
[a] Section on Gastroenterology, Wake Forest School of Medicine, Medical Center Boulevard, Winston-Salem, NC 27157, USA; [b] Section on Endocrinology, MetroHealth Regional, Case Western Reserve University School of Medicine, 2500 Metrohealth Drive, Cleveland, OH 44109, USA
* Corresponding author.
E-mail address: kkoch@wakehealth.edu

itself elicits gastric dysrhythmias and slows gastric emptying.[4,5] Patients frequently are seen in emergency rooms for low glucose levels, severe hyperglycemia, or ketoacidosis. Gastroparesis as an underlying condition needs to be considered in these cases.

In addition to antinauseant and prokinetic drug therapies, patients with diabetic gastroparesis also need to change their diet and the timing and dosing of insulin to better match the slow emptying of ingested food. The epidemiology, pathophysiology, clinical presentation, diagnostic testing, and treatments for diabetic gastroparesis are reviewed in this article.

EPIDEMIOLOGY

A recent update reported that there are more than 36 million individuals with diabetes in North America and the Caribbean[6] and most are cases of T2DM. The estimates of prevalence of gastroparesis in T1DM vary widely. Although in tertiary centers, up to 40% of patients with T1DM have gastroparesis,[7] surveys in Olmsted County, Minnesota, indicated a prevalence of 5%.[8]

Similarly, in specialized centers, 10% to 30% of patients with T2DM have gastroparesis[9]; in Olmsted County, the prevalence was 1%.[10] These differences likely reflect a selection bias, because more patients with diabetes and complications are seen in tertiary medical centers compared with surveys of patients in the community. Nevertheless, because of the increasing numbers of patients with T2DM, this population represents the largest group of patients with gastroparesis.

The number of patients with diabetes worldwide continues to increase. The World Health Organization estimated that in 2013 almost 350 million individuals had diabetes (mainly T2DM), and predicted mortality from diabetes will double by 2030 (http://www.who.int/mediacentre/factsheets/fs312/es/). Assuming a low estimate of gastroparesis incidence in T2DM of 1%, at least 5 million individuals with diabetes complicated with gastroparesis will require specialized diagnosis and care.

Gastroparesis evolves over time, presumably as acute and chronic hyperglycemia and reduced insulin and insulinlike growth factor 1 (IGF-1) signaling results in damage to the interstitial cells of Cajal (ICCs) and enteric neurons of the stomach.[11,12] Over a 10-year period, approximately 5.2% of patients with T1DM developed gastroparesis, whereas 5 times fewer (1%) patients with T2DM developed gastroparesis over that same period.[8] Although good control of glycemia prevents or delays many of the chronic complications of T1DM,[13] the effect of good glucose control on the onset or progression of gastroparesis in T1DM is unknown. Diabetic patients with gastroparesis often have many of the chronic complications of diabetes (retinopathy, nephropathy) and increased hospital use. In a few patients, gastroparesis is the first diabetic, neuropathic complication.

Compared with T2DM, patients with T1DM with gastroparesis are younger, thinner, and tend to have more severe delays in gastric emptying.[14] Mortality is increased in diabetic patients when they develop gastroparesis and is usually related to cardiovascular events[15] when compared with diabetic patients without gastroparesis.

NORMAL POSTPRANDIAL GASTRIC NEUROMUSCULAR ACTIVITY

The normal stomach performs a series of complex neuromuscular activities in response to the ingestion of solid foods.[16] First, the fundus relaxes to accommodate the volume of ingested food (**Fig. 1**). Normal fundic relaxation requires an intact vagus nerve and is mediated by enteric neurons containing nitric oxide. The relaxation of the fundus allows food to be accommodated without excess stretch on the fundic walls.

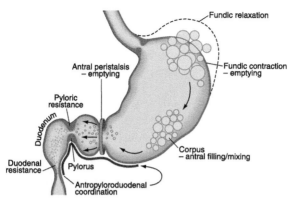

Fig. 1. Gastric neuromuscular responses to the ingestion of solid food. The fundus, corpus, antrum, pylorus, and duodenum are shown. The fundus relaxes to accommodate the ingested solid food. The fundus presses the food into the corpus-antrum, the mixing chambers of the stomach. Recurrent peristaltic waves triturate the solids into 1-mm to 2-mm particles (termed chyme), which are emptied from the antrum through the pylorus into the duodenum. The sequence requires antral-pyloroduodenal coordination. (*Adapted from* Koch KL. Gastric neuromuscular function and neuromuscular disorders. In: Feldman M, Friedman LS, Brandt LJ, editors. Sleisenger and Fordtran's gastrointestinal and liver disease: pathophysiology/diagnosis/management. Philadelphia: Elsevier; 2010. p. 789–815.)

Second, the corpus and antrum produce recurrent peristaltic waves that mix or triturate the ingested solids into fine particles termed chyme. The waves mix together the food particles, pepsin, and acid to prepare the ingested food for emptying. Peristaltic waves in the corpus-antrum occur at a frequency of 3 contractions per minute, a frequency that is dictated by the gastric pacemaker cells (the ICCs), which normally depolarize and repolarize at a rate of 3 cycles per minute (cpm) (see **Fig. 1**; **Fig. 2**).[17,18] The slow waves (pacesetter potentials) originate at the greater curvature of the stomach between the fundus and proximal corpus (see **Fig. 2**) and migrate in a circumferential and aboral direction at increasing velocity in the distal antrum.[16] The slow waves bring the circular muscle of the stomach to depolarization threshold and contractions, which occur in response to the release of acetylcholine. The action and plateau potentials are synchronized to the 3-cpm slow wave, thus resulting in the coordinated 3-per-minute peristaltic contractions.

Third, emptying of chyme contents begins when the ingested solid foods are sufficiently triturated. The peristaltic waves at 3 per minute empty aliquots of chyme through the pylorus into the duodenum (see **Fig. 1**). The pylorus acts as a sieve and can regulate the particle size as well as the volume of chyme that is emptied into the duodenum with each peristaltic wave. In the normal condition, the number of calories emptied per minute is consistent, at about 5 calories per minute in humans.[19] The emptying of food from the stomach is altered by the nature of the constituents (carbohydrate, protein, and fat) and the fiber and indigestible components. Carbohydrates are emptied faster than proteins, which are emptied faster than fats, which delay gastric emptying. Soluble and insoluble fibers are emptied after the nutrients.[20] Gastric emptying is also regulated by postpyloric influences. The release of cholecystokinin slows gastric emptying.[21] Intraluminal content with high concentration stimulates the release of peptide YY from the ileum to slow gastric emptying.[22] Normal postprandial neuromuscular activity is associated with a sense of comfortable fullness. In contrast, the ingestion of food elicits early satiety, nausea, and epigastric discomfort or pain in diabetic patients with gastroparesis.

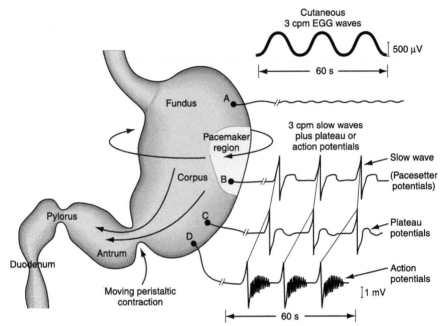

Fig. 2. Electrophysiology of gastric peristalsis. From the gastric pacemaker area on the greater curvature of the stomach to the pylorus, slow waves (pacesetter potentials) migrate circumferentially and distally as a myoelectric wave front. Electrodes placed on the fundus (A) show that there is little or no electric rhythmicity present. Electrodes B, C, and D record slow waves with plateau or spike potentials in the corpus-antrum. The plateau or spike potentials occur when enteric neurons release acetylcholine, resulting in circular muscle depolarization and contractions. The plateau and spike potentials, linked to the slow waves, result in 3 peristaltic contractions per minute controlled by the normal 3-cpm gastric slow wave. Gastric myoelectric activity recorded from cutaneous electrodes reflect the 3-cpm myoelectric events. (*Adapted from* Koch KL. Gastric neuromuscular function and neuromuscular disorders. In: Feldman M, Friedman LS, Brandt LJ, editors. Sleisenger and Fordtran's gastrointestinal and liver disease: pathophysiology/diagnosis/management. Philadelphia: Elsevier; 2010. p. 789–815.)

PATHOPHYSIOLOGY OF DIABETIC GASTROPARESIS
Gastric Neuropathy and Cajalopathy in Diabetic Gastroparesis

Full-thickness biopsies of the gastric corpus from patients with T1DM and T2DM and gastroparesis indicate that the disease is primarily a disease of gastric enteric neurons and ICCs.[11,12] We know that ICCs are depleted (<5/hpf compared with controls) in the diabetic gastroparesis stomach.[11,17] Gastric enteric neurons are decreased in numbers of cell bodies and processes are truncated. These neurons are surrounded by an immune infiltrate composed primarily of type 2 macrophages, suggesting a role for the immune system and carbon monoxide in the pathogenesis of diabetic gastroparesis.[23] The circular and longitudinal smooth muscle layers are normal or have very mild fibrosis. ICCs are depleted in diabetic mice with gastric emptying abnormalities.[24] Hyperglycemia in these animals is associated with dedifferentiation of ICCs into immature myoblasts, and intense insulin therapy restores ICC numbers to normal. It is postulated that platelet-derived growth factor (+) myoblasts have the potential to evolve into ICCs.[25]

Abnormalities of Fundic Relaxation

Relaxation of the fundus during ingestion of food requires normal vagus nerve function and the release of nitric oxide from inhibitory neurons.[26] In patients with diabetes, the fundus fails to relax normally (**Fig. 3**).[27] The ICCs function also as stretch receptors.[28] The loss of nitrergic neurons plus the absence of ICCs may account for the poor fundic relaxation and decreased gastric capacity seen in gastroparesis.[29]

Disorders of the Corpus-Antrum

The corpus and antrum perform the mixing and emptying activities of the stomach. In diabetic gastroparesis, corpus-antral contractions are ineffective, although the smooth muscle layers seem to be normal.[11,12] Thus, the depletion of ICCs and presence of abnormal enteric neurons are the mechanisms of gastric neuromuscular dysfunction. Loss of enteric neurons results in less acetylcholine release for contractions and less nitric oxide for relaxation of smooth muscle. Depletion of ICCs is associated with the presence of gastric dysrhythmias and loss of the normal 3-cpm myoelectric rhythm.[17,30] Gastric dysrhythmias range from tachygastrias to bradygastrias and a variety of aberrant conduction pathways in the corpus-antrum.[17] Gastric dysrhythmias reduce efficiency and the occurrence of normal gastric peristaltic waves and, thus, lead to slow gastric emptying and gastroparesis (see **Fig. 3**). Correction of gastric dysrhythmias with domperidone, a peripheral dopamine 2 antagonist, improved upper gastrointestinal (GI) symptoms, suggesting dysrhythmias correlate with symptoms.[31]

Disorders of Pyloric Relaxation

The pyloric sphincter also regulates gastric emptying.[16] The pylorus provides resistance to flow and a sieving function for particles as antral peristaltic waves propel

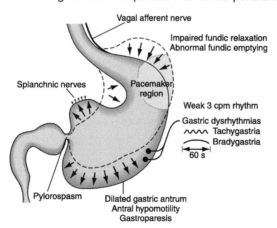

Fig. 3. Neuromuscular disorders of the stomach in diabetic gastroparesis. The fundus fails to relax normally to accommodate food. The gastric electric rhythm is abnormal because of the loss of ICCs, resulting in weak or absent 3-cpm activity and tachygastria and bradygastria. The antrum may dilate, and antral contractions are weak and uncoordinated, all of which lead to delayed gastric emptying. In a subset of patients with gastroparesis, 3-cpm myoelectric activity is present, but gastroparesis occurs because of pyloric dysfunction. Abnormalities of vagal afferent nerve or splanchnic nerve innervation may also be present in patients with diabetic gastroparesis. (*Adapted from* Koch KL. Gastric neuromuscular function and neuromuscular disorders. In: Feldman M, Friedman LS, Brandt LJ, editors. Sleisenger and Fordtran's gastrointestinal and liver disease: pathophysiology/diagnosis/management. Philadelphia: Elsevier; 2010. p. 789–815.)

chyme from the antrum into the duodenum (see **Fig. 1**). Relaxation of the pyloric sphincter to allow flow is mediated by nitric oxide released from enteric neurons.[16] In a subset of patients with idiopathic and diabetic gastroparesis, pylorospasm (failure of pyloric relaxation in coordination with antral peristaltic waves) results in gastroparesis (see **Fig. 3**).[32,33] Mechanical obstruction at the pylorus or post bulbar duodenum caused by ulcer disease or cancer must be excluded in patients with gastroparesis.[33]

Clinical Presentation

Symptoms associated with diabetic gastroparesis are early satiety, prolonged fullness, bloating, nausea and vomiting, and abdominal discomfort and pain. These symptoms are vague and nonspecific. Approximately 20% of patients develop these symptoms acutely and with a febrile illness.[34] A variety of diseases may cause these symptoms, and abdominal pain and causes of symptoms other than gastroparesis must be considered.

Nausea is the most bothersome and predominant symptom in diabetic patients with gastroparesis. Nevertheless, the nausea caused by gastroesophageal reflux disease (GERD) or constipation or gallbladder disease, common disorders in patients with diabetes, must be considered.[16] Nausea related to gastroparesis is typically located in the epigastrium and usually increases in severity after ingestion of meals. Vomitus contains chewed food. Prolonged stomach fullness and vague epigastric discomfort are common. Symptoms are similar in patients with T1DM and T2DM, although patients with T2DM tend to have more fullness and bloating.[34] **Table 1** lists demographic parameters and symptoms in patients with T1DM and T2DM and

Table 1
Demographic and clinical differences in patients with gastroparesis and T1DM and T2DM from the gastroparesis clinical research consortium

	T1DM (n = 78)	T2DM (n = 59)	P Value
Female (%)	70	76	
Age (y)	39 ± 11	53 ± 11	P<.001
Married (%)	54	64	
Ever smoked (%)	29	39	
Time from diabetes mellitus onset to initial symptom (y)	14 ± 11	8.4 ± 8	P<.005
Symptom duration (y)	6.2 ± 6	4.1 ± 3	
BMI	26 ± 6	33 ± 8	P<.001
Normal BMI (%)	47	14	
HbA$_{1c}$	8.3 ± 2	7.4 ± 1.7	P<.003
Major depression (%)	28	32	
GCSI	2.8 ± 1.1	3.0 ± 1.0	
GET at 4 h (%)	47 ± 27	33 ± 24	P<.001
Severe GET (%)	54	32	P<.001
Number of hospitalizations in past year	5.1 ± 6.4	3.2 ± 6.6	P<.003

Abbreviations: BMI, body mass index, calculated as weight in kilograms divided by the square of height in meters; GCSI, Gastroparesis Clinical Severity Index; GET, gastric emptying test; HbA$_{1c}$, hemoglobin A$_{1c}$.

Adapted from Koch KL, Hasler WL, Yates KP, et al, for the Gastroparesis Clinical Research Consortium. Contrasting gastroparesis in type 1 (T1DM) vs. type 2 (T2DM) diabetes: clinical course after 48 weeks of follow-up and relation to comorbidities and health resource utilization. Gastroenterology 2013;144(5 Suppl):S926-7.

gastroparesis.[15] In contrast to patients with idiopathic gastroparesis, fewer diabetic patients with gastroparesis report pain as a predominant symptom.[34]

In some patients (20%) with gastroparesis, abdominal pain is the predominant symptom.[34] The pain should be evaluated separately from other symptoms associated with gastroparesis in an attempt to determine a specific cause for the pain. Chronic cholecystitis, peptic ulcer diseases, and the abdominal wall syndrome need to be excluded. Stomach pain can be caused by pylorospasm or gastric sensitivity to stretch in patients with gastroparesis. Mechanical obstruction at the pylorus caused by ulcer or cancer must be excluded in patients with gastroparesis.

Physical examination may be normal or show obesity or undernutrition, retinopathy, neuropathy, or vitamin deficiency (cheilosis). Obesity in patients with T2DM is a risk factor for gastroparesis.[35] Abdominal examination may show distension, a succession splash, or positive Carnett sign. A positive Carnett sign indicates that abdominal pain is from an abdominal wall syndrome secondary to nerve entrapment or inflammation, often located at a healed incision site.[36,37]

Standard laboratory studies are usually normal. Hemoglobin A_{1c} levels have a wide range. Thyroid-stimulating hormone levels and fasting cortisol should be measured to screen for Addison disease and hypothyroidism. Vitamin D levels are frequently low.

TESTS FOR GASTROPARESIS AND GASTRIC DYSRHYTHMIAS
Solid-Phase Gastric Emptying Test

Tests for gastroparesis and gastric dysrhythmias are nuclear medicine scintigraphy, wireless capsule endoscopy, and electrogastrography (EGG). These tests should be performed after upper endoscopy to rule out mechanical obstruction, which produces symptoms similar to gastroparesis. The most standardized test for gastric emptying is the technetium-labeled low-fat egg albumin-based meal.[38,39] The patient must stop prokinetic agents 7 days before the test, fast after midnight, and blood glucose level on the day of the test should be less than 270 mg/dL. Immediately after the patient ingests the 257-calorie meal, a 1-minute scintigram is obtained with the patient in a sitting position and then for 1 minute every hour for 4 hours. Normal gastric emptying is 39% or less of the meal retained at 2 hours and 9% or less retained at 4 hours. Thus, gastroparesis is diagnosed by a documented retention of 40% or more at 2 hours or 10% or more at 4 hours.

The solid-phase gastric emptying test is also important, because some patients who have the symptoms associated with gastroparesis have rapid gastric emptying or dumping syndrome. In dumping syndrome, less than 30% of the test meal is retained at 60 minutes.[38]

Wireless Capsule Motility Test

The wireless capsule motility test measures intraluminal pH and pressure.[40] The capsule is swallowed during ingestion of a nutrient bar that contains the same number of calories as the Egg Beaters test meal. No further food intake is allowed for 5 hours. If the capsule does not empty from the stomach into the duodenum in 5 hours, then delayed gastric emptying is diagnosed. Small bowel and colon transit time are also measured, and results may help in determining the underlying pathophysiology of other GI symptoms.

Electrogastrography

Electrogastrography is the method of recording gastric myoelectric activity with a noninvasive method.[41,42] Electrocardiography-type electrodes are placed on the epigastrium, and the myoelectric signal is recorded before and after a water load or a nutrient load test. Normal gastric myoelectric activity (2.5–3.7 cpm) normally increases after the water load test.[42] Gastric dysrhythmias are defined as tachygastrias (3.5–10 cpm) or bradygastrias (1–2.5 cpm).[42] Tachygastrias and bradygastrias are associated with loss of ICCs; on the other hand, a normal 3-cpm rhythm is associated with the presence of normal numbers of ICCs.[21,34] A subset of patients with gastroparesis has normal or increased 3-cpm electric activity, a discordant finding that indicates the possibility of obstructive gastroparesis secondary to pyloric stenosis or pyloro-spasm (**Fig. 4**).[33,43]

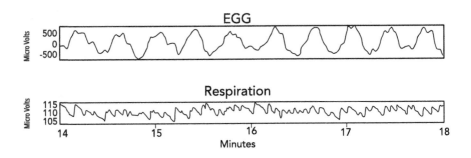

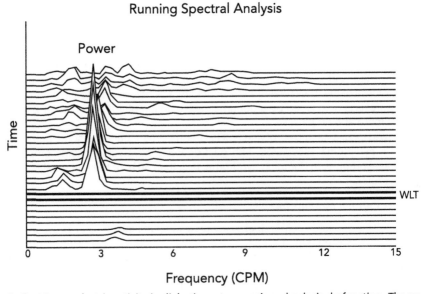

Fig. 4. Gastric myoelectric activity in diabetic gastroparesis and pyloric dysfunction. The upper tracings show an EGG rhythm strip and respiration rate signal. Time in minutes is shown. Clear 3-cpm EGG waves are present. The running spectral analysis shows frequency on the x-axis, time on the y-axis, and the power of the various frequencies in the EGG rhythm strip on the z-axis. After ingestion of the water load (WLT), most of the frequency peaks are in the normal range (2.5–3.5 cpm). This normal finding, in conjunction with delayed gastric emptying, suggests gastric outlet obstruction.

TREATMENTS
Diet for Diabetic Gastroparesis

Acute dietary management of exacerbation of symptoms associated with gastroparesis

Patients who have frequent vomiting episodes that may lead to dehydration are coached to sip small volumes (Step 1 of **Table 2**; eg, 56.6 g [2 oz] over 30–60 minutes every hour) of electrolyte-containing liquids and bouillonlike soup broths throughout the day; this may be accomplished with commercially available sports drinks. The purpose is to restore hydration with salt and water. Nausea and vomiting often improve with hydration, and the patient may then advance to steps 2 and 3, as outlined in **Table 2**.[16]

Chronic dietary management of symptoms associated with gastroparesis

One of the keys in the American Diabetes Association recommended medical nutrition therapy for patients with diabetes is an increase in consumption of complex carbohydrate-rich food items, such as salads, fresh raw fruits, and fresh raw vegetables.[44] These foods, although excellent for the diabetic patient with normal gastric emptying, are some of the most difficult foods for the weakened gastroparetic stomach to triturate and empty.

Table 2
Diet for nausea and vomiting in patients with diabetic gastroparesis

Diet	Goal	Avoid
Step 1: Sports Drinks and Bouillon		
For severe nausea and vomiting: Small volumes of salty liquids, with some caloric content to avoid volume depletion Chewable multiple vitamin each day	1000–1500 mL/d in multiple servings (eg, 12 120-mL servings over 12–14 h) Patient can sip 30–60 mL at a time to reach approximately 120 mL/h	Citrus drinks of all kinds; highly sweetened drinks
Step 2: Soups and Smoothies		
If step 1 is tolerated: Soup with noodles or rice and crackers Smoothies with low-fat dairy Peanut butter, cheese, and crackers in small amounts Caramels or other chewy confections Ingest above foods in at least 6 small-volume meals/d Chewable multiple vitamin each day	Approximately 1500 calories/d to avoid volume depletion and maintain weight (often more realistic than weight gain)	Creamy, milk-based liquids
Step 3: Starches, Chicken, Fish		
If step 2 is tolerated: Noodles, pastas, potatoes (mashed or baked), rice, baked chicken breast, fish (all easily mixed and emptied by the stomach) Ingest solids in at least 6 small-volume meals/d Chewable multiple vitamin each day	Common foods that patient finds interesting and satisfying and that provoke minimal nausea/vomiting symptoms	Fatty foods that delay gastric emptying; red meats and fresh vegetables that require considerable trituration; pulpy fibrous foods that promote formation of bezoars

Therefore, nutritious liquids, such as soups or smoothies, which require less gastric neuromuscular work to empty, are advised for patients with gastroparesis. Solid foods such as potatoes and pastas require less trituration and are emptied with less gastric neuromuscular work compared with red meats and fibrous foods. Starches are usually limited for the patient with diabetes, because of the high glycemic index, but these solid foods may be the only foods tolerated by patients with gastroparesis. The 3-step diet for patients with gastroparesis is a guide to help patients select foods that both limit postprandial GI symptoms and maintain hydration and nutrition (see **Table 2**).

These dietary changes require reeducation of the patient with diabetes and gastroparesis and their physicians. Less than 40% of diabetic patients with gastroparesis have had a dietary or nutrition consultation.[45] (See article elsewhere in this issue regarding diet counseling for patients with gastroparesis.) Consultation by a dietician who is knowledgeable in gastroparesis is invaluable. The goal is good nutrition and minimal postprandial symptoms, selecting foods appropriate for the severity of gastroparesis.

Glucose Control in the Diabetic Patient with Gastroparesis

Glucose control in the patient with diabetic gastroparesis can be difficult. The rate of gastric emptying of ingested nutrients is compromised by the severity of gastroparesis. Symptoms of nausea and vomiting affect appetite, and vomiting reduces absorption of anticipated calories. Liquid nutrients and solid foods may be retained in the stomach longer than expected by the patient or by the treating physician. Thus, postprandial hypoglycemia may develop if insulin is given in a preprandial time frame in patients with gastroparesis. A comprehensive approach to glucose control for patients with gastroparesis is reviewed later.

Patients with T1DM require insulin replacement, as do most (if not all) of the patients with T2DM and gastroparesis.[46] We do not recommend oral agents or noninsulin injectables for management of glycemia in patients with T2DM and gastroparesis. First, as a result of gastroparesis, oral medications may not empty from the stomach for hours, resulting in erratic pharmacokinetics and pharmocodynamics. The sulfonylureas are associated with hypoglycemia in these patients. The incretin mimetics slow stomach peristalsis and are associated with nausea and vomiting themselves and hence are not recommended.[47] Inhibitors of the enzyme dipeptidyl peptidase 4 depend on good insulin reserve, and most patients with T2DM and gastroparesis have had long duration of diabetes and likely have severely decreased capacity to secrete insulin. Besides the latter, no clinical trials have been published on the possible safety or efficacy of the use of these agents in patients with gastroparesis. The use of the peroxisome proliferator-activated receptor agonists in diabetes (without gastroparesis) is highly controversial and other agents (sodium-glucose cotransporter 2 inhibitors) have not been tested in these patients or may cause diarrhea and abdominal distension (disaccharidase inhibitors). Thus, we favor the use of insulin in the patient with T2DM and gastroparesis.

Basal and Meal Administration of Insulin by Injections

The current paradigm of insulin administration in the patient with T1DM or T2DM is based on the basal-bolus model, which is easier to model with pumps rather than multiple shots.[48] Basal is the amount of insulin estimated to be produced by the β cells to maintain glycemia in the postabsorptive state and hence independent of meal ingestion. Bolus is the insulin required to maintain postprandial glycemic excursion within an acceptable range. Basal insulin has to be administered via the subcutaneous route.

The boluses for meal insulin can be administered via the subcutaneous route or with the recently approved pulmonary route (via inhalation).

Basal and Meal Administration of Insulin by Pump

Insulin can be administered subcutaneously using a pump (continuous subcutaneous insulin infusion [CSII] delivery). CSII uses one type of insulin (fast acting), which is delivered continuously for the basal component. The pump can also deliver boluses of insulin in anticipation of or coincident with food ingestion.

A basic assumption (implicit and also explicit) of meal bolus is that gastric emptying of the ingested meal is completed within 4 hours and intestinal absorption of nutrients is completed within 4 to 6 hours. Thus, patients are recommended to use the new fast analogues of insulin, because they are absorbed from the subcutaneous tissue within 5 to 15 minutes after injection or delivery, peak in concentration in 1 to 2 hours, and decline in blood thereafter for a duration of 4 (kinetics) or 6 (pharmacodynamics) hours. Thus, these insulins are timed or administered to match anticipated nutrient absorption. This factor is problematic for patients with gastroparesis, because the onset and duration of the small intestinal absorption phase is critically dependent on the rate of gastric emptying, solid foods usually empty slowly, and the day-to-day variability in gastric emptying of common foods is unknown.

Sensor-Augmented Control of Glucose

Glucose sensors measure glucose continuously in the subcutaneous tissue, show the prevailing average results every 5 minutes, and allow patients to identify up or down trends and take preventive steps to avoid hypoglycemia or hyperglycemia.[49] This technique is now known as sensor-augmented management of glycemia.[50] The US Food and Drug Administration approved the first step in the evolution of technology toward an artificial pancreas, a software enhancement that allows for auto shut-off of insulin delivery by the pump if the glucose sensor detects hypoglycemia.[51]

Insulin Administration for the Patient with Gastroparesis

We recommend continuous insulin infusion for managing glycemia in patients with diabetes and gastroparesis, based not only on our experience but also on a small but positive trial that found improvement in glycemia and decreased hospitalizations.[52] If insurance coverage and patients' costs are an obstacle; then multiple shots are the next best option. In general terms, we do not favor the use of premixed insulin preparations. Monitoring of glycemia for insulin adjustment is preferably established with a system based on finger sticks augmented with continuous glucose monitoring.

Basal insulin administration

The estimated initial dose of basal insulin can be calculated using a formula of 0.2 to 0.3 units/kg/d for a patient with T2DM and 0.15 units/kg/d for someone with T1DM. Traditional adjustment of the basal is based on the glycemia measured before breakfast, which assumes postabsorptive state (some 11–14 hours after last meal). However, in patients with diabetic gastroparesis, the postabsorptive state is not so easy to define, because gastric emptying may be delayed all day, and an unknown amount of food (from accumulated breakfast, lunch, or dinner) is emptied during the night. Thus, the prebreakfast glycemia may not reflect real basal glycemia but ongoing postprandial glycemic excursions.

There are approaches to attempt to better estimate the postabsorptive glycemia in these patients. First, the patient may skip breakfast for 2 to 3 days and measure capillary glycemia every 1 to 2 hours after waking up until lunchtime to determine if glycemia remains stable or decreases slightly, reflecting the postabsorptive state. Second, the patient may substitute dinner (or even skip it) and measure capillary glycemia frequently through the night. Third, a better approach is to use a glucose sensor to detect trends. Analysis of trends can determine if meals are being retained in the stomach until a large trigger distorts nighttime glucose excursions that extend into the next morning or if the glycemia reflects the need for more basal insulin. The identification of these trends is demanding, but patients may find it useful to avoid hypoglycemia and severe hyperglycemia.

Bolus insulin administration for meals

The challenges are more complex for the meal bolus than for the basal insulin, as discussed earlier and recently documented.[53] Instead of discrete postprandial peaks of increased and decreased of glucose level, patients with gastroparesis show almost constant hyperglycemia interrupted by unpredictable dips into normal or low glucose ranges. The day-to-day variations in food choices and in the gastric emptying rates of those foods (and thus time of nutrient absorption) are completely unknown in patients with gastroparesis. Despite these caveats, some general recommendations can be made regarding the insulin meal bolus for patients with gastroparesis.

If using injections, then we suggest:

1. Use regular insulin (rather than insulin analogues), which has a longer duration effect
2. Administer insulin after the meal (not before)
3. Give dose fractionated insulin in 2 to 3 minishots spaced within 4 to 6 hours after meal ingestion (ie, instead of a single shot of 9 units, use 3 shots of 3 units each)

If using pumps, then we suggest:

1. Start meal bolus approximately 15 minutes after meal ingestion
2. Encourage patient to use the dual-wave feature and program a small initial first wave (ie, 10% to 20%) and program second wave for the next 5 to 6 hours

We recommend that whenever feasible a glucose sensor should be used. The patterns of the 24-hour readings of preprandial and postprandial glycemia in the individual patient should be carefully examined. In our experience, patients who use CSII augmented with a glucose sensor attain better control of their glycemia compared with a regimen based on injections.

Prokinetic Agents for Gastroparesis

Drugs that increase the rate of gastric emptying (prokinetic agents) have been the goal for treatment of diabetic gastroparesis for many years. This approach has not proved to be fruitful. The only prokinetic drugs available to treat gastroparesis are metoclopramide (Reglan) and erythromycin (**Table 3**). Metoclopramide is a drug with effects on several receptors: dopamine 2 receptors, $5-HT_3$ receptor antagonists, and acetylcholinesterase inhibitors.[54] Gastric emptying is increased by metoclopramide, but the drug also crosses the blood-brain barrier and causes a variety of central nervous system symptoms, ranging from nervousness to Parkinson disease to irreversible tardive dyskinesia.[55] Erythromycin is a macrolide antibiotic that stimulates motilin receptors and contractions in the corpus and antrum, which increases the rate of gastric emptying.[56]

Many drugs designed to improve the rate of gastric emptying have not improved the symptoms associated with gastroparesis. Studies of prokinetics and gastric stimulation have shown that the rate of gastric emptying does not correlate with the symptoms

Table 3
Drug and nondrug therapies used to treat upper GI symptoms in patients with diabetic gastroparesis

Therapy	Mechanisms and Sites of Action	Dosage	Adverse Effects
Prokinetic Therapy			
Macrolides			
Erythromycin	Motilin receptor agonist	125–250 mg 4 times daily	Nausea, diarrhea abdominal cramps, rash
Substituted Benzamides			
Metoclopramide	D_2 receptor antagonist; 5-HT$_3$-receptor antagonist; 5-HT$_4$ receptor agonist	5–20 mg before meals and at bedtime	Extrapyramidal symptoms, dystonic reactions, anxiety, depression, hyperprolactinemia, tardive dyskinesia
Domperidone[a]	D_2 receptor antagonist (peripheral)	10–20 mg before meals and at bedtime	Hyperprolactinemia, breast tenderness, galactorrhea
Antinauseant Therapy			
Serotonin Antagonists			
Ondansetron	5-HT$_3$ receptor antagonist	4–8 mg twice daily, either orally or intravenously	Headache, increased liver enzymes
Granisetron	5-HT$_3$ receptor antagonist	2 mg once daily or 3.1-mg patch	Headache, increased liver enzymes
Phenothiazines			
Prochlorperazine	CNS sites	5–10 mg 3 times daily	Hypotension, extrapyramidal symptoms
Antihistamines			
Promethazine	CNS, H$_1$ receptor antagonist	25 mg twice daily	Drowsiness
Dimenhydrinate	H$_1$ receptor antagonist	50 mg 4 times daily	Drowsiness
Cyclizine	H$_1$ receptor antagonist	50 mg 4 times daily	Drowsiness
Butyrophenones			
Droperidol	Central dopamine receptor antagonist	2.5–5 mg intravenously every 2 h	Sedation, hypotension
Antidepressants			
Mirtazapine	CNS sites	15 mg at bedtime	Weight gain
Benzodiazepines			
Lorazepam	CNS sites	0.5–1 mg 4 times daily	Drowsiness, lightheadedness
Alprazolam	CNS sites	0.25–0.5 mg 3 times daily	Drowsiness, lightheadedness
Dronabinol	CNS	5–10 mg 2 times daily	Sedation

(*continued on next page*)

Therapy	Mechanisms and Sites of Action	Dosage	Adverse Effects
Table 3 *(continued)*			
Electric Therapies			
Gastric electric stimulation	?Vagal afferents	12 cpm, 330 μs, 5 mÅ	Pocket infection
Gastric pacing	Control dysrhythmias, improve gastric emptying	3 cpm, 300 μs, 4 mÅ	Pocket infection
Endoscopic Therapies			
Botulinum toxin A injection into pylorus	Relax pyloric muscle	25–50 units per quadrant of pylorus	None
Balloon dilation of pylorus	Stretch pyloric muscle	20-mm balloon, 2 min	None
Radiofrequency ablation at LES	Improve gastric emptying and gastric myoelectric activity	NA	Transient dysphagia
Diet Therapies			
Gastroparesis diet	Diet based on gastric emptying physiology	See **Table 2**	None
High-protein drinks	Decreases gastric dysrhythmias	Unknown	None
Gastrostomy	Venting paretic stomach	As needed	
Jejunostomy	Enteral nutritional support	As needed	
Total parenteral nutrition	Bypass paretic stomach	As needed	Sepsis, thrombosis of central veins

Abbreviations: ?, questionably; 5-HT, 5-hydroxytryptamine; CNS, central nervous system; D_2, dopamine 2; H_1, histamine 1; LES, lower esophageal sphincter; NA, not applicable.
  [a] Compassionate clearance use only.

associated with gastroparesis.[57,58] Domperidone is a dopamine 2 receptor agonist that does not cross the blood-brain barrier, improves nausea and gastric dysrhythmias, and may improve the rate of gastric emptying in some patients with diabetic gastroparesis.[31] Pathophysiologic mechanisms, such as gastric dysrhythmias, gastric relaxation (or stretch), or pyloric dysfunction, may be more relevant to the postprandial nausea, early satiety, prolonged fullness, and discomfort than the rate of gastric emptying.

Antinauseant Drugs

Patients with diabetic gastroparesis often have daily nausea and vomiting. The quality of life during these times is poor. These symptoms may lead to dehydration, which requires frequent emergency room visits or hospitalizations. **Table 3** lists several drugs that are used empirically to treat nausea for patients with gastroparesis. There is no way to predict which medication will decrease nausea in an individual patient. Each drug may be tried for 4 to 8 weeks to see if nausea and vomiting improve. These drugs have not been specifically approved for use in patients who have symptoms associated with diabetic gastroparesis. In unremitting nausea and vomiting, normal weight cannot be maintained. A jejunostomy tube may be required for enteral feedings if small bowel motility is normal. Total parenteral nutrition may be needed in a few patients to support nutrition.

Pyloric Therapies

An important subset of patients with gastroparesis has normal or more than normal 3-cpm (EGG) signals, as shown in **Fig. 4**. In these patients, pyloric dysfunction secondary to pyloric stenosis or pylorospasm should be suspected, because most patients with gastroparesis have gastric dysrhythmias rather than normal electric rhythm.[33] Fixed mechanical obstruction at the pylorus or postbulbar areas that may require surgery must be excluded. If no mechanical obstruction is present, then injection of botulinum toxin A (BTA) into the pylorus or balloon dilation of the pylorus often relieves the symptoms associated with gastroparesis.[43,59] Pyloroplasty improves gastric emptying and symptoms in highly selected patients with gastroparesis and normal 3-cpm EGG signals who have previously responded well to BTA or dilation.[60]

Gastric Electric Stimulation

Gastric electric stimulation (GES) refers to therapeutic stimulation of the stomach with electric pulses. The stomach is typically stimulated at 12 cpm, 5 mA, 330 microseconds, and 50 Hz to decrease symptoms associated with gastroparesis.[61] The incidence of vomiting in patients with diabetic gastroparesis is reduced with GES, with improvement in symptoms and emptying at 1 year.[61] The mechanisms of action of GES are not known, but increased fundic accommodation or vagal afferent nerve stimulation with central nervous system effects have been suggested. GES may help patients who have failed diet and drug therapies.

Future Directions

The number of patients with diabetes and, thus, the number of patients with gastroparesis, is increasing dramatically in the United States and around the world. Gastroparesis should be suspected in diabetic patients with glucose excursions that are difficult to control and early satiety, nausea and vomiting, and abdominal discomfort. Gastric emptying and gastric electric rhythm tests are needed to confirm gastroparesis and define the obstructive subgroup of gastroparesis. Novel approaches are needed for the treatment of gastric dysrhythmias and abnormalities of gastric compliance and for GES paradigms. Patients with gastroparesis secondary to pyloric dysfunction should be identified and treated with pyloric therapies.

The insightful and careful management of diet therapy and administration of insulin, based on detailed assessment of postprandial glucose excursions in patients with diabetic gastroparesis, are critical areas on which to focus. Understanding the rate of gastric emptying of nutrients and subsequent glucose excursions is key to better management of postprandial glucose and symptoms in patients with diabetic gastroparesis. Continuous glucose monitoring with insulin pump therapy, progress toward the artificial pancreas, and teams of dedicated gastroenterologists, diabetologists, and dieticians are needed to improve glycemia and symptoms for patients with diabetic gastroparesis.

REFERENCES

1. Camilleri M, Parkman H, Shafi M, et al. Clinical guideline: management of gastroparesis. Am J Gastroenterol 2013;108:18–37.
2. Jorváth VJ, Izbéki F, Lengyel C, et al. Diabetic gastroparesis: functional/morphologic background, diagnosis, and treatment options. Curr Diab Rep 2014;14(9):527.

3. Koch KL. Diabetic gastropathy: gastric neuromuscular dysfunction in diabetes mellitus. A review of symptoms, pathophysiology, and treatment. Dig Dis Sci 1999;44:1061–75.

4. Coleski R, Hasler WL. Coupling and propagation of normal and dysrhythmic gastric slow waves during acute hyperglycemia in healthy humans. Neurogastroenterol Motil 2009;21:492–9.

5. Fraser R, Horowitz M, Maddox A, et al. Hyperglycemia slows gastric emptying in type 1 diabetes mellitus. Diabetologia 1990;33:675–80.

6. Yisahak SF, Beagley J, Hambleton IR, et al. IDF diabetes atlas. Diabetes in North America and the Caribbean: an update. Diabetes Res Clin Pract 2014;103: 223–30.

7. Horowitz M, O'Donovan D, Jones KL, et al. Gastric emptying in diabetes: clinical significance and treatment. Diabet Med 2002;19:177–94.

8. Choung RS, Locke GR, Schleck CD, et al. Risk of gastroparesis in subjects with type 1 and type 2 diabetes in the general population. Am J Gastroenterol 2012; 107:82–8.

9. Intagliata N, Koch KL. Gastroparesis in type 2 diabetes mellitus: prevalence, etiology, diagnosis, and treatment. Curr Gastroenterol Rep 2007;9:270–9.

10. Jung HK, Choung RS, Locke GR, et al. The incidence, prevalence, and outcomes of patients with gastroparesis in Olmstead County, Minnesota, from 1996 to 2006. Gastroenterology 2009;136:1225–33.

11. Grover M, Farrugia G, Lurken MS, et al. Cellular changes in diabetic and idiopathic gastroparesis. Gastroenterology 2011;140:1575–85.

12. Faussone-Pellegrini MS, Grover M, Pasricha PJ, et al. Ultrastructural differences between diabetic and idiopathic gastroparesis. J Cell Mol Med 2012;16:1573–81.

13. The Diabetes Control and Complications Trial Research Group. The effect of intensive diabetes therapy on measures of autonomic nervous system function in the Diabetes Control and Complications Trial (DCCT). Diabetologia 1998;4: 416–23.

14. Koch KL, Hasler WL, Yates KP, et al, for the Gastroparesis Clinical Research Consortium. Contrasting gastroparesis in type 1 (T1DM) vs. type 2 (T2DM) diabetes: clinical course after 48 weeks of follow-up and relation to comorbidities and health resource utilization. Gastroenterology 2013;144(5 Suppl):S926–7.

15. Hyett B, Martinez FJ, Gill BM, et al. Delayed radionucleotide gastric emptying studies predict morbidity in diabetics with symptoms of gastroparesis. Gastroenterology 2009;137:445–52.

16. Koch KL. Gastric neuromuscular function and neuromuscular disorders. In: Feldman M, Friedman LS, Brandt LJ, editors. Sleisenger and Fordtran's gastrointestinal and liver disease: pathophysiology/diagnosis/management. Philadelphia: Elsevier; 2010. p. 789–815.

17. O'Grady G, Angeli TR, Du P, et al. Abnormal initiation and conduction of slow wave activity in gastroparesis, defined by high-resolution electrical mapping. Gastroenterology 2012;143:589–98.

18. Koch KL. Electrogastrography for evaluation of patients with suspected gastroparesis. In: Parkman H, McCallum R, editors. Gastroparesis: pathophysiology, presentation, diagnosis and treatment. New York: Springer; 2011. p. 153–61.

19. Moran TH, Wirth JB, Schwartz GJ, et al. Interactions between gastric volume and duodenal nutrients in the control of liquid gastric emptying. Am J Physiol 1999; 276:R997–1002.

20. Camilleri M. Integrated upper gastrointestinal response to food intake. Gastroenterology 2006;131:640–58.

21. Woods SC. Gastrointestinal satiety signals. I. An overview of gastrointestinal signals that influence food intake. Am J Physiol Gastrointest Liver Physiol 2004; 286:G7–13.
22. Degan L, Oesch S, Casanova M, et al. Effect of peptide YY3-36 on food intake in humans. Gastroenterology 2005;129:1430–6.
23. Gibbons SJ, Verhulst PJ, Bharucha A, et al. Review article: carbon monoxide in gastrointestinal physiology and its potential in therapeutics. Aliment Pharmacol Ther 2013;38:689–702.
24. Ordog T. Interstitial cells of Cajal in diabetic gastroenteropathy. Neurogastroenterol Motil 2008;20:8–18.
25. Horvath VJ, Vittal H, Ordog T. Reduced insulin and IGF-1 signaling, not hyperglycemia, underlies the diabetes-associated depletion of interstitial cells of Cajal in the murine stomach. Diabetes 2005;54:1528–33.
26. Iwasaki H, Kajimura M, Osawa S, et al. A deficiency of gastric interstitial cells of Cajal accompanied by decreased expression of neuronal nitric oxide synthase and substance P in patients with type 2 diabetes mellitus. J Gastroenterol 2006;41:1076–87.
27. Rayner CK, Verhagen MA, Hebbard GG, et al. Proximal gastric compliance and perception of distension in type 1 diabetes mellitus: effects of hyperglycemia. Am J Gastroenterol 2000;95:1175–83.
28. Won KJ, Sanders KM, Ward SM. Interstitial cells of Cajal mediate mechanosensitive responses in the stomach. Proc Natl Acad Sci U S A 2005;102:14913–8.
29. He CL, Soffer EE, Ferris CD, et al. Loss of interstitial cells of Cajal and inhibitory innervation in insulin-dependent diabetes. Gastroenterology 2001;121: 427–34.
30. Lin Z, Sarosiek I, Forster J, et al. Association of the status of interstitial cells of Cajal and electrogastrogram parameters, gastric emptying, and symptoms in patients with gastroparesis. Neurogastroenterol Motil 2010;22(1):56–61.
31. Koch KL, Stern RM, Stewart WR, et al. Gastric emptying and gastric myoelectrical activity in patients with symptomatic diabetic gastroparesis: effect of long-term domperidone treatment. Am J Gastroenterol 1989;84:1069–75.
32. Mearin F, Camilleri M, Malagelada JR. Pyloric dysfunction in diabetics with recurrent nausea and vomiting. Gastroenterology 1986;90:1919–25.
33. Brzana RJ, Bingaman S, Koch KL. Gastric myoelectrical activity in patients with gastric outlet obstruction and idiopathic gastroparesis. Am J Gastroenterol 1998;93:1083–9.
34. Parkman HP, Yates K, Hasler WL, et al. Similarities and differences between diabetic and idiopathic gastroparesis. Clin Gastroenterol Hepatol 2011;9:1056–64.
35. Dickman R, Kislov J, Boaz M, et al. Prevalence of symptoms suggestive of gastroparesis in a cohort of patients with diabetes mellitus. J Diabetes Complications 2013;27:376–9.
36. Carnett JB. Intercostal neuralgia as a cause of abdominal pain and tenderness. Surg Gynecol Oncol 1926;12:625–34.
37. Srinivasan R, Greenbaum DS. Chronic abdominal wall pain: a frequently overlooked problem. Practical approach to diagnosis and management. Am J Gastroenterol 2002;97(4):824–30.
38. Tougas G, Eaker EY, Abell TL, et al. Assessment of gastric emptying using a low fat meal: establishment of international control values. Am J Gastroenterol 2000; 95:1456–62.
39. Abell TL, Camilleri M, Donohoe K, et al. Consensus recommendations for gastric emptying scintigraphy. A joint report of the Society of Nuclear Medicine and The

American Neurogastroenterology and Motility Society. Am J Gastroenterol 2008; 103:753–63.

40. Kuo B, McCallum RW, Koch KL, et al. Comparison of gastric emptying of a non-digestible capsule to a radio-labeled meal in healthy and gastroparetic subjects. Aliment Pharmacol Ther 2008;27:186–96.
41. Koch KL, Hong SP, Xu L. Reproducibility of gastric myoelectrical activity and the water load test in patients with dysmotility-like dyspepsia symptoms and in control subjects. J Clin Gastroenterol 2000;31(2):125–9.
42. Koch KL, Stern RM, editors. Handbook of electrogastrography. New York: Oxford University Press; 2003.
43. Kundu S, Koch KL. Effect of balloon distention or botulinum toxin A injection of the pylorus on symptoms and body weight in patients with gastroparesis and normal 3 cycle per minute gastric electrical activity. Am J Gastroenterol 2011;106:S35.
44. American Diabetes Association. Clinical practice guidelines 2014. Diabetes Care 2014;37(Suppl 1):S28–30.
45. Parkman HP, Yates KP, Hasler WL, et al. Dietary intake and nutritional deficiencies in patients with diabetic or idiopathic gastroparesis. Gastroenterology 2011;141: 486–98.
46. Bolen S, Feldman L, Vassy J, et al. Systematic review: comparative effectiveness and safety of oral medications for type 2 diabetes mellitus. Ann Intern Med 2007; 147:386–99.
47. Amori RE, Lau J, Pittas AG. Efficacy and safety of incretin therapy in type 2 diabetes: systematic review and meta-analysis. JAMA 2007;298(2):194–206.
48. Jeitler K, Horvath K, Berghold A, et al. Continuous subcutaneous insulin infusion versus multiple daily insulin injections in patients with diabetes mellitus: systematic review and meta-analysis. Diabetologia 2008;51:941–51.
49. Guerci B, Floriot M, Böhme P, et al. Clinical performance of CGMS in type 1 diabetic patients treated by continuous subcutaneous insulin infusion using insulin analogs. Diabetes Care 2003;26:582–9.
50. Bergenstal RM, Tamborlane WV, Ahmann A, et al. Effectiveness of sensor-augmented insulin-pump therapy in type 1 diabetes. N Engl J Med 2010;363: 311–20.
51. Danne T, Kordonouri O, Holder M, et al. Prevention of hypoglycemia by using low glucose suspend function in sensor-augmented pump therapy. Diabetes Technol Therapeutics 2011;11:1129–34.
52. Sharma D, Morrison G, Joseph F, et al. The role of continuous subcutaneous insulin infusion therapy in patients with diabetic gastroparesis. Diabetologia 2011; 54:2768–70.
53. Calles-Escandon J, Hasler WL, Koch KL, et al. Continuous blood glucose patterns in diabetic patients with gastroparesis: baseline findings from the GpCRC GLUMIT-DG study. Gastroenterology 2014;146(1 Suppl):S616.
54. Lata PF, Pigarelli DL. Chronic metoclopramide therapy for diabetic gastroparesis. Ann Pharmacother 2003;37:122–6.
55. Ganzini L, Casey DE, Haffman WF, et al. The prevalence of metoclopramide-induced tardive dyskinesia and acute extrapyramidal movements. Arch Intern Med 1993;153:1469–75.
56. Rayner CK, Su YC, Doran SM, et al. The stimulation of antral motility by erythromycin is attenuated by hyperglycemia. Am J Gastroenterol 2000;95:2233–41.
57. Janssen P, Harris MS, Jones M, et al. The relation between symptom improvement and gastric emptying in the treatment of diabetic and idiopathic gastroparesis. Am J Gastroenterol 2013;108(9):1382–91.

58. Thazhath SS, Jones KL, Horowitz M, et al. Diabetic gastroparesis: recent insights into pathophysiology and implications for management. Expert Rev Gastroenterol Hepatol 2013;7(2):127–39.
59. Friedenberg FK, Palit A, Parkman HP, et al. Botulinum toxin A for the treatment of delayed gastric emptying. Am J Gastroenterol 2008;103:416–23.
60. Scott BK, Koch KL, Westcott CJ. Pyloroplasty for patients with medically-refractory functional obstructive gastroparesis. Gastroenterology 2014;146(1 Suppl):S615.
61. McCallum RW, Snape W, Brody F, et al. Gastric electrical stimulation with Enterra therapy improves symptoms from diabetic gastroparesis in a prospective study. Clin Gastroenterol Hepatol 2010;8:947–54.

Idiopathic Gastroparesis

Henry P. Parkman, MD

KEYWORDS

- Gastroparesis • Gastric emptying • Idiopathic gastroparesis

KEY POINTS

- Idiopathic gastroparesis is a common form of gastroparesis, being among the three main causes of gastroparesis: diabetic, postsurgical, and idiopathic gastroparesis.
- Patients with idiopathic gastroparesis have a constellation of symptoms including nausea; vomiting; early satiety; postprandial fullness; and in some patients, upper abdominal pain.
- The presentation of idiopathic gastroparesis is similar to diabetic gastroparesis, although abdominal pain occurs more often in idiopathic gastroparesis, whereas nausea and vomiting are more severe in diabetic gastroparesis.
- Treatment of the symptoms may use agents used for diabetic gastroparesis and functional dyspepsia.
- Idiopathic gastroparesis significantly impacts on the quality of life of patients and development of new effective therapies for symptomatic control is needed.

INTRODUCTION

Gastroparesis is a chronic symptomatic disorder of the stomach manifested by delayed emptying without evidence of mechanical obstruction.[1,2] The common causes of gastroparesis include diabetic, postsurgical, and idiopathic.[1,2] Idiopathic gastroparesis (IG) refers to gastroparesis of unknown cause; that is, not from diabetes, not from prior gastric surgery, and not related to other endocrine, neurologic, or rheumatologic causes of gastroparesis. In addition, it is not related to medications that can delay gastric emptying, such as opiate narcotic analgesics and anticholinergics.[1]

In most series, IG is the most common category for gastroparesis. In the series reported by Soykan and colleagues[3] the causes in 146 patients were 36% idiopathic, 29% diabetic, 13% postgastric surgery, 7.5% Parkinson disease, 4.8% collagen vascular disorders, 4.1% intestinal pseudo-obstruction, and 6% miscellaneous causes. Miscellaneous causes of gastroparesis include other neurologic diseases, eating disorders, other metabolic or endocrine conditions (hypothyroidism), and critical illness.

Gastroenterology Section, Temple University School of Medicine, Parkinson Pavilion 8th Floor, 3401 North Broad Street, Philadelphia, PA 19140, USA
E-mail address: henry.parkman@temple.edu

Gastroenterol Clin N Am 44 (2015) 59–68
http://dx.doi.org/10.1016/j.gtc.2014.11.015
0889-8553/15/$ – see front matter © 2015 Elsevier Inc. All rights reserved.

gastro.theclinics.com

This article discusses IG, symptomatic gastroparesis not from other known etiologies. This article updates the present status of the understanding of this disorder and reviews recent studies from the National Institutes of Health (NIH) National Institute of Diabetes and Digestive and Kidney Diseases (NIDDK) Gastroparesis Consortium.

EPIDEMIOLOGY

Gastroparesis occurs more often in women than men, often by a 3:1 margin. This is true not only for IG, but also for the other main causes of gastroparesis (diabetic and postsurgical). Patients with IG are typically young or middle-aged women. Even after adjusting for gender differences in gastric emptying, because females in general have slower gastric emptying than males,[4] gastroparesis occurs more commonly in women.[5]

Outside of gender issues and cause, the epidemiology of gastroparesis has not been systematically studied. This is because for proper diagnosis, a gastric emptying test is needed, one that presently cannot be done in population studies. Data from the Rochester Epidemiology Project, a database of linked medical records of residents of Olmsted County, Minnesota, showed that the age-adjusted incidence of definite gastroparesis per 100,000 person-years for the years 1996 to 2006 was 9.8 for women and 2.4 for men.[6] Definite gastroparesis was defined as diagnosis of delayed gastric emptying by standard scintigraphy and symptoms of nausea and/or vomiting, postprandial fullness, early satiety, bloating, or epigastric pain for more than 3 months. The age-adjusted prevalence of definite gastroparesis per 100,000 persons was 37.8 for women and 9.6 for men. More recent estimates have suggested that the prevalence of gastroparesis was an underestimation and the prevalence is greater, approaching 2% of the general population.[7]

SYMPTOMS

Common symptoms of gastroparesis include nausea (>90% of patients), vomiting (84% of patients), and early satiety (60% of patients).[1–3] Other symptoms include postprandial fullness and upper abdominal pain.[8] There is slight variation in symptoms depending on the cause of gastroparesis: abdominal pain occurs more often in IG than in diabetic gastroparesis (DG),[8] whereas nausea and vomiting are more severe in DG than in IG.[9] In patients with gastroparesis, weight loss, malnutrition, and dehydration may be prominent in severe cases.

There is overlap in the symptoms of IG and functional dyspepsia. Abdominal pain or discomfort may be present to varying degrees in patients with gastroparesis, but it is not usually the predominant symptom, as it can be in functional dyspepsia.[10] A substantial minority of patients (20%–40%) with functional dyspepsia can have delayed gastric emptying,[10] blurring the distinction between IG and functional dyspepsia. Patients with IG often have a constellation of symptoms including nausea, vomiting, early satiety, postprandial fullness, and upper abdominal pain.

Symptoms may fluctuate, with episodes of pronounced symptoms interspersed with relatively symptom-free intervals. Thus it can be difficult to differentiate IG from cyclic vomiting syndrome, especially in the latter when there can be a "coalescence of symptoms," such that they can occur nearly daily rather than as typical for cyclic vomiting syndrome with the vomiting episodes more sporadic on a monthly or less frequent basis.[11] In cyclic vomiting syndrome, gastric emptying is normal or often, it can be rapid[11]

The symptom profile and symptom severity of gastroparesis can be assessed with the Gastroparesis Cardinal Symptom Index (GCSI),[12] a subset of the Patient

Assessment of Upper Gastrointestinal Symptoms.[13] The GCSI comprises three sub-scales (nausea and vomiting, postprandial fullness and early satiety, and bloating) that the patient scores with reference to the preceding 2 weeks.[12] The GCSI daily diary can be used to record symptoms on a daily basis and may be more accurate in recording symptoms.[14] This daily diary of symptoms captures symptoms of early satiety, nausea, vomiting, postprandial fullness, and upper abdominal pain. This questionnaire has been shown to capture relevant symptoms of gastroparesis in patients with DG and IG.

Although it has been a common assumption that the gastrointestinal symptoms can be attributed to the delay in gastric emptying characteristic of the disorder, most investigations have observed only weak correlations between symptom severity and the degree of gastric stasis.[15,16] In general, the symptoms that seem to be best correlated (significant, but low correlation coefficients of 0.2–0.3) with a delay in gastric emptying include nausea, vomiting, early satiety, and postprandial fullness.[17,18] Some symptoms present in patients with gastroparesis, such as bloating and upper abdominal pain, are not correlated with delayed gastric emptying and might be related to sensory alterations that might also be present in patients with gastroparesis.[18]

Most patients with gastroparesis are underweight, probably because of frequently experienced early satiety, nausea, and vomiting. Some patients with gastroparesis, however, are overweight, for reasons that are not well understood. In a recent study, the factors that influence bodyweight in patients with IG and in healthy control subjects were investigated.[19] Thirty-nine healthy control subjects and 29 subjects with IG underwent resting energy expenditure (indirect calorimetry), body composition (bioelectrical impedance), dietary intake (Block Food Frequency Questionnaire), symptoms (Patient Assessment of Upper GI Symptoms), and physical activity (Paffen-barger exercise survey) assessment. Both median caloric intake (1242 vs 1804 kcal; $P = .005$) and caloric expenditure (486 vs 2172 kcal; $P<.01$) were significantly lower in patients with gastroparesis as compared with control subjects, although body mass index (25.8 ± 5.8 vs 24.3 ± 4.0 kg/m^2) and resting energy expenditure (1327 ± 293 vs 1422 ± 243 kcal) were similar. Interestingly, the 12 patients with gastroparesis who had gained weight since diagnosis had lower symptom severity (12.9 ± 4.4 vs 19.3 ± 6.3; $P<.05$), consumed more calories (1342 vs 1134 kcal; $P = .08$), and expended fewer calories for activity per week (406 vs 644 median kcal; $P = .45$) compared with the 17 patients with gastroparesis who had lost weight or remained weight neutral. Thus, patients with gastroparesis consumed and expended fewer calories than healthy control subjects. A subgroup of patients with gastroparesis who were less symptomatic gained weight because of increased caloric intake and reduced energy expenditure.

National Institutes of Health Gastroparesis Consortium Registry Studies in Idiopathic Gastroparesis

The NIDDK Gastroparesis Clinical Research Consortium is a cooperative network of seven clinical centers and one Data Coordinating Center funded through the NIDDK of the NIH. The Gastroparesis Clinical Research Consortium Gastroparesis (GpC) Registry was implemented as an observational study of patients with gastroparesis enrolled prospectively at seven centers.[20] Several of the published studies have addressed IG.

The characteristics of 243 patients with IG enrolled in the GpC Registry were recently described.[20] This study is the largest study of patients with IG. Patients' mean age was 41 years, and most (88%) were female. The most common presenting symptoms were nausea (34%), vomiting (19%), and abdominal pain (23%). Severe delay in gastric emptying (>35% retention at 4 hours) was present in 28% of patients and was associated with more severe symptoms of nausea and vomiting and loss of appetite compared with patients with mild or moderate delay. Of these patients with IG, 86% met criteria for functional dyspepsia, predominately postprandial distress syndrome. Of interest, 46% of the patients were overweight. Thus, this study shows that IG is a heterogeneous syndrome that primarily affects young women and can also affect overweight or obese individuals.

Although gastroparesis can be diabetic or idiopathic, little is known about differences in their presentation. The GpC compared clinical characteristics, symptoms, and gastric emptying in patients with IG with patients with type 1 or type 2 diabetes mellitus DG.[21] A total of 416 patients with gastroparesis were analyzed; 254 had IG, and 137 had DG (78 had type 1 and 59 had type 2 diabetes mellitus). Symptoms that prompted evaluation more often included vomiting for DG and abdominal pain for IG. Patients with DG had more severe retching and vomiting than those with IG, whereas patients with IG had more severe early satiety and postprandial fullness subscores. Compared with IG, gastric retention was greater in patients with type 1 diabetes mellitus. Thus, there are many similarities and some differences in clinical characteristics of DG and IG. Gastroparesis is a heterogeneous disorder; the cause of the gastroparesis impacts symptoms and severity.

Abdominal pain can be present in patients with IG. Factors associated with abdominal pain in gastroparesis have not been well studied. The NIH GpC studied the symptom of abdominal pain and how it relates to other clinical factors in 393 patients with gastroparesis.[22] Upper abdominal pain was moderate-severe in 261 (66%) patients. Pain and discomfort were predominant in 81 (21%); nausea and vomiting were predominant in 172 (44%). Moderate-severe pain was more prevalent with IG than in DG and correlated with scores for nausea and vomiting and opiate use, but not gastric emptying. Gastroparesis severity, quality of life, and depression and anxiety were worse with moderate-severe pain. Predominant pain and discomfort were associated with impaired quality of life. Thus, moderate-severe abdominal pain is prevalent in gastroparesis, impairs quality of life, and is associated with idiopathic etiology and opiate use. Pain was predominant in one-fifth of gastroparetics. Predominant pain has at least as great an impact on disease severity and quality of life as compared with the more classic symptoms of predominant nausea and vomiting.

Bloating is commonly reported in gastroparesis, but is an underappreciated symptom of gastroparesis. The prevalence of bloating in gastroparesis and its severity was assessed in 335 patients with gastroparesis.[23] Bloating severity of at least severe (GCSI ≥4) grades was reported by 41% of patients. Bloating severity related to female gender and overweight status and correlated with intensity of nausea, postprandial fullness, visible distention, abdominal pain, and altered bowel function. Antiemetics, probiotics, and antidepressants with significant norepinephrine reuptake inhibitor activity may affect reports of bloating. Disease-specific quality of life and general measures of well-being were progressively impaired with increasing bloating severity. Thus, the symptom of bloating impairs quality of life but is not influenced by gastric emptying rates.

Many patients with gastroparesis have had their gallbladders removed; how this impacts on gastroparesis is not known. The clinical presentations of patients with gastroparesis were compared in those with prior cholecystectomy with patients who have not had their gallbladder removed.[24] Of 391 subjects with DG or IG, 142 (36%) had a prior cholecystectomy. Patients with prior cholecystectomy were more often female, older, and overweight or obese. Cholecystectomy had been performed in 46% of type 2 diabetes mellitus compared with 24% of type 1 diabetes mellitus and

38% of IG. Patients with cholecystectomy had more comorbidities, particularly chronic fatigue syndrome, fibromyalgia, depression, and anxiety. Postcholecystectomy patients with gastroparesis had increased health care use and had a worse quality of life. Etiology was not independently associated with a prior cholecystectomy. Thus, symptom profiles in patients with and without cholecystectomy differ: postcholecystectomy patients with gastroparesis had more severe upper abdominal pain and retching and less severe constipation. These data suggest that prior cholecystectomy is associated with selected manifestations of gastroparesis.

PATHOPHYSIOLOGY

A potential cause in some patients with IG has been suggested to be viral injury to the nerves or muscles of the stomach, known as postviral gastroparesis. It has been suggested that IG of acute onset with infectious prodrome could constitute postviral or viral injury to the neural innervation of the stomach or the interstitial cells of Cajal in the stomach. In the NIH GpC study of IG, half the patients had an acute onset of symptoms and a minority of patients (19%) reported an initial infectious prodrome, such as gastroenteritis or respiratory infection.[20] In the McCallum series, postviral gastroparesis was suspected in 23% of patients with IG.[25] This clinical diagnosis of postviral gastroparesis is suggested in previously healthy persons with an acute onset of viral illness with nausea, vomiting, diarrhea, fever, and cramps who have persistence of symptoms (nausea, vomiting, early satiety) for more than 3 months with a delay in gastric emptying. Viruses suspected as potential causes are cytomegalovirus, Epstein-Barr virus, and herpes varicella-zoster. Symptoms of IG after a presumed viral illness tend to be less severe than in gastroparesis from other causes. Overall, these patients seem to have a good prognosis, with many patients having a slow resolution of their symptoms.[25]

Gastric emptying is mediated by the vagus nerve, which helps regulates fundic accommodation, antral contraction, and pyloric relaxation.[1] These regional gastric motility changes with food ingestion are then mediated through smooth muscle cells, which control stomach contractions; interstitial cells of Cajal, which regulate gastric pacemaker activity; and enteric neurons, which initiate smooth muscle cell activity.[1] The pathophysiology of gastroparesis has not been fully elucidated but seems to involve abnormalities in functioning of several elements including autonomic nervous system, smooth muscle cells, enteric neurons, and interstitial cells of Cajal. Histologic studies in patients with gastroparesis demonstrate defects in the morphology of enteric neurons, smooth muscle cells, and interstitial cells of Cajal and increased concentrations of inflammatory cells in gastric tissue.[26]

National Institutes of Health Gastroparesis Consortium Studies on Pathology

Cellular changes associated with DG and IG have recently been described from patients with gastroparesis by the NIH GpC. Full-thickness gastric body biopsy specimens were obtained from 40 patients with gastroparesis (20 diabetic) and matched control subjects.[27] Histologic abnormalities were found in 83% of patients. The most common defects were loss of interstitial cell of Cajal with remaining ICC showing injury, an abnormal immune infiltrate containing macrophages, and decreased nerve fibers. On light microscopy, no significant differences were found between DG and IG with the exception of neuronal nitric oxide synthase expression, which was decreased in more patients with IG (40%) compared with patients with diabetes (20%) by visual grading. On electron microscopy, a markedly increased connective tissue stroma was present in both disorders. This study suggests that on full-thickness biopsy specimens, cellular abnormalities are found in most patients with gastroparesis. The most common findings were loss of Kit expression, suggesting loss of ICC, and an increase in CD45 and CD68 immunoreactivity. These findings suggest that examination of tissue can lead to valuable insights into the pathophysiology and possibly treatments for the patient.

The association of these cellular changes in patients with gastroparesis with gastroparesis symptoms and gastric emptying was recently reported.[28] IG with a myenteric immune infiltrate scored higher on the average GCSI and nausea score as compared with those without an infiltrate. Interstitial cells of Cajal counts inversely correlated with 4-hour gastric retention in DG but not in IG. There was also a significant correlation between loss of ICC and enteric nerves in DG but not in IG. Thus, in DG, loss of ICC is associated with delayed gastric emptying. Interstitial cells of Cajal or enteric nerve loss did not correlate with symptom severity. Overall clinical severity and nausea in IG is associated with a myenteric immune infiltrate. Thus, full-thickness gastric biopsies can help define specific cellular abnormalities in gastroparesis, some of which are associated with physiologic and clinical characteristics of gastroparesis.

MANAGEMENT

Management of gastroparesis is guided by the goals of correcting fluid, electrolyte, and nutritional deficiencies; identifying and treating the cause of delayed gastric emptying (eg, diabetes); and suppressing or eliminating symptoms.[1,2] Treatment of the symptoms may include agents used for DG and functional dyspepsia. Care of patients generally relies on dietary modification, prokinetics medications that stimulate gastric motor activity, antiemetic drug therapy to suppress symptoms of nausea and vomiting, and symptom modulators (psychotropic agents) that reduce symptom expression. Narcotic analgesics should be avoided. Although narcotic analgesics may acutely improve abdominal pain, with chronic use, they delay gastric emptying, may themselves lead to symptoms of nausea and vomiting, may upregulate abdominal pain, and lead to dependence. Total parenteral nutrition, although used in some refractory patients, is associated with complications of infections and thrombosis. Aspects on treatment are discussed in detail elsewhere in this issue. Particulars of treatment in IG are discussed next.

Dietary Aspects in Gastroparesis

Gastroparesis can lead to food aversion, poor oral intake, and subsequent malnutrition. In the NIH GpC gastroparesis registry, dietary intake and nutritional deficiencies were characterized in 305 patients with DG and IG[29] who completed diet questionnaires (Block Food Frequency Questionnaire). Caloric intake averaged 1168 $\pm$ 801 kcal/day, amounting to 58% $\pm$ 39% of daily total energy requirements. A total of 194 patients (64%) reported caloric-deficient diets. Only five patients (2%) followed a diet suggested for patients with gastroparesis. Deficiencies were present in several vitamins and minerals; patients with idiopathic disorders were more likely to have diets with estimated deficiencies in vitamins A, B_6, C, and K, iron, potassium, and zinc than patients with diabetes. Only one-third of patients were taking multivitamin supplements. More severe symptoms (bloating and constipation) were characteristic of patients who reported an energy-deficient diet. Surprisingly, only 32% of patients had nutritional consultation after the onset of gastroparesis; consultation was more likely among patients with longer duration of symptoms and more hospitalizations and patients with diabetes. Multivariable logistic regression analysis indicated that nutritional consultation increased the chances that daily total energy requirements were met (odds ratio, 1.51; $P = .08$). Thus, many patients with gastroparesis have diets deficient in calories, vitamins, and minerals. Most patients are not following a "gastroparesis diet." Nutritional consultation is obtained infrequently, especially in IG. A nutritional consultation may be helpful for instructions on dietary therapy and to address nutritional deficiencies.

Psychotropic Medications As Symptom Modulators

Gastroparesis is a challenging syndrome to manage, with few effective treatments and lack of rigorously controlled trials. Symptom modulators (psychotropic agents, such as tricyclic antidepressants) are often used to treat refractory symptoms of nausea, vomiting, and abdominal pain. Evidence from well-designed studies for this use is lacking. Tricyclic antidepressants may have benefits in suppressing symptoms in some patients with nausea and vomiting and patients with abdominal pain. Doses of tricyclic antidepressants are lower than used to treat depression. A reasonable starting dose for a tricyclic drug is 10 to 25 mg at bedtime. If benefit is not observed in several weeks, doses are increased by 10- to 25-mg increments up to 75 mg. Side effects are common with use of tricyclic antidepressants and can interfere with management and lead to a change in medication in some patients. The secondary amines, nortriptyline and desipramine, may have fewer side effects than amitriptyline, which itself may delay gastric emptying. The recent NIH gastroparesis consortium study with nortriptyline in IG did not show an effect on overall symptoms of gastroparesis.[30] However, there was a suggestion that low nortriptyline doses (10–25 mg at bedtime) might decrease nausea, whereas higher doses might decrease fullness. The recently completed NIH functional dyspepsia treatment trial showed a favorable effect for amitriptyline for functional dyspepsia; this was seen in patients with normal gastric emptying, but not in those with delayed gastric emptying.[31]

Gastric Electric Stimulation

Gastric electric stimulation is a treatment of refractory gastroparesis involving implantation of a neurostimulator. The currently approved stimulator delivers a high-frequency (12 cpm), low-energy signal with short pulses to the gastric muscle along the greater curvature. Based on initial studies that have shown symptom benefit with low complications, the gastric electric neurostimulator was granted humanitarian approval from the Food and Drug Administration for the treatment of chronic, refractory nausea and vomiting secondary to IG or DG.[32] Symptoms of vomiting improved with gastric stimulation. This symptomatic benefit was primarily seen in patients with DG than in IG.[32] In the study by Maranki and colleagues,[33] three predictive factors for clinical improvement with gastric electric stimulation were found: (1) diabetic rather than idiopathic etiology, (2) predominant symptoms of nausea and/or vomiting rather than abdominal pain, and (3) lack of the use of regular narcotic pain medications. In this series, gastric electric stimulation significantly improved symptoms of nausea and vomiting, but not abdominal pain. In a recently reported, prospective study of gastric electric stimulation for IG,[34] there was a reduction in vomiting during the initial 6-week open label "on" treatment period. A double-blind 3-month period showed a nonsignificant reduction in vomiting in the "on" versus "off" period, the primary outcome variable. At 12 months with open label "on" stimulation, there was a sustained decrease in vomiting and days of hospitalizations.

SUMMARY

IG refers to gastroparesis of unknown cause not from diabetes; not from prior gastric surgery; and not related to other endocrine, neurologic, or rheumatologic causes of gastroparesis. Patients with IG often have a constellation of symptoms including nausea, vomiting, early satiety, postprandial fullness, and upper abdominal pain. Although the presentation of IG is relatively similar to DG, abdominal pain occurs more often in IG, whereas nausea and vomiting are more severe in DG. Treatment may include agents used for DG and functional dyspepsia, including dietary management, prokinetics agents, antiemetic agents, and symptom modulators. IG significantly impacts on the quality of life of patients through its chronic symptoms of nausea, vomiting, and abdominal pain. Unfortunately, current approved treatment options do not adequately address clinical need. Development of new effective therapies for symptomatic control is needed.

REFERENCES

1. Camilleri M, Parkman HP, Shafi MA, et al. Clinical guideline: management of gastroparesis. Am J Gastroenterol 2013;108:18–37.
2. Parkman HP, Hasler WL, Fisher RS. American Gastroenterological Association technical review on the diagnosis and treatment of gastroparesis. Gastroenterology 2004;127:1592–622.
3. Soykan I, Sivri B, Sarosiek I, et al. Demography, clinical characteristics, psychological and abuse profiles, treatment, and long-term follow-up of patients with gastroparesis. Dig Dis Sci 1998;43:2398–404.
4. Knight LC, Parkman HP, Brown KL, et al. Delayed gastric emptying and decreased antral contractility in normal premenopausal women compared to men. Am J Gastroenterol 1997;92:968–75.
5. Stanghellini V, Tosetti C, Paternico A, et al. Risk indicators of delayed gastric emptying of solids in patients with functional dyspepsia. Gastroenterology 1996;110:1036–42.
6. Jung HK, Choung RS, Locke GR III, et al. The incidence, prevalence, and outcomes of patients with gastroparesis in Olmsted County, Minnesota, from 1996 to 2006. Gastroenterology 2009;136:1225–33.
7. Rey E, Choung RS, Schleck CD, et al. Prevalence of hidden gastroparesis in the community: the gastroparesis "iceberg". J Neurogastroenterol Motil 2012;18:34–42.
8. Cherian D, Sachdeva P, Fisher RS, et al. Abdominal pain is a frequent symptom of gastroparesis. Clin Gastroenterol Hepatol 2010;8:676–81.
9. Cherian D, Parkman HP. Nausea and vomiting in diabetic and idiopathic gastroparesis. Neurogastroenterol Motil 2012;24:217–22.
10. Tack J, Talley NJ, Camilleri M, et al. Functional gastroduodenal disorders. Gastroenterology 2006;130:1466–79.
11. Abell TL, Adams KA, Boles RG, et al. Cyclic vomiting syndrome in adults. Neurogastroenterol Motil 2008;20:269–84.
12. Revicki DA, Rentz AM, Dubois D, et al. Development and validation of a patient-assessed gastroparesis symptom severity measure: the Gastroparesis Cardinal Symptom Index. Aliment Pharmacol Ther 2003;18:141–50.
13. Rentz AM, Kahrilas P, Stanghellini V, et al. Development and psychometric evaluation of the patient assessment of upper gastrointestinal symptom severity index (PAGI-SYM) in patients with upper gastrointestinal disorders. Qual Life Res 2004;13:1737–49.
14. Revicki DA, Camilleri M, Kuo B, et al. Development and content validity of a gastroparesis cardinal symptom index daily diary. Aliment Pharmacol Ther 2009;30:670–80.

15. Horowitz M, Maddox AF, Wishart JM, et al. Relationships between oesophageal transit and solid and liquid gastric emptying in diabetes mellitus. Eur J Nucl Med 1991;18:229–34.

16. Pasricha PJ, Colvin R, Yates K, et al. Characteristics of patients with chronic unexplained nausea and vomiting and normal gastric emptying. Clin Gastroenterol Hepatol 2011;9:567–76.e1-4.

17. Pathikonda M, Sachdeva P, Malhotra N, et al. Gastric emptying scintigraphy: is four hours necessary? J Clin Gastroenterol 2012;46:209–15.

18. Cassilly DW, Wang YR, Friedenberg FK, et al. Symptoms of gastroparesis: use of the gastroparesis cardinal symptom index in symptomatic patients referred for gastric emptying scintigraphy. Digestion 2008;78:144–51.

19. Homko CJ, Zamora LC, Boden G, et al. Body weight in patients with idiopathic gastroparesis: roles of symptoms, caloric intake, physical activity and body metabolism. Neurogastroenterol Motil 2014;26:283–9.

20. Parkman HP, Yates K, Hasler WL, et al. Clinical features of idiopathic gastroparesis vary with sex, body mass, symptom onset, delay in gastric emptying, and gastroparesis severity. Gastroenterology 2011;140:101–15.

21. Parkman HP, Yates K, Hasler WL, et al, National Institute of Diabetes and Digestive and Kidney Diseases Gastroparesis Clinical Research Consortium. Similarities and differences between diabetic and idiopathic gastroparesis. Clin Gastroenterol Hepatol 2011;9:1056–64.

22. Hasler WL, Wilson LA, Parkman HP, et al. Factors related to abdominal pain in gastroparesis: contrast to patients with predominant nausea and vomiting. Neurogastroenterol Motil 2013;25:427–38.

23. Hasler WL, Wilson LA, Parkman HP, et al. Bloating in gastroparesis: severity, impact, and associated factors. Am J Gastroenterol 2011;106:1492–502.

24. Parkman HP, Yates K, Hasler WL, et al. Cholecystectomy and clinical presentations of gastroparesis. Dig Dis Sci 2013;58:1062–73.

25. Bityutskiy LP, Soykan I, McCallum RW. Viral gastroparesis: a subgroup of idiopathic gastroparesis–clinical characteristics and long-term outcomes. Am J Gastroenterol 1997;92:1501–4.

26. Harberson J, Thomas R, Harbison S, et al. Gastric neuromuscluar pathology of gastroparesis: analysis of full-thickness antral biopsies. Dig Dis Sci 2010;55:359–70.

27. Grover M, Farrugia G, Lurken MS, et al, NIDDK Gastroparesis Clinical Research Consortium. Cellular changes in diabetic and idiopathic gastroparesis. Gastroenterology 2011;140:1575–85.

28. Grover M, Bernard CE, Pasricha PJ, et al, NIDDK Gastroparesis Clinical Research Consortium (GpCRC). Clinical-histological associations in gastroparesis: results from the Gastroparesis Clinical Research Consortium. Neurogastroenterol Motil 2012;24:531–9.

29. Parkman HP, Yates KP, Hasler WL, et al, NIDDK Gastroparesis Clinical Research Consortium. Dietary intake and nutritional deficiencies in patients with diabetic or idiopathic gastroparesis. Gastroenterology 2011;141:486–98.

30. Parkman HP, Van Natta ML, Abell TL, et al. Effect of nortriptyline on symptoms of idiopathic gastroparesis: the NORIG randomized clinical trial. JAMA 2013;310:2640–9.

31. Locke GR, Bouras EP, Howden CW, et al. The NIH functional dyspepsia treatment trial (FDTT) [abstract]. Gastroenterology 2013;145:S145.

32. Abell T, McCallum R, Hocking M, et al. Gastric electrical stimulation for medically refractory gastroparesis. Gastroenterology 2003;125:421–8.

33. Maranki JL, Lytes V, Meilahn JE, et al. Predictive factors for clinical improvement with Enterra gastric electric stimulation treatment for refractory gastroparesis. Dig Dis Sci 2008;53:2072–8.

34. McCallum RW, Sarosiek I, Parkman HP, et al. Gastric electrical stimulation with Enterra therapy improves symptoms of idiopathic gastroparesis. Neurogastroenterol Motil 2013;25:815–21.

Other Forms of Gastroparesis

Postsurgical, Parkinson, Other Neurologic Diseases, Connective Tissue Disorders

Eamonn M.M. Quigley, MD, FRCP, FRCPI

KEYWORDS

- Gastroparesis • Parkinson disease • Multiple sclerosis • Motor neuron disease
- Neurologic • Post-surgical • Fundoplication • Scleroderma

KEY POINTS

- Fundoplication, bariatric procedures, and pancreatic surgeries are nowadays the surgical approaches most commonly complicated by gastroparesis.
- Virtually any neurologic disorder may be complicated by gastroparesis, and its development may affect nutrition and drug availability.
- Gastroparesis is a common feature of gastrointestinal involvement in scleroderma and other connective tissue disorders.

POSTSURGICAL GASTROPARESIS

Although acute gastroparesis may be a component of the ileus syndrome that can complicate many surgical procedures and of the acute pseudo-obstruction syndrome that may accompany severe sepsis and multiorgan failure, this review focuses on chronic manifestations of gastric dysmotility.[1] In contrast to chronic gastroparesis, whose pathophysiology is often poorly understood, inflammatory processes seem fundamental to the inhibition of motility in the acute form.

Gastroparesis and other disorders of gastric sensorimotor function may complicate specific surgical procedures.[2] In the important Olmstead County study of the community prevalence of gastroparesis, 7.2% of all cases of definite gastroparesis were related to prior gastrectomy or fundoplication.[3] Rates of postsurgical gastroparesis vary widely depending on many factors, including the site and nature of the surgical procedure. For example, in their comprehensive review, Dong and colleagues[4] noted

The author has nothing to disclose.

Division of Gastroenterology and Hepatology, Houston Methodist Hospital, Well Cornell Medical College, 6550 Fannin Street, SM 1001, Houston, TX 77030, USA

E-mail address: equigley@tmhs.org

Gastroenterol Clin N Am 44 (2015) 69–81

http://dx.doi.org/10.1016/j.gtc.2014.11.006

gastro.theclinics.com

that rates ranged from 0.4% to 5% following gastrectomy, from 20% to 50% after pylorus-preserving pancreaticoduodenectomy, and from 50% to 70% after cryoablation therapy for pancreatic cancer.

Vagotomy

Although vagotomy is infrequently performed nowadays in the management of acid-peptic disease, inadvertent vagal injury may complicate other interventions, rendering an understanding of the complex effects of vagotomy on gastric motor function still relevant. Receptive relaxation, a vagally mediated reflex, is impaired. As a consequence, the early phase of liquid emptying is accelerated. This acceleration causes rapid emptying of hyperosmolar solutions into the proximal small intestine and may result in the early dumping syndrome. By contrast, and as a consequence of impaired antropyloric function, the later phases of liquid and solid emptying are prolonged by vagotomy. Other motor effects of vagotomy include an impairment of the motor response to feeding (which contributes to the pathophysiologic mechanisms of postvagotomy diarrhea) and a suppression of the antral component of the migrating motor complex. The latter phenomenon is particularly prevalent among individuals who have symptomatic postvagotomy gastroparesis.

The now standard addition of a drainage procedure, such as a pyloroplasty or gastroenterostomy, has tended to negate the effects of vagotomy alone. In most patients, the net result of the combined procedure is little alteration in the gastric emptying of liquids or solids. Thus, prolonged postoperative gastroparesis (ie, lasting longer than 3–4 weeks) is, in fact, rare (<2.5% of patients after either vagotomy and pyloroplasty or vagotomy and antrectomy).[5] Significant postoperative gastroparesis may occur, however, in patients who have a prior history of prolonged gastric outlet obstruction. In this circumstance, normal gastric emptying may not return for several weeks.

Longitudinal studies suggest that vagotomy-related gastroparesis tends to resolve over time, with one study suggesting gastric emptying rates in those who had undergone either a truncal or a highly selective vagotomy being similar by 12 months after the procedure.[6]

Persisting postsurgical gastric motor dysfunction often presents a formidable management challenge. Therapeutic responses to prokinetic agents have proved particularly disappointing in this group. In these resistant cases, a completion gastrectomy may be the best alternative. It should be noted, however, that in one large series this approach was deemed successful in only 43% of patients.[7]

Gastrectomy

Antral resection by removing the antral mill renders the stomach incontinent to solids and leads to accelerated emptying, and symptomatic "dumping" may occur in up to 50% of patients after Billroth I or II gastrectomy.[8] Late dumping symptoms occur 90 to 120 minutes after a meal and are a consequence of reactive hypoglycemia. The accommodation reflex is impaired among symptomatic patients.[9] By contrast, delayed gastric emptying sometimes occurs after a Billroth II gastrectomy as a result of a large atonic gastric remnant.[8] Meng and colleagues[10] reported a 6.9% frequency of gastroparesis among 563 patients who underwent radical gastrectomy for gastric cancer in their unit in Shanghai, China. Preoperative gastric outlet obstruction and the performance of a Billroth II anastomosis were the principal risk factors for the occurrence of gastroparesis. Of note, they documented a similar rate of gastroparesis (3.7%) among a smaller group of patients who underwent a laparoscopic gastrectomy.[10] Laparoscopy-assisted, pylorus-preserving gastrectomy represents a less radical operative approach to early gastric cancer; gastric stasis is the most common complication of this procedure, occurring in 6.2% of cases.[11] In one series, and in contrast to the aforementioned experience with this procedure following vagotomy, completion gastrectomy resulted in significant symptomatic improvement among subjects with postgastrectomy gastroparesis.[12]

Roux-en-Y Syndrome

The creation of a Roux-en-Y gastroenterostomy may be associated with a specific clinical entity, the Roux syndrome.[13] Severe symptoms of postprandial abdominal pain, bloating, and nausea many develop. Studies have variably described impaired gastric motor function[14] and a functional obstruction within the duodenal Roux limb as a result of motor asynchrony.[13,15] The latter can be revealed by manometry, but the status of these motility patterns in the pathophysiologic processes of this syndrome remains unclear.[16]

Pancreatectomy

Pancreatectomy and pylorus-preserving pancreaticoduodenectomy, in particular, have been associated with a high incidence of postoperative gastric stasis. The principal predictor of gastric emptying delay after these operations is the occurrence of other postoperative complications.[17,18] Operative technique seems, in general, to be of less importance, although there is a suggestion that an antecolic anastomosis may be associated with less emptying delay. Accordingly in what has been, perhaps, the largest series (N = 711) to date, Parmar and colleagues[19] documented an overall rate of delayed gastric emptying following pancreaticoduodenectomy of 20%. The occurrence of gastroparesis did not seem to be influenced by such technical factors as pylorus preservation or whether the gastrojejunostomy was antecolic or retrocolic, but was associated with fistula formation, postoperative sepsis, and reoperation. These results contrast with those of a prior systematic review, which found that antecolic reconstruction was linked to lower rates of gastroparesis.[20] Furthermore, others have suggested that the use of a Billroth II rather than a gastrojejunostomy for reconstruction following this procedure may reduce the risk of gastric emptying delay.[21] Preoperative diabetes has been identified as an additional risk factor.[22] Gastroparesis has also been reported following pancreas transplantation.[23]

Antireflux Operations

The physiology of the lower esophageal sphincter and the proximal stomach are intimately related in health; it should come as no surprise, therefore, that a variety of antireflux procedures can influence gastric sensorimotor function.[24] Fundoplication, as expected, affects sensorimotor function of the proximal stomach.[25–27] Most, but not all,[28] studies have demonstrated impaired relaxation of the proximal stomach, in response to meal ingestion, following this surgical procedure. Although the usual effect of fundoplication is to accelerate, rather than delay, gastric emptying,[26] instances of gastroparesis have been described following antireflux surgery and endoscopic antireflux procedures.[29] Given the high frequency with which the procedure is now performed, it should come as no surprise that Nissen fundoplication was the most common cause of postsurgical gastroparesis in the audit performed by the National Institute of Diabetes and Digestive and Kidney Diseases gastroparesis consortium.[30] The pathophysiologic process leading to these occurrences is unclear. In some, postsurgical gastroparesis may represent the overt appearance of an unrecognized preoperative disorder; in others there is compelling evidence to incriminate vagal injury, which is especially likely in relation to redo procedures and may contribute to persistent gas-bloat symptoms.[31] In rare instances, postfundoplication gastroparesis may be persistent and severe. Although gastric resection does not seem to offer much help for these unfortunate patients,[32] some success has been reported with an approach that combines conversion to a partial fundoplication with a pyloroplasty.[33]

Bariatric Surgery

Ardila-Hani and Soffer[34] comprehensively reviewed the impact of bariatric (or metabolic) surgical procedures on gastrointestinal motor function. Esophageal problems were by far the most common. Gastric emptying did not appear to be affected by laparoscopic adjustable gastric banding and tended to accelerate following Roux-en-Y gastric bypass. However, instances of gastroparesis, at times severe and persistent, have been reported following the latter procedure. Salameh and colleagues,[35] for example, described successful treatment of 6 patients with intractable gastroparesis following Roux-en-Y gastric bypass for morbid obesity using gastric electrical stimulation. In an uncontrolled trial, endoscopic injection of the pylorus with botulinum toxin A produced symptomatic improvement in a small series of patients with postvagotomy gastroparesis, which was thought to result from fundoplication in the vast majority.[36]

Other Procedures

Virtually any procedure that could compromise the vagi or affect upper gastrointestinal motor function could result in gastroparesis. Clinically significant gastroparesis has, therefore, been reported not only in association with a wide range of gastric procedures but also in relation to esophageal resection,[37] botulinum toxin injection for achalasia,[38] lung transplantation, and even hepatic surgery. Sutcliffe and colleagues[37] noted a 12% rate of gastric emptying delay following esophagectomy in their series; in another report, gastroparesis was more common after minimally invasive than open esophagectomy.[39] Gastroparesis in relation to lung transplantation is especially ominous, as its presence preoperatively has been associated with an increased risk for the development of bronchiolitis obliterans syndrome.[40] Though common before surgery,[40] new-onset gastroparesis was documented in 6% of subjects after transplantation in one large series.[41] In the lung transplant patient gastroparesis may trigger or exacerbate gastroesophageal reflux, from which these patients have no protection. For this reason there is a low threshold for the performance of fundoplication in this patient population, and gastric electrical stimulation has been added to address concomitant gastroparesis.[42]

Although cholecystectomy, per se, has not been incriminated as a cause of gastroparesis,[43] a prior cholecystectomy seems to negatively affect the natural history of both diabetic and idiopathic gastroparesis.[44]

PARKINSON DISEASE AND OTHER NEUROLOGIC DISORDERS

As populations age the prevalence of neurologic disease in the community continues to increase, and consultations relating to gastrointestinal motility problems in the patient afflicted with a neurologic disorder become ever more common.

The high prevalence of gastroparesis and other disturbances of gut motor function in neurologic diseases is based on similarities in morphology and function between the neuromuscular apparatus of the gut and that of the somatic nervous system. First, it is now recognized that the enteric and central nervous systems share many similarities, both morphologic and functional. The basic organization of the enteric nervous system

(ENS) (neurons, ganglia, glia, and ENS-blood barrier), and the ultrastructure of its components, are similar to those of the central nervous system (CNS), and almost all neurotransmitters identified within the CNS are also found in enteric neurons; the concept of ENS involvement in neurologic disease should not, therefore, come as a great surprise. Second, given the prevalence of dysfunction in the autonomic nervous system (an important modulator of enteric neuromuscular function) in several neurologic syndromes, in addition to the existence of several primary and secondary disorders of autonomic function, disturbed autonomic modulation of gut motor function may be an important contributory factor to symptomatology in some scenarios. Third, it is now evident that the gut has important sensory functions; though usually subconscious, gut sensation may be relayed to and perceived within the CNS. Sensory input is also fundamental to several reflex events in the gut, such as the viscerovisceral reflexes that coordinate function along the gut. However, the role of sensory dysfunction in the mediation of common symptoms, such as abdominal pain and nausea, in the patient with CNS disease with gastrointestinal manifestations has not been extensively investigated.

PATHOGENESIS OF GASTROINTESTINAL DYSFUNCTION IN NEUROLOGIC DISEASE

Although a whole range of disease processes affecting central, peripheral, and autonomic nervous systems may affect gut motor function, the 2 predominant neurologic disorders encountered in gastrointestinal practice are cerebrovascular disease and parkinsonism.

Cerebrovascular Disease

In contrast to swallowing function, gastric, small intestinal, colonic, and anorectal motor or sensory function have been little studied in the context of stroke and, therefore, the pathophysiology of complications involving these parts of the gastrointestinal tract is less clearly understood. Nevertheless, there is some indirect evidence to suggest that gastric emptying may be delayed following an acute stroke[45] and may have implications for feeding and drug administration.

Parkinson Disease

Idiopathic Parkinson disease (PD) causes widespread and sometimes severe derangement of gastrointestinal motility.[46–49] There are 2 basic contributors to gastrointestinal dysfunction in PD. First, striatal muscle dysfunction in the oropharynx, proximal esophagus, and anal canal is based on the same neurologic abnormalities that cause the cardinal manifestations of this disorder. The second component, namely dysfunction in the smooth muscle parts of the gastrointestinal tract, is less well understood but may reflect abnormality in the autonomic and/or enteric nervous systems.[50–53] Indeed, neuropathologic changes reminiscent of CNS Parkinson features, such as dopamine depletion[52] and the presence of Lewy neuritis[53] and α-synuclein,[54,55] has been demonstrated in the myenteric and submucosal plexi.

The pathophysiology of dysphagia and constipation in PD has received some attention, but little is known of the pathogenesis of symptoms arising from the stomach and small intestine, despite their high prevalence.[56] The contribution of autonomic dysfunction is illustrated by the higher prevalence of gastrointestinal symptoms and postural instability among patients with a PD variant, multiple system atrophy, in whom autonomic dysfunction is especially common.[57,58] For some symptoms, such as nausea, the contribution of antiparkinsonian medications and dopaminergics, in particular, must be borne in mind.

Delayed gastric emptying has been well documented in PD[59–65] and delayed emptying of solids has been linked, in some studies, to the severity of motor impairment.[60,62] Here again, the impact of levodopa must be accounted for.[62] The association between gastric emptying delay and the presence of levodopa response fluctuations,[61] coupled with irregular patterns of drug absorption[66] and the documentation of improved symptom control with intrajejunal[67] or transdermal[68] administration of antiparkinsonian drugs, underlines the potential clinical relevance of gastric emptying delay: by retarding drug delivery and absorption, gastroparesis could induce or further exacerbate response fluctuations. Several factors, however, limit the interpretation of reports of delayed gastric emptying and its association with upper gastrointestinal symptoms in PD.[60] These factors include variations in the patient population studied (eg, age, gender, disease severity, study location), the definition of gastroparesis, and the methodology used to assess the gastric emptying rate (meal, test technique, study protocol, and manner of interpretation). Variations between studies in these parameters make it very difficult to attempt real comparisons or draw firm conclusions. Nevertheless, delayed gastric emptying may occur in as many as 70% to 100% of PD patients attending specialist neurology clinics; the prevalence of symptomatic gastroparesis, in PD, however, remains unknown. Indeed, there has been a lack of a consistent correlation between gastric emptying rate and upper gastrointestinal symptoms in PD. While it is reasonable to assume that gastroparesis may contribute to the weight loss that has been so well documented in PD,[69] it is unclear as to whether nutrient delivery is affected by delayed gastric emptying, and a relationship between delayed gastric emptying and weight loss is yet to be demonstrated. Electrogastrography has also been used to study gastric motor activity in PD, but correlations with symptoms have been poor.[70,71] Parenthetically, it is of interest to note the suggestion that *Helicobacter pylori* and *Helicobacter heilmannii* infection are implicated in contributing to, not only gastrointestinal symptoms and weight loss in PD[72], but also systemic proinflammatory cytokine activation,[73] and even the pathogenesis of PD itself.[74]

Multiple Sclerosis

Delayed gastric emptying,[75] isolated cases of gastroparesis,[76–79] and even an instance of gastric perforation[80] have been reported in multiple sclerosis, with their cause attributed to autonomic dysfunction of central origin.[81] In one small series, parallel improvements in neurologic and gastric emptying function were documented in response to corticosteroid therapy.[79]

Autonomic and Peripheral Neuropathies

Given its ever increasing worldwide prevalence, diabetic autonomic neuropathy is by far the most common autonomic neuropathy encountered in clinical practice; diabetic gastroparesis is dealt with in detail by Koch and Calles-Escandón, elsewhere in this issue. Gastrointestinal involvement occurs to a variable extent in the many other types of autonomic peripheral neuropathies.[82] Upper gastrointestinal symptoms (early satiety, nausea and vomiting) are common in autoimmune autonomic neuropathies.[83]

Autonomic dysfunction is commonly detectable in Guillain-Barré syndrome (GBS) but is usually of minor clinical importance.[84] Delayed gastric emptying, gastroparesis, constipation, diarrhea, and fecal incontinence have all been described in GBS.[85] The gastrointestinal tract has a role in the pathogenesis of GBS; 15% to 40% of cases of GBS in the West have followed infection with *Campylobacter jejuni*.[86]

Muscle Disease

Myopathy and muscular dystrophy

Gastrointestinal involvement has been described in several muscular dystrophies,[87–90] but has been most extensively documented in myotonic dystrophy and Duchenne muscular dystrophy. Symptoms suggestive of gastroparesis, such as early satiety, nausea, vomiting, and epigastric pain, are common in myotonic dystrophy.[91,92] Of these, abdominal pain, dysphagia, vomiting, diarrhea, coughing while eating, and fecal incontinence were the most common in one survey[92]; up to 25% of patients consider gastrointestinal involvement as the most disabling feature of their disease.[93] Delayed gastric emptying and gastroparesis have indeed been well documented,[94–96] and instances of gastric volvulus described.[97] In Duchenne dystrophy, gastric motor dysfunction is an early feature,[98] resulting in hypomotility and gastroparesis,[99] which can be profound and result in acute gastroparesis and gastric dilatation.[100,101]

MANAGEMENT OF GASTROPARESIS IN PARKINSON DISEASE AND OTHER NEUROLOGIC DISORDERS

A multidisciplinary team (neurologist/neurosurgeon, gastroenterologist, nutritionist, therapist, specialist nurse), aware of the wishes and needs of the family and their carers, and mindful of the nature and the natural history of the underlying disease process, is best placed to assess and manage gastroparesis and other gastrointestinal problems in the patient with neurologic disease.

For the patient with PD and gastric emptying delay it is critical to avoid metoclopramide, in view of its central antidopaminergic effects; domperidone and mosapride, if available, may provide some potential therapeutic solutions. The main aim of pharmacologic therapy in correcting delayed gastric emptying in PD is primarily to reduce response fluctuations rather than deal with upper gastrointestinal symptoms. If pharmacologic approaches do not work, jejunal or transdermal delivery of L-dopa is an interesting option, although jejunal delivery may be technically challenging. The role of gastric electrical stimulation has not been defined in this population.

CONNECTIVE TISSUE DISORDERS

Gastroparesis and related symptoms may be prominent features of any disorder associated with autonomic neuropathy, and may also be components of both primary and secondary intestinal pseudo-obstruction syndromes. In scleroderma, one of the most common causes of pseudo-obstruction, gastroparesis is common, and gastric involvement tends to parallel that of the esophagus.[102] In the Olmstead County study, 10.8% of all cases of definite gastroparesis were associated with the presence of a connective tissue disorder.[2] In scleroderma, gastric involvement has been documented in anywhere from 10% to 75% of all patients and delayed gastric emptying in 50% to 75% of those with scleroderma who have gastrointestinal symptoms. Gastroparesis has important clinical consequences in scleroderma, including malnutrition and exacerbation of gastroesophageal reflux. The latter is of critical importance, given the predilection of these patients to severe and complicated reflux resulting from severe lower esophageal sphincter hypotension and markedly impaired esophageal peristaltic amplitude. Using the relatively noninvasive ^{13}C-octonoic acid breath test, Marie and colleagues[103] documented delayed gastric emptying in 47% of 57 consecutive scleroderma patients. Furthermore, they described a close correlation between a gastrointestinal symptom score and gastric emptying delay.[103]

Using the same approach, Hammar and colleagues[104] discovered gastroparesis in 29% of their 28 patients with primary Sjögren syndrome.

Most recently, a reported association between Ehlers-Danlos syndrome type III (the joint hypermobility syndrome) and a variety of functional gastrointestinal symptoms, including those that may be based on gastric emptying delay, has begun to emerge.[105–107] In some studies, gastroparesis has been documented.[105]

REFERENCES

1. Aderinto-Adike AO, Quigley EM. Gastrointestinal motility problems in critical care: a clinical perspective. J Dig Dis 2014;15:335–44.
2. Shafi MA, Pasricha PJ. Post-surgical and obstructive gastroparesis. Curr Gastroenterol Rep 2007;9:280–5.
3. Jung HK, Choung RS, Locke GR 3rd, et al. The incidence, prevalence, and outcomes of patients with gastroparesis in Olmsted County, Minnesota, from 1996 to 2006. Gastroenterology 2009;136:1225–33.
4. Dong K, Yu XJ, Li B, et al. Advances in mechanisms of postsurgical gastroparesis syndrome and its diagnosis and treatment. Chin J Dig Dis 2006;7:76–82.
5. Fich A, Neri M, Camilleri M, et al. Stasis syndromes following gastric surgery: clinical and motility features of sixty symptomatic patients. J Clin Gastroenterol 1990;12:505–12.
6. Chang TM, Chen TH, Tsou SS, et al. Differences in gastric emptying between highly selective vagotomy and posterior truncal vagotomy combined with anterior seromyotomy. J Gastrointest Surg 1999;3:533–6.
7. Forstner-Barthell AW, Murr MM, Nitecki S, et al. Near-total completion gastrectomy for severe postvagotomy gastric stasis: analysis of early and long-term results in 62 patients. J Gastrointest Surg 1999;3:15–21.
8. Akkermans LM, Hendrikse CA. Post-gastrectomy problems. Dig Liver Dis 2000; 32(Suppl 3):S263–4.
9. Le Blanc-Louvry I, Savoye G, Maillot C, et al. An impaired accommodation of the proximal stomach to a meal is associated with symptoms after distal gastrectomy. Am J Gastroenterol 2003;98:2642–7.
10. Meng H, Zhou D, Jiang X, et al. Incidence and risk factors for postsurgical gastroparesis syndrome after laparoscopic and open radical gastrectomy. World J Surg Oncol 2013;11:144.
11. Jiang X, Hiki N, Nunobe S, et al. Postoperative pancreatic fistula and the risk factors of laparoscopy-assisted distal gastrectomy for early gastric cancer. Ann Surg Oncol 2012;19:115–21.
12. Speicher JE, Thirlby RC, Burggraaf J, et al. Results of completion gastrectomies in 44 patients with postsurgical gastric atony. J Gastrointest Surg 2009;13: 874–80.
13. Mathias JR, Fernandez A, Sninsky CA, et al. Nausea, vomiting and abdominal pain after Roux-en-Y anastomosis: motility of the jejunal limb. Gastroenterology 1985;88:101–7.
14. Hinder RA, Esser MB, DeMeester TR. Management of gastric emptying disorders following the Roux-en-Y procedure. Surgery 1988;104:765–72.
15. Vantrappen G, Coremans G, Janssens J, et al. Inversion of the slow wave frequency gradient in symptomatic patients with Roux-en-Y anastomosis. Gastroenterology 1991;101:1282–8.
16. Miedema BW, Kelly KA, Camilleri M, et al. Human gastric and jejunal transit and motility after Roux gastrojejunostomy. Gastroenterology 1992;103:1133–43.

17. Fabre JM, Burgel JS, Navarro F, et al. Delayed gastric emptying after pancrea-ticoduodenectomy and pancreaticogastrostomy. Eur J Surg 1999;165:560–5.
18. Horstmann O, Becker H, Post S, et al. Is delayed gastric emptying following pancreaticoduodenectomy related to pylorus preservation? Langenbecks Arch Surg 1999;384:354–9.
19. Parmar AD, Sheffield KM, Vargas GM, et al. Factors associated with delayed gastric emptying after pancreaticoduodenectomy. HPB (Oxford) 2013;15:763–72.
20. Su AP, Cao SS, Zhang Y, et al. Does antecolic reconstruction for duodenojeju-nostomy improve delayed gastric emptying after pylorus-preserving pancreati-coduodenectomy? a systematic review and meta-analysis. World J Gastroenterol 2012;18:6315–23.
21. Shimoda M, Kubota K, Katoh M, et al. Effect of Billroth II or Roux-en-Y recon-struction for the gastrojejunostomy on delayed gastric emptying after pan-creaticoduodenectomy: a randomized controlled study. Ann Surg 2013;257:938–42.
22. Qu H, Sun GR, Zhou SQ, et al. Clinical risk factors of delayed gastric emptying in patients after pancreaticoduodenectomy: a systematic review and meta-anal-ysis. Eur J Surg Oncol 2013;39:213–23.
23. Ben-Youssef R, Baron PW, Franco E, et al. Intrapyloric injection of botulinum toxin a for the treatment of persistent gastroparesis following successful pancreas transplantation. Am J Transplant 2006;6:214–8.
24. Penagini R, Alloca M, Cantu P, et al. Relationship between motor function of the proximal stomach and transient lower oesophageal sphincter relaxation after morphine. Gut 2004;53:1227–31.
25. Vu MK, Straathof JW, van der Schaar PJ, et al. Motor and sensory function of the proximal stomach in reflux disease and after laparoscopic Nissen fundoplica-tion. Am J Gastroenterol 1999;94:1481–9.
26. Vu MK, Ringers J, Arndt JW, et al. Prospective study of the effect of laparo-scopic hemifundoplication on motor and sensory function of the proximal stom-ach. Br J Surg 2000;87:338–43.
27. Lindeboom MY, Vu MK, Ringers J, et al. Function of the proximal stomach after partial versus complete laparoscopic fundoplication. Am J Gastroenterol 2003;98:284–90.
28. Scheffer RC, Tatum RP, Shi G, et al. Reduced tLESR elicitation in response to gastric distention in fundoplication patients. Am J Physiol Gastrointest Liver Physiol 2003;284:G815–20.
29. Richards WO, Scholz S, Khaitan L, et al. Initial experience with the Stretta pro-cedure for the treatment of gastroespohageal reflux disease. J Laparoendosc Adv Surg Tech A 2001;11:267–73.
30. Sarosiek I, Yates KP, Abell PL, et al. Interpreting symptoms suggesting gastro-paresis in patients after gastric and esophageal surgeries. Gastroenterology 2011;140:S-813.
31. Richter JE. Gastroesophageal reflux disease treatment: side effects and compli-cations of fundoplication. Clin Gastroenterol Hepatol 2013;11:465–71.
32. Clark CJ, Sarr MG, Arora AS, et al. Does gastric resection have a role in the management of severe postfundoplication gastric dysfunction? World J Surg 2011;35:2045–50.
33. Masqusi S, Velanovich V. Pyloroplasty with fundoplication in the treatment of combined gastroesophageal reflux disease and bloating. World J Surg 2007;31:332–6.

34. Ardila-Hani A, Soffer EE. Review article: the impact of bariatric surgery on gastrointestinal motility. Aliment Pharmacol Ther 2011;34:825–31.

35. Salameh JR, Schmieg RE Jr, Runnels JM, et al. Refractory gastroparesis after Roux-en-Y gastric bypass: surgical treatment with implantable pacemaker. J Gastrointest Surg 2007;11:1669–72.

36. Reddymasu SC, Singh S, Sankula R, et al. Endoscopic pyloric injection of botulinum toxin-A for the treatment of postvagotomy gastroparesis. Am J Med Sci 2009;337:161–4.

37. Sutcliffe RP, Forshaw MJ, Tandon R, et al. Anastomotic strictures and delayed gastric emptying after esophagectomy: incidence, risk factors and management. Dis Esophagus 2008;21:712–7.

38. Radaelli F, Paggi S, Terreni N, et al. Acute reversible gastroparesis and megaduodenum after botulinum toxin injection for achalasia. Gastrointest Endosc 2010;71:1326–7.

39. Nafteux P, Moons J, Coosemans W, et al. Minimally invasive oesophagectomy: a valuable alternative to open oesophagectomy for the treatment of early oesophageal and gastro-oesophageal junction carcinoma. Eur J Cardiothorac Surg 2011;40:1455–63.

40. Raviv Y, D'Ovidio F, Pierre A, et al. Prevalence of gastroparesis before and after lung transplantation and its association with lung allograft outcomes. Clin Transplant 2012;26:133–42.

41. Paul S, Escareno CE, Clancy K, et al. Gastrointestinal complications after lung transplantation. J Heart Lung Transplant 2009;28:475–9.

42. Filichia LA, Baz MA, Cendan JC. Simultaneous fundoplication and gastric stimulation in a lung transplant recipient with gastroparesis and reflux. JSLS 2008; 12:303–5.

43. Vignolo MC, Savassi-Rocha PR, Coelho LG, et al. Gastric emptying before and after cholecystectomy in patients with cholecystolithiasis. Hepatogastroenterology 2008;55:850–4.

44. Parkman HP, Yates K, Hasler WL, et al. Cholecystectomy and clinical presentations of gastroparesis. Dig Dis Sci 2013;58:1062–73.

45. Schaller BJ, Graf R, Jacobs AH. Pathophysiological changes of the gastrointestinal tract in ischemic stroke. Am J Gastroenterol 2006;101:1655–65.

46. Quigley EM. Gastrointestinal dysfunction in Parkinson's disease. Semin Neurol 1996;16:245–50.

47. Jost WH. Gastrointestinal dysfunction in Parkinson's disease. J Neurol Sci 2010; 289:69–73.

48. Gallagher DA, Lees AJ, Schrag A. What are the most important nonmotor symptoms in patients with Parkinson's disease? Mov Disord 2010;25:2493–500.

49. Pfeiffer RF. Gastrointestinal dysfunction in Parkinson's disease. Parkinsonism Relat Disord 2011;17:10–5.

50. Lebouvier T, Chaumette T, Paillusson S, et al. The second brain and Parkinson's disease. Eur J Neurosci 2009;30:735–41.

51. Natale G, Pasquali L, Ruggieri S, et al. Parkinson's disease and the gut: a well known clinical association in need of an effective cure and explanation. Neurogastroenterol Motil 2008;20:741–9.

52. Singaram C, Ashraf W, Gaumnitz EA, et al. Depletion of dopaminergic neurons in the colon in Parkinson's disease. Lancet 1995;346:861–86.

53. Lebouvier T, Neunlist M, Bruley des Varannes S, et al. Colonic biopsies to assess the neuropathology of Parkinson's disease and its relationship with symptoms. PLoS One 2010;5:e12728.

54. Shannon KM, Keshavarzian A, Mutlu E, et al. Alpha-synuclein in colonic submu-cosa in early untreated Parkinson's disease. Mov Disord 2012;27:709–15.

55. Gold A, Turkalp ZT, Munoz DG. Enteric alpha-synuclein expression is increased in Parkinson's disease but not Alzheimer's disease. Mov Disord 2013;28: 237–40.

56. Edwards L, Pfeiffer RF, Quigley EM, et al. Incidence of gastrointestinal symp-toms in Parkinson's disease. Mov Disord 1991;6:151–6.

57. Colosimo C, Morgante L, Antonini A, et al, PRIAMO Study Group. Non-motor symptoms in atypical and secondary parkinsonism: the PRIAMO study. J Neurol 2010;257:5–14.

58. Antonini A, Barone P, Marconi R, et al. The progression of non-motor symptoms in Parkinson's disease and their contribution to motor disability and quality of life. J Neurol 2012;259:2621–31.

59. Marrinan S, Emmanuel AV, Burn DJ. Delayed gastric emptying in Parkinson's disease. Mov Disord 2014;29:23–32.

60. Heetun ZS, Quigley EM. Gastroparesis and Parkinson's disease: a systematic review. Parkinsonism Relat Disord 2012;18:433–40.

61. Djaldetti R, Baron J, Ziv I, et al. Gastric emptying in Parkinson's disease: patients with and without response fluctuations. Neurology 1996;46:1051–4.

62. Hardoff R, Sula M, Tamir A, et al. Gastric emptying time and gastric motility in patients with Parkinson's disease. Mov Disord 2001;16:1041–7.

63. Goetze O, Wieczorek J, Mueller T, et al. Impaired gastric emptying of a solid test meal in patients with Parkinson's disease using ^{13}C-sodium octanoate breath test. Neurosci Lett 2005;375:170–3.

64. Thomaides T, Karapanaayiotides T, Zoukos Y, et al. Gastric emptying after semi-solid food in multiple system atrophy and Parkinson disease. J Neurol 2005;25:1055–9.

65. Goetze O, Nikodem AB, Wiezcorek J, et al. Predictors of gastric emptying in Parkinson's disease. Neurogastroenterol Motil 2006;18:369–75.

66. Nyholm D, Lennernas H. Irregular gastrointestinal drug absorption in Parkinson's disease. Expert Opin Drug Metab Toxicol 2008;4:193–203.

67. Eggert K, Schrader C, Hahn M, et al. Continuous jejunal levodopa infusion in patients with advanced Parkinson disease: practical aspects and outcome of motor and non-motor complications. Clin Neuropharmacol 2008;31:151–66.

68. Steiger M. Constant dopaminergic stimulation by transdermal delivery of dopa-minergic drugs: a new treatment paradigm in Parkinson's disease. Eur J Neurol 2008;15:6–15.

69. Kashihara K. Weight loss in Parkinson's disease. J Neurol 2006;253(Suppl 7): VII38–41.

70. Naftali T, Gadoth N, Huberman M, et al. Electrogastrography in patients with Parkinson's disease. Can J Neurol Sci 2005;32:82–6.

71. Chen CL, Lin HH, Chen SY, et al. Utility of electrogastrography in differentiating Parkinson's disease with or without gastrointestinal symptoms: a prospective controlled study. Digestion 2005;71:187–91.

72. Dobbs RJ, Dobbs SM, Weller C, et al. Role of chronic infection and inflam-mation in the gastrointestinal tract in the etiology and pathogenesis of idio-pathic parkinsonism. Part 1: eradication of *Helicobacter* in the cachexia of idiopathic parkinsonism. Helicobacter 2005;10:267–75.

73. Bjarnason IT, Charlett A, Dobbs RJ, et al. Role of chronic infection and inflam-mation in the gastrointestinal tract in the etiology and pathogenesis of idiopathic parkinsonism. Part 2: response of facets of clinical idiopathic parkinsonism

to *Helicobacter pylori* eradication. A randomized, double-blind, placebo-controlled efficacy study. Helicobacter 2005;10:276–87.

74. Weller C, Charlett A, Oxlade NL, et al. Role of chronic infection and inflammation in the gastrointestinal tract in the etiology and pathogenesis of idiopathic parkinsonism. Part 3: predicted probability and gradients of severity of idiopathic parkinsonism based *H. pylori* antibody profile. Helicobacter 2005;10:288–97.

75. El-Maghraby TA, Shalaby NM, Al-Tawdy MH, et al. Gastric motility dysfunction in patients with multiple sclerosis assessed by gastric emptying scintigraphy. Can J Gastroenterol 2005;19:141–5.

76. Gupta YK. Gastroparesis with multiple sclerosis. JAMA 1984;252:42.

77. Read SJ, Leggett BA, Pender MP. Gastroparesis with multiple sclerosis. Lancet 1995;346:1228.

78. Raghav S, Kipp D, Watson J, et al. Gastroparesis in multiple sclerosis. Mult Scler 2006;12:243–4.

79. Reddymasu SC, Bonino J, McCallum RW. Gastroparesis secondary to a demyelinating disease: a case series. BMC Gastroenterol 2007;7:3.

80. Ben-Zvi JS, Daniel SJ. Painless gastric perforation in a patient with multiple sclerosis. Am J Gastroenterol 1988;83:1008–11.

81. Haensch CA, Jorg J. Autonomic dysfunction in multiple sclerosis. J Neurol 2006; 253(Suppl 1):I3–9.

82. Freeman R. Autonomic peripheral neuropathy. Lancet 2005;365:1259–70.

83. Klein CM, Vernino S, Lennon VA, et al. The spectrum of autoimmune autonomic neuropathies. Ann Neurol 2003;53:752–8.

84. Van Doorn PA, Ruts L, Jacobs BC. Clinical features, pathogenesis, and treatment of Guillain-Barré syndrome. Lancet Neurol 2008;7:939–50.

85. McDougall AJ, McLeod JG. Autonomic neuropathy, I. Clinical features, investigation, pathophysiology, and treatment. J Neurol Sci 1996;137:79–88.

86. Sivadon-Tardy V, Orlokowski D, Rozenberg F, et al. Guillain-Barré syndrome, greater Paris area. Emerg Infect Dis 2006;12:990–3.

87. Simpson AJ, Khilnani MT. Gastrointestinal manifestations of the muscular dystrophies. Am J Roentgenol Radium Ther Nucl Med 1975;125:948–55.

88. Nowak TV, Ionasescu V, Anuras S. Gastrointestinal manifestations of the muscular dystrophies. Gastroenterology 1982;82:800–10.

89. Karasick D, Karasick S, Mapp E. Gastrointestinal radiologic manifestations of proximal spinal muscular atrophy (Kugelberg-Welander syndrome). J Natl Med Assoc 1982;74:475–8.

90. Staiano A, Del Giudice E, Romano A, et al. Upper gastrointestinal tract motility in children with progressive muscular dystrophy. J Pediatr 1992;121:720–4.

91. Bellini M, Biagi S, Stasi S, et al. Gastrointestinal manifestations in myotonic muscular dystrophy. World J Gastroenterol 2006;12:1821–8.

92. Ronnblom A, Forsberg H, Danielsson A. Gastrointestinal symptoms in myotonic dystrophy. Scand J Gastroenterol 1996;31:654–7.

93. Tieleman AA, van Vliet J, Jansen JB, et al. Gastrointestinal involvement is frequent in myotonic dystrophy type 2. Neuromuscul Disord 2008;18:646–9.

94. Bellini M, Alduini P, Costa F, et al. Gastric emptying in myotonic dystrophy patients. Dig Liver Dis 2002;34:484–8.

95. Ronnblom A, Andersson S, Hellstrom PM, et al. Gastric emptying in myotonic dystrophy. Eur J Clin Invest 2002;32:570–4.

96. Horowitz M, Maddox A, Maddern GJ, et al. Gastric and esophageal emptying in dystrophia myotonica. Effect of metoclopramide. Gastroenterology 1987;92:570–7.

97. Kusunoki M, Hatada T, Ikeuchi H, et al. Gastric volvulus complicating myotonic dystrophy. Hepatogastroenterology 1992;39:586–8.
98. Borrelli O, Salvia G, Mancini V, et al. Evolution of gastric electrical features and gastric emptying in children with Duchenne and Becker muscular dystrophy. Am J Gastroenterol 2005;100:695–702.
99. Barohn RJ, Levine EJ, Olson JO, et al. Gastric hypomotility in Duchenne's muscular dystrophy. N Engl J Med 1988;319:15–8.
100. Bensen ES, Jaffe KM, Tarr PI. Acute gastric dilatation in Duchenne muscular dystrophy: a case report and review of the literature. Arch Phys Med Rehabil 1996;77:512–4.
101. Chung BC, Park HJ, Yoon SB, et al. Acute gastroparesis in Duchenne's muscular dystrophy. Yonsei Med J 1998;39:175–9.
102. Marie I, Levesque H, Ducrotté P, et al. Gastric involvement in systemic sclerosis: a prospective study. Am J Gastroenterol 2001;96:77–83.
103. Marie I, Gourcerol G, Leroi AM, et al. Delayed gastric emptying determined using the 13C-octanoic acid breath test in patients with systemic sclerosis. Arthritis Rheum 2012;64:2346–55.
104. Hammar O, Ohlsson B, Wollmer P, et al. Impaired gastric emptying in primary Sjögren's syndrome. J Rheumatol 2010;37:2313–8.
105. Zarate N, Farmer AD, Grahame R, et al. Unexplained gastrointestinal symptoms and joint hypermobility: is connective tissue the missing link? Neurogastroenterol Motil 2010;22:252–252.e78.
106. Fikree A, Grahame R, Aktar R, et al. A prospective evaluation of undiagnosed joint hypermobility syndrome in patients with gastrointestinal symptoms. Clin Gastroenterol Hepatol 2014;12:1680–7.
107. Kovacic K, Chelimsky TC, Sood MR, et al. Joint hypermobility: a common association with complex functional gastrointestinal disorders. J Pediatr 2014; 165:973–8.

Nutritional Considerations in the Patient with Gastroparesis

Carol Rees Parrish, MS, RD

KEYWORDS

• Diet • Nutrition • Nutritional assessment • Enteral • Nutritional support

KEY POINTS

- Patients with gastroparesis (GP) are at high risk for nutritional compromise, not only because of chronic nausea and vomiting, which can result in poor intake, but also because of potential anatomic changes such as gastric resection or bypass.
- Target weight should be set for patient and intervention provided before a patient becomes severely malnourished.
- Use of parenteral nutrition (PN) should be reserved only for those patients who fail enteral feedings.

INTRODUCTION

A 57-year-old woman presents to the gastrointestinal (GI) clinic with myositis, poorly controlled diabetes mellitus (DM), nausea, vomiting, dehydration, and a 10-lb (4.5-kg) unintentional weight loss. GP is confirmed by gastric emptying study. Oral diet modification failed with continued nausea, vomiting, further weight loss, and aggravated glycemic control due to steroid therapy. On her third admission and a weight loss of 30 lb (210 to 180 lb [95.3 to 81.6 kg]), the decision was made to place a percutaneous endoscopic gastrostomy (PEG) with a jejunal extension (PEG/J) for enteral nutrition (EN), hydration, and medication delivery. Feedings went well initially in the hospital, but the patient continued to eat and drink after discharge when she felt better, resulting in 2 more admissions due to failed therapy and poor glycemic control. In an effort to give her some relief and keep her hospital free, the patient was strongly encouraged to stop eating and drinking anything other than a few ice chips, and she was miserable enough that she agreed. Tube feeding goals were met nocturnally, glycemic control improved, and she was discharged without readmission. She then followed up in GI nutrition clinic to ensure nutritional goals continued to be met.

Department of Nutrition Services, University of Virginia Health System, PO Box 800673, Charlottesville, VA 22908-0673, USA
E-mail address: crp3a@virginia.edu

Gastroenterol Clin N Am 44 (2015) 83–95
http://dx.doi.org/10.1016/j.gtc.2014.11.007
0889-8553/15/$ – see front matter © 2015 Elsevier Inc. All rights reserved.

gastro.theclinics.com

Gastroparesis

GP, defined as delayed gastric emptying for greater than 3 months, is documented by a delayed gastric emptying study in a patient devoid of mechanical or functional obstruction, can be profoundly incapacitating. This debilitating process alters one's ability to work, attend school, or carry out other normal daily activities. GP can affect the patient's emotional, mental, and social well-being, as well as the body's ability to function normally; basically, it compromises life.[1] Eating becomes a chore and is not pleasurable, and as a result, weight loss and compromised nutritional status are common in moderate to severe cases. Furthermore, in those with DM, glycemic control can become difficult.[2] The following outlines a practical approach to nutritional care of the patient with GP from nutritional assessment and oral dietary intervention to, finally, nutritional support.

NUTRITIONAL ASSESSMENT

Initial and ongoing nutritional assessment and intervention are critical aspects of care of the patient with GP.[3,4] Thorough assessment distinguishes those patients who need simple dietary changes from those who are so malnourished that nutritional support is justified. For example, a patient who develops nausea while eating the usual 3 large meals per day may not require supplemental calories, but rather smaller, more frequent meals. In contrast, the patient with severe GP who has significant vomiting after intake of clear liquids may require gastric decompression and jejunal feeding to provide not only nutrients, fluids, and medications but also symptom relief.

Unintentional Weight Loss

Unintentional weight loss over time is one of the most basic yet undeniable indicators that a patient's nutritional status is in trouble.[5] Comparing a current weight (once the patient has been rehydrated) with the patient's usual weight and documenting the percentage of total weight loss over time can stratify the degree of nutritional risk and help guide therapy. Use of an ideal body weight instead of a patient's actual weight is not recommended, as it may overestimate or underestimate the degree of nutritional risk.

Glycemic Control

In patients with DM, it is often difficult to sort out which came first, poor glucose control or GP. Regardless, good glycemic control (especially any wide swings in glucose control) is necessary for improving gastric emptying, nutrient utilization, and preventing catabolism.[6] In addition, out-of-control DM may be the primary reason the patient is losing weight. Glycemic control can be monitored by patient glycemic records and periodic measurement of glycosylated hemoglobin (HbA1C) level.

Bowel Habits

Constipation can worsen the symptoms of GP, and chronic constipation may be a sign of a more generalized intestinal dysmotility.[7] When practitioners justifiably pay so much attention to the upper gut in patients with chronic nausea and vomiting, they sometimes tend to overlook the lower tract; in fact, this author's experience is that while the gastroenterologist focuses on the GP, the primary care physician is taking care of the bowels, and sometimes their interventions are at odds with one another. For example, the addition of fiber bulking agents to help with constipation only exacerbates delayed gastric emptying. Identifying normal bowel habits is also important, particularly with inpatients who are on bed rest and perhaps pain medications, because during a hospitalization, physicians often prescribe nightly docusate to the patient who normally uses Miralax (polyethylene glycol 3350) twice a day at home.

NUTRITIONAL INTERVENTION—ORAL DIET

Prospective controlled trials regarding dietary contributions in this patient population are near nonexistent; hence, diet therapy has been devised based on known emptying characteristics of protein, fat, and carbohydrate and emptying of liquid foods versus solids.[6,8] Other than 2 small studies evaluating large versus small food particle size and symptom response in patients with insulin-treated DM, single-meal trials in heterogeneous populations with GP or normal volunteers and patient surveys are all that has been published to date.[8,9] Diet therapy and nutritional supplementation therefore must be individualized, taking into consideration the underlying cause of the GP such as postsurgical process versus underlying chronic disease course. See Appendix 1 for one institution's sample diet for GP (more complete and other versions available at www.ginutrition.virginia.edu under patient education materials).

Smaller, More Frequent Meals

The larger the volume of food ingested, the slower the emptying, and both caloric density and bulk (fiber) contribute to this.[10] Early satiety is a frequent complaint; hence, smaller amounts of food at frequent intervals during the day is the first nutritional intervention that should be implemented. Six or more small meals/snacks during the course of the day may be needed for patients to take in enough food to meet their nutritional needs.

Fat

Physiologically, it is well known that fat slows gastric emptying, and patients with GP are therefore often advised to restrict fat in their diet. However, eliminating fat also removes a significant calorie source and requires patients to eat larger volumes of food if they are to meet nutrient needs and stop weight loss. It may be that solid foods high in fat are the culprit; clinically, this author has found that fat-containing liquids are often well tolerated and can be a valuable source of nutrition for the patient with GP.

Decreasing Fiber

High-fiber foods and stool-bulking agents delay gastric emptying, leading to early satiety and symptom exacerbation in those with GP. Some patients may even present with a gastric bezoar as the first indication that they have GP. Small-bowel bacterial overgrowth (SBBO) is a known risk factor in those with dysmotility disorders, and frequent use of proton pump inhibitors, which is not uncommon in this population, further aggravates the problem. Consuming a high-fiber diet, or using a fiber-containing tube feeding formula in those requiring enteral nutritional support, can intensify abdominal distension, gas, bloating, reflux, and diarrhea. For those patients who have formed a bezoar, fiber avoidance is especially important.[11]

Another dietary intervention under investigation in dysmotility disorders is the avoidance of FODMAPs, or fermentable oligo-di-monosaccharides and polyols.[12,13] FODMAPs are highly fermentable by gut bacteria, as well as highly osmotic, and they too can further accentuate symptoms in those with GP. They are not only found in certain foods but are also added to some enteral formulas (fructooligosaccharides [FOS] are one of them) in addition to many liquid medications for flavorings, including sugar alcohols such as sorbitol and xylitol.[14] Their effect can be additive, so that a patient on enteral feedings with a fiber-containing formula and liquid medications may seem intolerant to the tube feeding, when in fact the problem is purely the FODMAP/fiber load they are receiving.[15]

Liquids Versus Solids

As liquid emptying is usually preserved in patients with GP, transitioning to more liquid calories in the diet may help patients meet their nutritional needs, especially during exacerbations. It may help in some patients to have them start the day with some solid food but then consume more liquid-type meals as the day progresses and the feeling of fullness increases. As mentioned earlier, fat-containing nutritional drinks are often well tolerated.

Particle Size

In the normal setting, a major function of the stomach is to grind food into smaller particles (trituration) initiating digestion. This function may be impaired or lost in the patient with GP, so a focus on chewing foods well may help to compensate and aid in this process to improve emptying. Two small studies[9,16] have demonstrated symptom improvement when ground foods versus solid food meals were provided. It should be noted that with good dentition, grinding food before ingesting would seem unnecessary, yet good dental care can be difficult for these patients. Not only can frequent vomiting alter enamel and weaken teeth but also when just getting off the couch is a chore, it can be hard enough just to make it to physician appointments and easy to delay dental treatment. Although pureed foods have not been studied, if grinding food into smaller particles has been shown to decrease symptoms, pureeing food may be an option for patients having difficulty tolerating even ground foods. With a good blender, anything can be pulverized if adequate liquid is added.

Patient Positioning

Positioning or use of gravity may also play a role in helping patients tolerate an oral diet. If turning on one's right side is necessary to undergo a barium swallow, then patients may get some relief by sitting upright for 1 to 2 hours after a meal or by even going for a gentle walk.

SPECIAL CONSIDERATION—VITAMINS AND MINERALS

Patients who have had prolonged nausea and vomiting leading to poor nutritional intake are at risk for multiple nutrient deficiencies. In a large multicenter study evaluating food frequency questionnaires, patients with GP from idiopathic or DM cause were found to have diets deficient in calories and numerous vitamins and minerals.[17] When eating nearly ceases, taking vitamins and minerals generally does too. Patients with GP due to a previous gastric surgery are at even greater risk for nutrient deficiencies because of anatomic changes and alterations in nutrient utilization.[18] For example, patients with a subtotal gastrectomy are more at risk for iron and vitamins B_{12}, D, and E deficiencies; gastric bypass surgery, a procedure that creates malabsorption, significantly increases the risk for an even wider range of nutrient deficiencies.[19] See **Box 1** for those nutrients that may warrant particular attention, although any patient with significant and unintentional weight loss is at risk for pan-nutrient deficiencies.

It may be prudent to provide supplements to patients with malnutrition or known poor nutritional intake with a therapeutic vitamin and mineral supplement for an empiric length of time ($\sim$4 weeks) until they are eating normally again, or, if requiring enteral feedings, until goal delivery rate is achieved. Chewable or liquid supplements may be better tolerated in some than the tablet form; for others, a smaller dose (such as one-half tablet, twice a day) may work better; remember, any is better than none in

---

Box 1
Nutrients that may warrant particular attention in the patient with gastroparesis

- Vitamin D (25-OH vitamin D)

- Serum vitamin B_{12}/methylmalonic acid (methylmalonic acid in those at high risk for small bowel bacterial overgrowth (SBBO), as vitamin B_{12} can be converted to biologically inactive form in the gut before absorption)

- Iron/ferritin (in non–acute phase setting)

- Folate: elevated serum folate level may be suggestive (but not diagnostic) of SBBO in patients with a dysmotility disorder. Bacteria in the small bowel synthesize folate, which is then absorbed into the bloodstream, resulting in elevated serum levels.[20]

- Vitamin E (gastric resection 2 years post-op)

- Thiamine: gastric bypass or others with vomiting greater than 3 weeks[19]

From University of Virginia Health System, Nutrition Support Traineeship Syllabus. Charlottesville (VA): University of Virginia; 2013; with permission.

---

those who need it. Avoid giving multiple, individual supplements, as this not only gets costly but is also time consuming and compliance may decrease.

NUTRITIONAL SUPPORT

Patients unable to maintain a healthy weight despite oral diet modifications are candidates for specialized nutritional support. A defined target weight should be set with the patient; if a patient is unable to achieve this or drops below this weight, nutritional support should be initiated. Indications for enteral access and nutritional support include the following[3]:

- Unintentional weight loss of greater than 5% to 10% over 3 to 6 months
- Inability to meet weight goals
- Weight falls to less than what was agreed on by patient and physician as time for intervention
- Need for gastric decompression
- Frequent hospitalizations, with or without weight loss
  - Dehydration
  - Diabetic ketoacidosis
  - Refractory nausea/vomiting
  - Requiring access for consistent delivery of medications, hydration, and nutrition
- Overall quality of life is unsustainable or plain failure to thrive

Enteral Nutrition

In patients who cannot consistently meet their nutritional requirements or regain the much needed lost weight, EN support is recommended. EN is associated with fewer infections and complications, is less expensive, and is less labor intensive for nursing staff and caregivers compared with PN. The selection of the best enteral access device varies between health care institutions and continues to be a source of debate owing to the lack of prospective trials evaluating the various approaches. Vented and nonvented options are available. For those with uncontrolled vomiting, a venting port indicates that there is a separate gastric port to drain off gastric secretions in an effort to give the patient relief from ongoing vomiting,[21] although careful monitoring is needed if this route is chosen because of the potential risk for hypochloremic metabolic alkalosis.[22] Nonvented tubes do not offer such an option. See **Box 2** for enteral access options. A more in-depth discussion on various enteral access techniques is available elsewhere.[3,6] Regardless of the type of access chosen, jejunal feeding has been shown to improve symptoms, glycemic control and reduce the need for hospitalization.[23–25]

The enteral feeding regimen

A standard, polymeric formula should be well tolerated by the vast majority of patients. Although a significant number of those with GP have DM, specialized formulas for those with DM have not demonstrated an outcome benefit to date, are considerably more expensive, and contain fiber as well as FOS, a FODMAP.[15,26] Fiber-containing formulas may cause abdominal discomfort in patients with GP and intestinal dysmotility (see section on fiber in the oral diet section earlier in the discussion). To avoid blaming unsuccessful enteral feeding on what might be exacerbation of SBBO due to fiber and FODMAP formulas, a nonfiber, non-FOS formula is recommended at the initiation of enteral feeding. Once a patient is well established and tolerating the regimen, different formulas can be trialed if desired.

To prevent clouding the issue of enteral tolerance versus persistent oral food intolerance, a strict period of withholding oral food should be enlisted for at least 48 hours during EN initiation or until the patient is clearly tolerating EN well. This method avoids blaming persistent symptoms of GP on enteral feeding intolerance, when it is the oral intake that is responsible. If a patient is to be cycled to either nocturnal or daytime feedings, this should be initiated at the outset, especially in those with insulin-dependent DM. Otherwise, the whole process of achieving glycemic control has to be undertaken twice: first on continuous feeding, then again when changing the patient to nocturnal feeding, resulting in a delay in discharge. Discharging a patient home on continuous EN, unless absolutely necessary, should be avoided. Continuous EN does not allow freedom from the pump or the return of a patient's quality of life. In those having to remain on continuous EN, an enteral backpack should be obtained for the patient before discharge; if the home care company says they do not have them, then another home care company should be chosen for the patient. For patients who require insulin and are going to be put on nocturnal EN delivery, blood glucose monitoring and short-acting insulin coverage should be done every 4 hours during EN infusion for the first 48 hours or until longer-acting insulin needs can be determined to maximize glycemic control. This procedure ensures nutrient repletion and also prevents further alteration to gastric emptying due to poor control. More in-depth discussion and trouble-shooting enteral feeding tolerance is available elsewhere.[3,8]

Parenteral Nutrition

The use of PN should be the exception in the patient with GP unless the patient suffers from a dysmotility that extends beyond the stomach into the small bowel or colon or has a pandysmotility disorder such as chronic intestinal pseudo-obstruction. In those patients with significant malnutrition, peripheral PN may be used short term as a bridge until enteral access is achieved, although some might argue that dextrose added to standing intravenous fluids can be an effective way to initiate the refeeding process. Transition to EN should be pursued when clinically feasible.

SUMMARY

GP potentially compromises not only one's nutritional status but also all aspects of life. Nutritional assessment and timely nutritional support are an important aspect of care in this patient population. Good glycemic control not only is essential for maximizing

Box 2
Enteral access options: short term and long term

Nonvented Tubes

- Gastric tube or percutaneous endoscopic gastrostomy (PEG): typically not done in a patient with severe GP given the delayed gastric emptying. In milder cases, because liquids empty differently than solids, gastric delivery may be acceptable.

- Nasogastric, nasoduodenal, or nasojejunal: tends to migrate back into stomach with persistent vomiting; not a long-term option.

- Direct percutaneous endoscopic jejunostomy: difficult to place; not commonly placed in most institutions.

- Surgical or laparoscopic jejunal tube: common to many facilities.

- Interventional radiologically (IR) placed: largest tube that can be placed is an 18F catheter; unless facility has investigated and chosen specific tubes meant for long term, many tubes placed are not meant to be used long term or be exposed to gastric acid for long. In addition, many IR departments may place feeding tubes but have nothing set up to prepare the patient for home in terms of teaching the patient how to care for the tube, how to use the tube for enteral feeding, equipment and formula needed, as well as set the patient up with home care; all of this is left up to the referring physician, and if the referring physician is not aware he/she needs to do this, the patient suffers in the mayhem that follows (this author has seen this happen numerous times at outside facilities).

Vented Tubes

- Separate G and J tubes: gastric venting may be improved as there is no internal J tube taking up lumen space within the larger tube to impair venting; 2 separate tube sites to care for, with potential infection and leakage issues, not to mention the cosmetic aspects.

- PEG with a jejunal extension (often called Jet-PEG): abdominal placement is important; author's experience, to the right of the spine, lower antrum (not too close to the pylorus), facing the pylorus, easier to place j-arm with less stomach to traverse, hence less "play" on the j-arm by movement of spine, decreasing migration of j-arm back into the stomach. Smaller j-arms are more prone to clogging; advise 12F j-arm with goal to put feeding ports past ligament of Treitz. Education about medications via j-arm is crucial. If j-arm clogs, gets kinked, cannot be repaired, then patient only needs a new j-arm.

- Long-term G-J tubes: one tube that has a gastric tube housing a smaller tube within. The outer gastric tube is smaller, hence the internal jejunal tube is too. These tubes may not vent as well and clog more often as a result. Tube failure means the tube needs replacing.

- Nasogastric-jejunal tube: these tubes are meant to be used short term; because the larger gastric tube needs to handle gastric decompression, it is made of harder plastic, and therefore comfort is an issue for patients. The jejunal tube within is also of small diameter (8–10F), hence the clog potential as well as kinking is high. Placement of these tubes often requires fluoroscopy, unless the endoscopist is experienced, as these tubes often come back up into the proximal small bowel or stomach when the endoscope is removed.

  o Examples include the following:

    ▪ Dobbhoff Naso-Jejunal Feeding and Gastric Decompression Tube, Covidien (Mansfield, MA) (16F)

      • www.kendallpatientcare.com/pageBuilder.aspx?webPageID=0&topicID=72623& xsl=xsl/productPagePrint.xsl

    ▪ Compat Stay-Put Nasojejunal Feeding Tube, Nestle (Nestle HealthCare Nutrition, Inc., Florham Park, NJ)

      • www.nestlehealthscience.us/products/compat-stay-put%E2%84%A2-nasojejunal-feeding-tube

- ■ Jejunal Feeding/Gastric Decompression Tube, Bard (Bard Access Systems, Inc., Salt Lake City, UT)
  - • www.bardaccess.com/feed-jejunal.php
- ■ Silicone Gastro-Duodenal Levin Tube, Vygon (Vygon Sa, Lansdale, PA), Alibaba, 3T-Medical
  - • www.hellotrade.com/vygon-sa/silicone-gastro-duodenal-tube.html

From University of Virginia Health System, Nutrition Support Traineeship Syllabus; Charlottesville, VA; 2013; with permission.

nutrient utilization in those with DM but is also critical for removing delayed gastric emptying from hyperglycemia. Nutritional intervention can decrease symptoms, replenish nutrient stores, reduced hospitalizations, and improve an individual's overall quality of life. See **Box 3** for further resources.

Box 3
Resources for physicians and for patients with gastroparesis

- • University of Virginia Health System, GI Nutrition Web site www.ginutrition.virginia.edu links to
  - ○ Patient education materials
    - ■ Several diets for gastroparesis and low FODMAPs
      - • Short version
      - • Long version
      - • Renal
      - • Diabetes
      - • Low FODMAP
  - ○ Nutrition Articles in Practical Gastroenterology
    - ■ Parrish CR, McCray S. Gastroparesis & nutrition: the art. Pract Gastroenterol 2011;XXXV(9):26.
    - ■ Parrish CR, Yoshida C. Nutrition intervention for the patient with gastroparesis: an update. Pract Gastroenterol 2005;XXIX(8):29.
- • Association of Gastrointestinal Motility Disorders, Inc
  - www.agmd-gimotility.org
- • Cyclic Vomiting Association
  - www.cvsaonline.org/
- • International Foundation for Functional Gastrointestinal Disorders
  - www.iffgd.org/
- • Gastroparesis Dysmotility Association
  - www.digestivedistress.com

REFERENCES

1. Camilleri M, Bharucha AE, Farrugia G. Epidemiology, mechanisms, and management of diabetic gastroparesis. Clin Gastroenterol Hepatol 2011;9(1):5–12.
2. Uppalapati SS, Ramzan Z, Fisher RS, et al. Factors contributing to hospitalization for gastroparesis exacerbations. Dig Dis Sci 2009;54:2404–9.
3. Parrish CR, Yoshida C. Nutrition intervention for the patient with gastroparesis: an update. Pract Gastroenterol 2005;XXIX(8):29. Available at: www.ginutrition.virginia.edu.
4. Abell TL, Bernstein RK, Cutts T, et al. Treatment of gastroparesis: a multidisciplinary clinical review. Neurogastroenterol Motil 2006;18:263–83.
5. Jensen GL, Hsiao PY, Wheeler D. Nutrition screening and assessment. In: Mueller CM, editor. The A.S.P.E.N. adult nutrition support core curriculum. 2nd edition. Silver Spring (MD): American Society for Parenteral and Enteral Nutrition; 2012. p. 155–69.
6. Camilleri M, Parkman HP, Shafi MA, et al. Clinical guideline: management of gastroparesis. Am J Gastroenterol 2013;108(1):18–37.
7. Schiller LR. Nutrients and constipation: cause or cure? Pract Gastroenterol 2008; XXXII(4):43. Available at: www.ginutrition.virginia.edu.
8. Parrish CR, McCray S. Gastroparesis & nutrition: the art. Pract Gastroenterol 2011;XXXV(9):26. Available at: www.ginutrition.virginia.edu.
9. Olausson EA, Störsrud S, Grundin H, et al. A small particle size diet reduces upper gastrointestinal symptoms in patients with diabetic gastroparesis: a randomized controlled trial. Am J Gastroenterol 2014;109(3):375–85.
10. Camilleri M. Integrated upper gastrointestinal response to food intake. Gastroenterology 2006;131:640–58.
11. Sanders MK. Bezoars: from mystical charms to medical and nutritional management. Pract Gastroenterol 2004;XXVIII(1):37. Available at: www.ginutrition.virginia.edu.
12. Barrett JS. Extending our knowledge of fermentable, short-chain carbohydrates for managing gastrointestinal symptoms. Nutr Clin Pract 2013;28(3):300–6.
13. Gibson PR, Shepherd SJ. Evidence-based dietary management of functional gastrointestinal symptoms: the FODMAP approach. J Gastroenterol Hepatol 2010;25(2):252–8.
14. Wolever TM, Piekarz A, Hollads M, et al. Sugar alcohols and diabetes: a review. Can J Diabetes 2002;26(4):356–62.
15. Halmos EP. Role of FODMAP content in enteral nutrition-associated diarrhea. J Gastroenterol Hepatol 2013;28(Suppl 4):25–8.
16. Olausson EA, Alpsten M, Larsson A, et al. Small particle size of a solid meal increases gastric emptying and late postprandial glycaemic response in diabetic subjects with gastroparesis. Diabetes Res Clin Pract 2008;80:231–7.
17. Parkman HP, Yates KP, Hasler WL, et al. Dietary intake and nutritional deficiencies in patients with diabetic or idiopathic gastroparesis. Gastroenterology 2011; 141(2):486–98.
18. Radigan A. Post-gastrectomy: Managing the nutrition fall-out. Pract Gastroenterol 2004;XXVIII(6):63. Available at: www.ginutrition.virginia.edu.
19. O'Donnell K. Severe micronutrient deficiencies in RYGB patients: rare but potentially devastating. Pract Gastroenterol 2011;XXXV(11):13. Available at: www.ginutrition.virginia.edu.
20. Hoffbrand AV, Tabaqchali S, Mollin DL, et al. High serum folate levels in intestinal blind-loop syndrome. Lancet 1966;1(7451):1339–42.

21. Kim CH, Nelson DK. Venting percutaneous gastrostomy in the treatment of refractory idiopathic gastroparesis. Gastrointest Endosc 1998;47:67–70.
22. Parrish CR, Quatrara B. Reinfusion of intestinal secretions: a viable option for select patients. Pract Gastroenterol 2010;XXXIV(4):26. Available at: www.ginutrition.virginia.edu.
23. Fontana RJ, Barnett JL. Jejunostomy tube placement in refractory diabetic gastroparesis: a retrospective review. Am J Gastroenterol 1996;91(10):2174–8.
24. Maple JT, Petersen BT, Baron TH, et al. Direct percutaneous endoscopic jejunostomy: outcomes in 307 consecutive attempts. Am J Gastroenterol 2005;100(12):2681–8.
25. Parkman HP, Hasler WL, Fisher RS. American Gastroenterological Association technical review on the diagnosis and treatment of gastroparesis. Gastroenterology 2004;127:1592–622.
26. Hise ME, Fuhrman MP. The effect of diabetic-specific formulae on clinical and glycemic indicators. Pract Gastroenterol 2009;XXXIII(5):20–36. Available at: www.ginutrition.virginia.edu.

APPENDIX 1: GASTROPARESIS DIET TIPS
Introduction

Gastroparesis means stomach (*gastro*) paralysis (*paresis*). In gastroparesis, the stomach empties too slowly. Gastroparesis can have many causes, so symptoms range from mild (but annoying) to severe and week-to-week or even day-to-day.

This handout is designed to give some suggestions for diet changes in the hope that symptoms will improve or even stop. Very few research studies have been done to guide one as to which foods are better tolerated by patients with gastroparesis. The suggestions are mostly based on experience and the understanding of how the stomach and different foods normally empty. Anyone with gastroparesis should see a doctor and a Registered Dietitian for advice on how to maximize their nutritional status.

The Basics

Volume
The larger the meal, the slower the stomach empties. It is important to decrease the amount of food eaten at a meal, so one has to eat more often. Smaller meals more often (6–8 or more if needed) may allow one to eat enough.

Liquids versus Solids
If decreasing the meal size and increasing the number of meals does not work, the next step is to switch to more liquid-type foods. Liquids empty the stomach more easily than solids do. Pureed foods may also be better.

Fiber
Fiber (found in many fruits, vegetables, and grains) may slow stomach emptying and fill the stomach up too fast; this does not leave room for foods that may be easier tolerated. A *bezoar* is a mixture of food fibers that may get stuck in the stomach and not empty well, like a hairball in a cat. For patients who have had a bezoar, fiber restriction is important. This restriction includes avoiding over-the-counter fiber/bulking medicines like Metamucil (psyllium husk) and others.

Fat
Fat may slow stomach emptying in some patients, but many can easily consume fat in beverages. Experience at the University of Virginia Health System is that fat in liquid forms, such as whole milk, milk shakes, and nutritional supplements, is often well tolerated. Unless a fat-containing food or fluid clearly causes worse symptoms, fat

should not be limited, because people with gastroparesis often need all the calories they can get, as eating enough may be very hard to do. Liquid fat is often well tolerated, pleasurable, and provides a great source of calories in smaller amounts.

Medications

There are a few medications that can slow stomach emptying. Patients should ask their doctor if any of the medicines they are taking could be slowing down stomach emptying.

Getting Started

- Set a goal weight you want to meet.
- Avoid large meals.
- Eat enough to meet your goal weight. It may be 4 to 8 smaller meals and snacks.
- Avoid solid foods that are high in fat, and avoid adding too much fat to foods. High-fat drinks are usually okay; try them and see.
- Eat nutritious foods first before filling up on empty calories such as candy, cakes, and sodas.
- Chew foods well, especially meats. Meats may be easier to eat if ground or puréed.
- Avoid high-fiber foods because they may be harder for your stomach to empty.
- Sit up while eating, and stay upright for at least 1 hour after you finish. Try taking a nice walk after meals.
- If you have diabetes, keep your blood sugar under control. Let your doctor know if your blood sugar runs greater than 200 mg/dL on a regular basis.

Getting your Calories

When getting enough calories is a daily struggle, make everything you eat and drink count:

- Take medications with calorie-containing beverages such as milk, juice, and sweet tea instead of water or diet drinks.
- High-calorie drinks are better than water because they provide calories and fluid. Use peach, pear, or papaya nectar; fruit juices and drinks; Hawaiian Punch; Hi C; lemonade; Kool-Aid; sweet tea; even soda.
- Fortify milk by adding dry milk powder: add 1 cup powdered milk to 1 quart milk.
- Drink whole milk if tolerated instead of skim or 2%. Use whole, condensed, or evaporated milk when preparing cream-based soups, custards, puddings, and hot cereals, smoothies, and milkshakes.
- Add Carnation Instant Breakfast, protein powder, dry milk powder, or other flavored powders or flavored syrups to whole milk or juices.
- Make custards and puddings with eggs or egg substitutes such as Eggbeaters.
- Try adding ice cream, sherbet, and sorbet to ready-made supplements such as Nutra-shakes, Ensure, or Boost. Peanut butter, chocolate syrup, or caramel sauce is also great in these.

Suggested Foods for Gastroparesis

Starches

Breads: white bread and "light" whole wheat bread (no nuts, seeds), including French/Italian, bagels (plain or egg), English muffin, plain roll, pita bread, tortilla (flour or corn), pancake, waffle, naan, and flat bread

Cereals: quick oats (plain), grits, cream of wheat, cream of rice, and puffed wheat and rice cereals, such as Cheerios, Sugar Pops, Kix, Rice Krispies, Fruit Loops, Special K, and Cocoa Crispies

Grains/potatoes: rice (plain), pasta, macaroni (plain), bulgur wheat (couscous), barley, sweet and white potatoes (no skin, plain), yams, French fries (baked)

Crackers/chips: arrowroot, breadsticks, matzoh, melba toast, oyster, saltines, soda, zwieback, water crackers, baked potato chips, pretzels

Meats, Fish, and Poultry, Ground or Pureed

Beef: baby beef, chipped beef, flank steak, tenderloin, plate skirt steak, round (bottom or top), rump

Veal: leg, loin, rib, shank, shoulder

Pork: lean pork, tenderloin, pork chops, ham

Poultry (skinless): chicken, turkey

Wild game (no skin): venison, rabbit, squirrel, pheasant, duck, goose

Fish/shellfish (fresh or frozen, plain, no breading): crab, lobster, shrimp, clams, scallops, oysters, tuna (in water)

Cheese: cottage cheese, grated parmesan

Other: eggs (no creamed or fried), egg white, egg substitute; tofu, strained baby meats (all)

Vegetables (cooked, and if necessary, blenderized/strained)

Beets, tomato sauce, tomato juice, tomato paste or purée, carrots, strained baby vegetables (all), mushrooms, vegetable juice

Fruits and Juices (cooked and, if necessary, blenderized/strained)

Fruits, applesauce, banana, peaches (canned), pears (canned), strained baby fruits (all), juices (all), fruit drinks, fruit flavored beverages

Milk Products (if tolerated)

Milk, any as tolerated, chocolate, buttermilk, yogurt (without fruit pieces), frozen yogurt, kefir (liquid yogurt), evaporated milk, condensed milk, milk powder, custard/pudding

Soups

Broth, bouillon, strained creamed soups (with milk or water)

Beverages

Hot cocoa (made with water or milk), Kool-Aid, lemonade, Tang, and similar powdered products, Gatorade or Powerade, soft drinks, coffee/coffee drinks, tea/chai

Seasonings/Gravies

Cranberry sauce (smooth), fat-free gravies, Molly McButter, Butter Buds

Mustard, ketchup, vegetable oil spray, soy sauce, teriyaki sauce, tabasco sauce, vanilla and other flavoring extracts, vinegar

Desserts/Sweets

Angel food cake, animal crackers, gelatin, ginger snaps, graham crackers, popsicles, plain sherbet, vanilla wafers, gum, gum drops, hard candy

Jelly beans, lemon drops, rolled candy (such as Lifesavers), marshmallows

Seedless jams and jellies

The following foods have been associated with bezoar formation and may need to be avoided (see Fiber section).

Apples, berries, coconut, figs, oranges, persimmons, brussels sprouts
Green beans, legumes, potato peels, sauerkraut

When Solids Do Not Seem to Be Working, Try Blenderized Food

Any food can be blenderized, but solid foods need to be thinned down with some type of liquid.

- If you do not have a blender, strained baby foods may be used and can be thinned down as needed with milk, soy or rice milk, water, or broth.
- Always clean the blender well. Any food left in the blender for more than 1 to 2 hours could cause food poisoning.
- Meats, fish, poultry, and ham: blend with broths, water, milk, vegetable or V-8 juice, tomato sauce, or gravies.
- Vegetables: blend with water, tomato juice, broth, strained baby vegetables.
- Starches: potatoes, pasta, rice: blend with soups, broth, milk, water, or gravies; add strained baby meats to add protein if needed. Consider using hot cereals, such as cream of wheat or rice, grits, as your starch at lunch and dinner.
- Fruits: blend with their own juices, other fruit juices, water, strained baby fruits.
- Cereals: make with caloric beverage such as whole milk (or even evaporated/condensed milk), soy or rice milk, juice, Ensure, Boost, or store brand equivalent, instead of water. Add sugars, honey, molasses, syrups, or other flavorings and butter or vegetable oil for extra calories.
- Mixed dishes: lasagna, macaroni and cheese, spaghetti, chili, chop suey: add adequate liquid of your choice, blend well, and strain.

From University of Virginia Health System, Digestive Health Center, Charlottesville, VA; 2014; with permission.

Prokinetics in Gastroparesis

Andres Acosta, MD, PhD, Michael Camilleri, MD*

KEYWORDS

- Domperidone • Erythromycin • Ghrelin • Metoclopramide • Pharmacology
- Pyridostigmine • Receptor • Relamorelin • Serotonin

KEY POINTS

- Prokinetic agents are medications that enhance coordinated gastrointestinal motility and transit of content in the gastrointestinal tract, mainly by amplifying and coordinating the gastrointestinal muscular contractions.
- Prokinetic therapy should be considered as a means to improve gastric emptying and symptoms of gastroparesis.
- Metoclopramide remains the first-line prokinetic therapy, because it is the only approved medication for gastroparesis in the United States.
- Other medications for gastroparesis should be used by balancing benefits and risks of treatment.
- There are newer agents being developed for the management of gastroparesis targeting different pathways: 5-hydroxytryptamine type 4 (receptor agonists), new motilin receptors agonists, and ghrelin agonists.

INTRODUCTION

Gastroparesis is defined as objectively delayed gastric emptying in the absence of mechanical obstruction and in the presence of upper gastrointestinal symptoms including early satiety, postprandial fullness, nausea, vomiting, bloating, and upper abdominal pain.[1,2] The most common causes of gastroparesis are diabetes mellitus, postsurgical, and idiopathic; less common causes are iatrogenic, extrinsic neuronal (such as parkinsonism and paraneoplastic disease), and infiltrative disorders (such as scleroderma).[1,3–7] The management of gastroparesis is based on dietary therapy;

Funding: Dr M. Camilleri is supported by grants R01-DK92179 and R01-DK67071 from National Institutes of Health.
Conflicts of interest: None.
Clinical Enteric Neuroscience Translational and Epidemiological Research (C.E.N.T.E.R.), Mayo Clinic, 200 First Street Southwest, Rochester, MN 55905, USA
* Corresponding author. Mayo Clinic, 200 First Street Southwest, Charlton Building, Room 8-110, Rochester, MN 55905.
E-mail address: camilleri.michael@mayo.edu

restoration of fluid and electrolyte balance; nutritional support; treating the underlying cause, such as optimization of glycemic control in diabetics; and stimulation of gastric emptying (**Fig. 1**).[2]

This article discusses in detail the prokinetic agents available or under evaluation for the treatment of gastroparesis.

PROKINETICS: DEFINITIONS AND CLASSIFICATIONS

Prokinetic agents are medications that enhance coordinated gastrointestinal motility and transit of content in the gastrointestinal tract, mainly by amplifying and

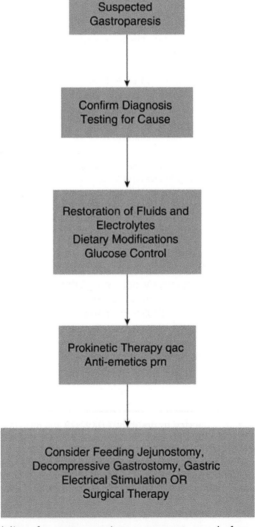

Fig. 1. Clinical guidelines for gastroparesis management. qac, before every meal; prn, as required or needed. (*From* Camilleri M, Parkman HP, Shafi MA, et al. Clinical guideline: management of gastroparesis. Am J Gastroenterol 2013;108(1):18–37; with permission.)

coordinating the gastrointestinal muscular contraction. Prokinetics enhance coordination among the segments of the gut, which is necessary for propulsion of luminal contents. Prokinetics may be either selective to certain areas of the gastrointestinal tract or more generalized, and this reflects the distribution of the receptor targets of the different compounds.

Acetylcholine (Ach), released from primary motor neurons in the myenteric plexus, is the principal excitatory transmitter mediating muscle contractility; other excitatory transmitters are the tachykinins (such as substance P), motilin, and ghrelin. To date, most of the clinically useful prokinetic agents act upstream of Ach, at receptor sites on the motor neuron, or on neurons or nonneuronal cells that synapse with cholinergic neurons. Prokinetic agents are pharmacologically and chemically diverse; they release excitatory neurotransmitters at the nerve-muscle junction without interfering with the normal physiologic patterns and rhythms of motility.

The gastric prokinetics (their main effect is to enhance gastric contractility) include dopamine receptor antagonists, motilin receptor agonists, serotonin (5-hydroxytryptamine [5-HT] type 4 [5-HT$_4$]) receptor agonists, cholinesterase inhibitors, and ghrelin agonists. This article categorizes medications as approved or under evaluation.

PROKINETICS IN MANAGEMENT GUIDELINES FOR GASTROPARESIS

The American College of Gastroenterology (ACG) guidelines, published in 2013, documented the evidence for the pharmacologic management of gastroparesis and used the GRADE (Grades of Recommendation Assessment, Development and Evaluation) system to evaluate the strength of the recommendations (strong, moderate, or weak if the desirable effects on an intervention clearly outweigh the undesirable effects, and as conditional if there is uncertainty) and the overall quality of evidence (high, moderate, low, or very low).[8]

The most recently published guidelines for the pharmacologic management of gastroparesis[2] are shown in **Box 1**.

APPROVED MEDICATIONS (INCLUDING OFF-LABEL USE)
Dopamine Receptor Antagonists

There are 2 dopamine receptor antagonists available for the management of gastroparesis: metoclopramide and domperidone. Metoclopramide should be the first-line treatment and is the only medication approved by the US Food and Drug Administration (FDA) for the indication of gastroparesis, with recommended use for less than 12 weeks. Domperidone can be prescribed through the FDA's Expanded Access to Investigational Drugs program. Both agents are dopamine2 (D2) receptor antagonists. Dopamine inhibits the release of Ach, thus decreasing gastric and proximal small bowel motility.[9] A D2 antagonist reverses the inhibitory effects of endogenous dopamine.

Metoclopramide
Chemistry and pharmacokinetics Metoclopramide, or 4-amino-5-chloro-N-(2-(diethylamino)ethyl)-2-methoxybenzamide, is a substituted benzamide derivative, with a chemical structure similar to procainamide, but without antiarrhythmic effects.[10] Metoclopramide is metabolized mainly by CYP2D6 and to a lesser extent by the CYP3A4 and CYP1A3[11]; up to 30% of the drug is excreted unchanged in the urine.[12]

Mechanism of action Metoclopramide has dual activity as a D2 receptor antagonist and a 5-HT$_4$ agonist, decreasing effects of dopamine and thereby stimulating the

---

Box 1
Recommendations in ACG 2013 guidelines for gastroparesis

- In addition to dietary therapy, prokinetic therapy should be considered to improve gastric emptying and gastroparesis symptoms, taking into account benefits and risks of treatment (strong recommendation, moderate level of evidence).

- Metoclopramide is the first line of prokinetic therapy and should be administered at the lowest effective dose in a liquid formulation to facilitate absorption. The risk of tardive dyskinesia has been estimated to be less than 1%. Patients should be instructed to discontinue therapy if they develop side effects including involuntary movements (moderate recommendation, moderate level of evidence).

- For patients unable to use metoclopramide, domperidone can be prescribed with investigational new drug clearance from the US Food and Drug Administration and has been shown to be as effective as metoclopramide in reducing symptoms without the propensity for causing central nervous system side effects; given the propensity of domperidone to prolong corrected QT interval on electrocardiogram, a baseline electrocardiogram is recommended and treatment withheld if the corrected QT is greater than 470 milliseconds in men and greater than 450 milliseconds in women. Follow-up electrocardiogram on treatment with domperidone is also advised (moderate recommendation, moderate level of evidence).

- Erythromycin improves gastric emptying and symptoms from delayed gastric emptying. Administration of intravenous erythromycin should be considered when intravenous prokinetic therapy is needed in hospitalized patients. Oral treatment with erythromycin also improves gastric emptying. However, the long-term effectiveness of oral therapy is limited by tachyphylaxis (strong recommendation, moderate level of evidence).

- Treatment with antiemetic agents should be given for improvement of associated nausea and vomiting, but does not result in improved gastric emptying (conditional recommendation, moderate level of evidence).

- Tricyclic antidepressants can be considered for refractory nausea and vomiting in gastroparesis, but do not result in improved gastric emptying and may potentially retard gastric emptying (conditional recommendation, low level of evidence).

From Camilleri M, Parkman HP, Shafi MA, et al. Clinical guideline: management of gastroparesis. Am J Gastroenterol 2013;108(1):18–37; with permission.

---

cholinergic receptors. This effect promotes the release of Ach, which increases lower esophageal sphincter and gastric tone, increases intragastric pressure, improves antroduodenal coordination, and accelerates gastric emptying.[10] The dual effects on gastric contractility and the centrally mediated antiemetic effect are considered responsible for the improved symptoms of gastroparesis (**Fig. 2**). The antiemetic effect is mainly mediated from inhibition of D2 and 5-HT$_3$ receptors within the nausea or vomiting centers in the brainstem, especially the chemoreceptor trigger zone and the area postrema.

Pharmacodynamics and clinical pharmacology The effect of metoclopramide on gastric emptying has been shown in short-term (less than 4 weeks) studies (**Table 1**).[13–18] Metoclopramide significantly increased gastric motor activity in patients with gastroparesis, often triggering an intense burst of motor activity in the stomach.[19] Metoclopramide improved gastric emptying by 56% in patients with gastroparesis compared with 37% in the placebo group.[20] These short-term studies showed generally poor correlation of acceleration of gastric emptying with symptom improvement.

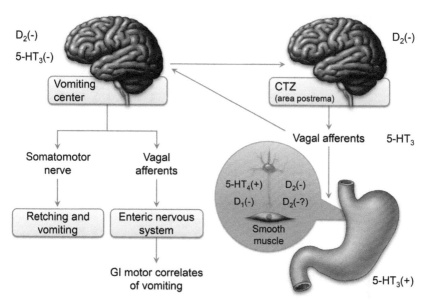

Fig. 2. Dual mechanism of action of metoclopramide. GI, gastrointestinal. (*From* Lee A, Kuo B. Metoclopramide in the treatment of diabetic gastroparesis. Expert Rev Endocrinol Metab 2010;5(5):653–62; with permission.)

Formulations Metoclopramide is available in multiple formulations: oral, orally disintegrating sublingual, intranasal, subcutaneous injections, and intravenous. The last 3 formulations have the advantage of bypassing the first-pass elimination in the liver and are ideal in patients with limited absorption caused by recurrent vomiting.[10]

Dosing The current guidelines recommend starting with liquid formulation at 5 mg orally, 30 minutes before meals and at bedtime. If needed, the doses can be increased to 10 mg, up to 4 times per day, but it is recommended to avoid doses higher than 40 mg daily to avoid side effects.

Adverse effects Metoclopramide is associated with reversible or irreversible side effects, and the FDA has placed a Black Box warning on the use of metoclopramide (http://www.fda.gov/newsevents/newsroom/pressannouncements/ucm149533.htm). Metoclopramide's central nervous system (CNS) side effects are secondary to easy crossing of the blood-brain barrier and are observed in up to 30% of patients.[2] Thus the most common side effects are related to the dopaminergic effects on the CNS. The reversible side effects, which resolve once the drug is discontinued, are mainly drowsiness, fatigue, lethargy, hyperprolactinemia, and worsening depression.[10]

The extrapyramidal reactions associated with metoclopramide are acute dystonic reactions, such as facial spasms, torticollis, oculogyric crisis, trismus, abdominal rigidity, or spasm of the entire body; these effects usually are reversible.[21] The irreversible and most concerning side effect is tardive dyskinesia, which typically occurs at doses higher than 40 mg daily. The overall frequency of all extrapyramidal side effects associated with metoclopramide is 0.2%.[10,22,23] Treatment recommendations and careful monitoring are described by Rao and Camilleri.[23]

In addition, metoclopramide may increase the half-life of other drugs metabolized by CYP2D6. Hence, the use of metoclopramide in combination with other neuroleptic

Table 1
Trials of metoclopramide for gastroparesis

Reference #	Design	#, Cause	Dose	Duration	Results
20	DB, PC, XO, RCT	10 DG	10 mg QID	3 wk/arm	Improved symptoms and vomiting; ~60% acceleration in GE liquid 150-kcal meal
13	DB, PC, PG, RCT	28: 5 DM, 4 PSG, 19 IG	10 mg QID	3 wk	Improved symptoms by 29%
15	PC, RCT	18 DG	10 mg QID	3 wk	Improved symptom score by 29%, improved GE by 25%
16	DB, PC, XO, RCT	13 DG with GE accelerated by metoclopramide	10 mg QID	3 wk/arm	Improved symptoms with mean reduction of 52.6%
17	DB, RCT, domperidone controlled	45 DG	10 mg QID	4 wk	Improved symptoms by 39%; similar efficacy with domperidone, which had fewer AEs
18	DB, XO, erythromycin-control RCT	13 DG	10 mg TID	3 wk/arm	Both treatments accelerated GE compared with baseline and improved symptoms score
56	Open	1 DG	15 mg QID	6 mo	Improved symptoms, GE liquids, antral contraction frequency
57	Open	10 GI symptomatic (N,V) type 1 DM; 6 asymptomatic T1DM, 18 controls	10 mg once	acute	Improved GE solids

Abbreviations: AE, adverse events; DB, double-blind; DG, diabetic gastroparesis; DM, diabetes mellitus; GE, gastric emptying; GI, gastrointestinal; IG, idiopathic gastroparesis; N, nausea; PC, placebo-controlled; PG, parallel group; PSG, postsurgical gastroparesis; QID, 4 times a day; RCT, randomized controlled trial; TID, 3 times a day; T1DM, type 1 diabetes mellitus; V, vomitting; XO, crossover.

From Camilleri M, Parkman HP, Shafi MA, et al. Clinical guideline: management of gastroparesis. Am J Gastroenterol 2013;108(1):18–37; with permission.

drugs, such as haloperidol, thioridazine, chlorpromazine, perphenazine, and risperidone, can increase the risk of extrapyramidal symptoms. Polymorphisms in CYP2D6, KCNH2, and HTR4 genes were associated with side effects, whereas polymorphisms in KCNH2 and ADRA1D genes were associated with clinical response.[24]

Domperidone

Chemistry and pharmacokinetics Domperidone is a D2 receptor antagonist with similar efficacy to metoclopramide as an antiemetic and prokinetic. However, domperidone has poor penetration of the blood-brain barrier with limited to no CNS side effects. Domperidone structure is based on butyrophenones, and the drug has a low oral bioavailability (15%) that can be further decreased by increasing gastric pH.[25] Domperidone has high affinity for gastrointestinal tissue, and high concentrations of the drug are found in the esophagus, stomach, and small intestine after oral administration.[26] Approximately 90% of domperidone is bound to plasma proteins. It has a half-life of 7.5 hours, is mainly metabolized by the liver, and 32% of the drug is excreted in the urine.[27]

Mechanism of action Domperidone increases the amplitude of esophageal motor function and antroduodenal contractions, coordinates peristalsis across the pylorus, and accelerates gastric emptying.[28,29] The effect of domperidone on gastric emptying has been shown in short-term studies (**Table 2**).

Dosing The current guidelines recommend starting with 10 mg 3 times a day, and increasing to 20 mg 3 times a day and at bedtime. Patients should have a baseline electrocardiogram and another when on medication, because domperidone can prolong the QTc interval. Domperidone should be avoided if the corrected QTc interval is greater than 470 milliseconds in men and greater than 450 milliseconds in women.

Although available for the past 25 years in most countries (and a recent recommendation from European Medicines Agency (EMA) made it also available over the counter in Europe), it is only available in the United States through compassionate clearance for patients with refractory gastroparesis (http://www.fda.gov/cder/news/domperidone.htm).

Adverse effects Side effects with oral administration of domperidone occur in less than 7% of patients and include headaches, dry mouth, diarrhea, anxiety, and hyperprolactinemia. As with metoclopramide, domperidone inhibits the CYP2D6 enzyme, and drug-drug interactions should be considered.[30] There are polymorphisms that predispose to potentially higher drug levels of domperidone and cardiac toxicity; nevertheless, the opinion of the European Medicines Agency's Pharmacovigilance Risk Assessment Committee was that the benefits outweighed risks when given in the short term and in low doses to treat nausea or vomiting, but not for bloating or heartburn. The recommended doses are 10 mg up to 3 times daily by mouth for adults and adolescents weighing 35 kg or more, and 0.25 mg/kg bodyweight up to 3 times daily for children or patients weighing less than 35 kg.[31]

Motilin Receptor Agonists

The most common motilin receptor agonists are the macrolides, a class of antibiotics that stimulates the motilin receptors in the gastrointestinal tract. Erythromycin is the most commonly studied macrolide. These agents improve gastric emptying and symptoms; however, in the medium or long term, they are associated with tachyphylaxis caused by downregulation of the motilin receptor, typically starting within 2 weeks of the onset of therapy.[32]

Table 2
Trials of domperidone in gastroparesis

Reference #	Type of Study	N, Cause	Duration	Symptom Improvement vs Baseline (Open) vs Placebo (RCT)	Δ Gastric Emptying	Adverse Effects
58	Open, 10 mg QID	3 DG	1 wk	Yes, not quantified	Improved, not quantified	NA
59	Open	12 IG; 3 DG, 2 PSG	48 mo	68.3% (P<.05)	34.5% (P<.05)	↑ Prolactin (100%), symptoms (17.6%)
60	Retrospective	57 DM	377 d	70% patients improved	NA	16%
61	Open	6 DG	6 mo	79.2% (P<.01)	26.9% (NS)	NA
62	Open	12 DG	Single oral dose	Chronic oral administration (35–51 d) reduced symptoms	↑ Solid and liquid emptying (P<.005)	NA
63	RCT, PG, withdrawal study	208 DG: 105 DOM, 103 PLA	4 wk	53.8% lower overall score with domperidone (P = .025)	NA	2%–3% ↑ prolactin, similar to placebo
64	RCT, PC, XO	13 DG	8 wk	↓ In symptom frequency and intensity vs placebo (P<.03)	NA	NA
65	RCT, PC, XO	6 DG	Single 10 mg IV	NA	↑ Homogenized solid emptying	NA
66	RCT, PC, XO	8 IG; 3 DG	4 wk	No overall benefit compared with placebo; 2 of 3 DM improved	NA	Gas pains, skin rash
67	RCT, PG vs cisapride, 14 per group	Total 31 pediatric DG; 3 excluded for poor compliance	8 wk	Domperidone improved vs baseline (P<.001); domperidone vs cisapride (P<.01)	Domperidone significantly more effective than placebo in reducing the gastric emptying time measured by ultrasonography	None recorded
17	RCT, PG, vs metoclopramide	95 DG	4 wk	41.19% improved vs baseline (NA); NS vs metoclopramide	NA	CNS effects more severe and common with metoclopramide: somnolence, mental acuity (49% metoclopramide vs 29% DOM)

Abbreviations: CNS, central nervous system; DG, diabetic gastroparesis; DM, diabetes-mellitus; DOM, domperidone; IG, idiopathic gastroparesis; IV, intravenously; NA, not assessed; NS, nonsignificant; PC, placebo-controlled; PG, parallel group; PLA, placebo; PSG, postsurgical gastroparesis; QID, 4 times a day; RCT, randomized controlled trial; XO, crossover.

From Camilleri M, Parkman HP, Shafi MA, et al. Clinical guideline: management of gastroparesis. Am J Gastroenterol 2013;108(1):18–37; with permission.

Erythromycin

Mechanism of action Erythromycin induces phasic contractions in the antrum by cholinergic activity and promotes pyloric relaxation through action on the inhibitory nerves of the pylorus.[33–35] High-dose erythromycin (eg, 2–3 mg/kg intravenously [IV]) stimulates migrating motor complex activities, whereas lower dosing (eg, 1 mg/kg IV) activates phasic stomach and small bowel motility similar to a fed pattern.[2,33,36] The lack of a long-term effect, mainly explained by tachyphylaxis,[32] precludes medium-term efficacy in clinical practice, and there have been no long-term, randomized, placebo-controlled trials.

Dosing

The current recommended doses are 1.5 to 3 mg/kg IV (by infusion over 45 minutes) every 6 hours in patients admitted to hospital with gastroparesis, and 125 mg, twice a day, orally in liquid formulation, for outpatient gastroparesis management. The oral regimen may provide benefit for a few weeks.

Adverse effects Side effects of erythromycin include abdominal pain, nausea, and diarrhea. Erythromycin also may induce drug interactions with agents that alter or are metabolized by CYP3A4, and they should be used carefully in combination with diltiazem or verapamil because of an increased risk for sudden cardiac death.[37]

Other macrolides, such as azithromycin and clarithromycin

Other macrolides, such as azithromycin and clarithromycin, accelerate gastric emptying.[38,39] However, there are no randomized controlled trials comparing these drugs with placebo or other medications, and their use should be balanced with the potential for tachyphylaxis, cardiac risk, and antibiotic resistance.

5-Hydroxytryptamine Type 4 Receptor Agonists

5-HT$_4$ receptors are distributed throughout the gastrointestinal tract and have been extensively studied in gastrointestinal motility disorders.

Cisapride and tegaserod

In the past, 2 5-HT$_4$ receptor agonists, cisapride and tegaserod, were on the market for indications of gastroparesis and chronic constipation, respectively. However, their poor receptor selectivity and cisapride's high affinity for the heart voltage-gated K$^+$ (hERG-K$^+$) channel caused drug-induced ventricular arrhythmias.

Prucalopride, naronapride, velusetrag, and YKP10811

A new generation of 5-HT$_4$ receptor agonists, such as prucalopride, naronapride, velusetrag, and YKP10811, have lower affinity for the hERG-K$^+$ channel and higher selectivity for the 5-HT$_4$ receptor.[40,41]

Prucalopride Prucalopride is approved by the EMA for the treatment of chronic constipation. In addition, prucalopride accelerates gastric emptying and small bowel transit in patients with chronic constipation[42] and could be considered as a potential agent for gastroparesis. However, the use of prucalopride for gastroparesis is not supported by any clinical evidence or trials to date. Prucalopride is currently not approved by the FDA for any indication.

YKP10811 YKP10811 accelerated gastrointestinal and colonic transit and gastric empting, and improved bowel functions, compared with placebo, in an 8-day study in patients with functional constipation.[41]

Cholinesterase Inhibitors

Neostigmine
Neostigmine is a cholinesterase inhibitor that induced an irregular increase in gastro-duodenal motor activity, sometimes characterized by propagated and nonpropagated clustered contractions,[43] and accelerated liquid gastric emptying in critically ill patients with delayed gastric emptying.[44] Neostigmine is only available in parenteral formulation and may be used in the hospital setting.

Pyridostigmine
Pyridostigmine may have similar efficacy to neostigmine; it is used off-label in liquid formulation at a dose of 60 mg, 3 times a day. However, there are no clinical trials to support its use in gastroparesis.

MEDICATIONS CURRENTLY UNDER EVALUATION
New Motilin Receptor Agonist

GSK962040 (Camicinal)
GSK962040 is a nonmotilide motilin receptor agonist with low molecular mass that increases gastrointestinal motility in dogs.[45] It selectively activates the motilin receptor in humans and specifically activates the antrum preferentially relative to the fundus, small intestine, or colon in human tissue in vitro.[46] This medication has been evaluated to determine safety and tolerability in humans.[47] It is currently being investigated in phase 2 clinical trials (ClinicalTrials.gov trial NCT01262898).

Ghrelin Agonists

Ghrelin is a 28-amino residue peptide secreted mainly in the stomach and, through the ghrelin receptor, it promotes gastric motility in mice, rats, dogs, and humans.[48–50] Synthetic ghrelin agonists, predominantly small molecules, are being developed as prokinetic agents that may prove useful in the treatment of gastrointestinal dysmotility disorders such as gastroparesis.[51] Actions and therapeutic pathways of ghrelin for gastrointestinal disorders have been reviewed elsewhere.[52]

Relamorelin
Relamorelin, a pentapeptide synthetic ghrelin agonist, has similar characteristics to native ghrelin but with improved stability, a longer plasma half-life, and greater potency. Results from 2 small, phase 1b, placebo-controlled, single-dose (100 μg), 2-period, crossover studies in patients with type 2 diabetes mellitus and type 1 diabetes mellitus and prior documentation of delayed gastric emptying indicated that relamorelin was generally well tolerated. Relamorelin significantly accelerated gastric emptying of solids at 1 and 2 hours (**Fig. 3**). The most common adverse events included hyperhidrosis, dizziness, fatigue, abdominal pain/cramping, decreased blood pressure, hunger, feeling cold, and muscular weakness.[53]

A subsequent randomized, double-blind, placebo-controlled, adaptive-design, parallel-group, 28-day, phase 2 study was conducted in patients with diabetic gastroparesis. Compared with baseline, relamorelin, 10 μg, twice a day, resulted in significant acceleration of gastric emptying ($P<.03$). There were also significant improvements in vomiting end points on relamorelin treatment compared with placebo; these effects were most evident in the 58.3% of patients who had vomiting during the baseline period.[54]

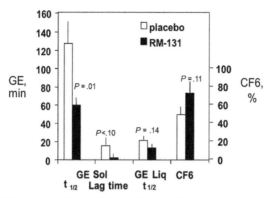

Fig. 3. Effects of Relamorelin (RM-131) in patients with type 2 diabetic gastroparesis with previously documented delayed gastric emptying (GE). CF6, colonic filling 6 hr; Liq, liquid; Sol, solid. (*From* Shin A, Camilleri M, Busciglio I, et al. The ghrelin agonist RM-131 accelerates gastric emptying of solids and reduces symptoms in patients with type 1 diabetes mellitus. Clin Gastroenterol Hepatol 2013;11(11):1453–59; with permission.)

Ulimorelin (TZP-102)

Ulimorelin is a ghrelin receptor agonist that accelerates gastric emptying and improves upper gastrointestinal symptoms in diabetic patients with gastroparesis.[55] In a phase 2a study, ulimorelin improved gastroparesis symptoms without correlation or improvement in gastric emptying. However, in a phase 2b study, ulimorelin efficacy was not shown compared with placebo.

SUMMARY

Prokinetic agents should be the first line of treatment of patients with gastroparesis. Metoclopramide remains the only approved medication in the United States for the indication of gastroparesis. The use of metoclopramide should be limited to less than 12 weeks; this limitation is a challenge for patients and their physicians, because gastroparesis often lasts several years. Other medications, including domperidone, require special FDA approval or off-label use. Promising new agents being developed for the management of gastroparesis include 5-HT$_4$ agonists and the ghrelin agonist, relamorelin.

REFERENCES

1. Camilleri M, Bharucha AE, Farrugia G. Epidemiology, mechanisms, and management of diabetic gastroparesis. Clin Gastroenterol Hepatol 2011;9(1):5–12 [quiz: e7].
2. Camilleri M, Parkman HP, Shafi MA, et al. Clinical guideline: management of gastroparesis. Am J Gastroenterol 2013;108(1):18–37 [quiz: 38].
3. Choung RS, Locke GR 3rd, Schleck CD, et al. Risk of gastroparesis in subjects with type 1 and 2 diabetes in the general population. Am J Gastroenterol 2012; 107(1):82–8.
4. Parkman HP, Yates K, Hasler WL, et al. Clinical features of idiopathic gastroparesis vary with sex, body mass, symptom onset, delay in gastric emptying, and gastroparesis severity. Gastroenterology 2011;140(1):101–15.
5. Camilleri M. Clinical practice. Diabetic gastroparesis. N Engl J Med 2007;356(8): 820–9.

6. Frantzides CT, Carlson MA, Zografakis JG, et al. Postoperative gastrointestinal complaints after laparoscopic Nissen fundoplication. JSLS 2006;10(1):39–42.
7. Bityutskiy LP, Soykan I, McCallum RW. Viral gastroparesis: a subgroup of idiopathic gastroparesis–clinical characteristics and long-term outcomes. Am J Gastroenterol 1997;92(9):1501–4.
8. Atkins D, Best D, Briss PA, et al. Grading quality of evidence and strength of recommendations. BMJ 2004;328(7454):1490.
9. Tonini M, Cipollina L, Poluzzi E, et al. Review article: clinical implications of enteric and central D2 receptor blockade by antidopaminergic gastrointestinal prokinetics. Aliment Pharmacol Ther 2004;19(4):379–90.
10. Lee A, Kuo B. Metoclopramide in the treatment of diabetic gastroparesis. Expert Rev Endocrinol Metab 2010;5(5):653–62.
11. Desta Z, Wu GM, Morocho AM, et al. The gastroprokinetic and antiemetic drug metoclopramide is a substrate and inhibitor of cytochrome P450 2D6. Drug Metab Dispos 2002;30(3):336–43.
12. Bateman DN. Clinical pharmacokinetics of metoclopramide. Clin Pharmacokinet 1983;8(6):523–9.
13. Perkel MS, Moore C, Hersh T, et al. Metoclopramide therapy in patients with delayed gastric emptying: a randomized, double-blind study. Dig Dis Sci 1979; 24(9):662–6.
14. Perkel MS, Hersh T, Moore C, et al. Metoclopramide therapy in fifty-five patients with delayed gastric emptying. Am J Gastroenterol 1980;74(3):231–6.
15. McCallum RW, Ricci DA, Rakatansky H, et al. A multicenter placebo-controlled clinical trial of oral metoclopramide in diabetic gastroparesis. Diabetes Care 1983;6(5):463–7.
16. Ricci DA, Saltzman MB, Meyer C, et al. Effect of metoclopramide in diabetic gastroparesis. J Clin Gastroenterol 1985;7(1):25–32.
17. Patterson D, Abell T, Rothstein R, et al. A double-blind multicenter comparison of domperidone and metoclopramide in the treatment of diabetic patients with symptoms of gastroparesis. Am J Gastroenterol 1999;94(5):1230–4.
18. Erbas T, Varoglu E, Erbas B, et al. Comparison of metoclopramide and erythromycin in the treatment of diabetic gastroparesis. Diabetes Care 1993;16(11):1511–4.
19. Malagelada JR, Rees WD, Mazzotta LJ, et al. Gastric motor abnormalities in diabetic and postvagotomy gastroparesis: effect of metoclopramide and bethanechol. Gastroenterology 1980;78(2):286–93.
20. Snape WJ Jr, Battle WM, Schwartz SS, et al. Metoclopramide to treat gastroparesis due to diabetes mellitus: a double-blind, controlled trial. Ann Intern Med 1982; 96(4):444–6.
21. Ganzini L, Casey DE, Hoffman WF, et al. The prevalence of metoclopramide-induced tardive dyskinesia and acute extrapyramidal movement disorders. Arch Intern Med 1993;153(12):1469–75.
22. Bateman DN, Rawlins MD, Simpson JM. Extrapyramidal reactions with metoclopramide. Br Med J (Clin Res Ed) 1985;291(6500):930–2.
23. Rao AS, Camilleri M. Review article: metoclopramide and tardive dyskinesia. Aliment Pharmacol Ther 2010;31(1):11–9.
24. Parkman HP, Mishra A, Jacobs M, et al. Clinical response and side effects of metoclopramide: associations with clinical, demographic, and pharmacogenetic parameters. J Clin Gastroenterol 2012;46(6):494–503.
25. Reddymasu SC, Soykan I, McCallum RW. Domperidone: review of pharmacology and clinical applications in gastroenterology. Am J Gastroenterol 2007;102(9): 2036–45.

26. Van Nueten JM, Ennis C, Helsen L, et al. Inhibition of dopamine receptors in the stomach: an explanation of the gastrokinetic properties of domperidone. Life Sci 1978;23(5):453–7.
27. Champion MC, Hartnett M, Yen M. Domperidone, a new dopamine antagonist. CMAJ 1986;135(5):457–61.
28. Weihrauch TR, Forster CF, Krieglstein J. Evaluation of the effect of domperidone on human oesophageal and gastroduodenal motility by intraluminal manometry. Postgrad Med J 1979;55(Suppl 1):7–10.
29. Valenzuela JE. Dopamine as a possible neurotransmitter in gastric relaxation. Gastroenterology 1976;71(6):1019–22.
30. Parkman HP, Jacobs MR, Mishra A, et al. Domperidone treatment for gastroparesis: demographic and pharmacogenetic characterization of clinical efficacy and side-effects. Dig Dis Sci 2011;56(1):115–24.
31. EMA-webpage. 2014. Available at: http://www.ema.europa.eu/docs/en_GB/document_library/Referrals_document/Domperidone_31/Recommendation_provided_by_Pharmacovigilance_Risk_Assessment_Committee/WC500162559.pdf. Accessed September 4, 2014.
32. Richards RD, Davenport K, McCallum RW. The treatment of idiopathic and diabetic gastroparesis with acute intravenous and chronic oral erythromycin. Am J Gastroenterol 1993;88(2):203–7.
33. Janssens J, Peeters TL, Vantrappen G, et al. Improvement of gastric emptying in diabetic gastroparesis by erythromycin. Preliminary studies. N Engl J Med 1990;322(15):1028–31.
34. Catnach SM, Fairclough PD. Erythromycin and the gut. Gut 1992;33(3):397–401.
35. Parkman HP, Pagano AP, Vozzelli MA, et al. Gastrokinetic effects of erythromycin: myogenic and neurogenic mechanisms of action in rabbit stomach. Am J Phys 1995;269(3 Pt 1):G418–26.
36. Hejazi RA, McCallum RW, Sarosiek I. Prokinetics in diabetic gastroparesis. Curr Gastroenterol Rep 2012;14(4):297–305.
37. Ray WA, Murray KT, Meredith S, et al. Oral erythromycin and the risk of sudden death from cardiac causes. N Engl J Med 2004;351(11):1089–96.
38. Larson JM, Tavakkoli A, Drane WE, et al. Advantages of azithromycin over erythromycin in improving the gastric emptying half-time in adult patients with gastroparesis. J Neurogastroenterol Motil 2010;16(4):407–13.
39. Bortolotti M, Mari C, Brunelli F, et al. Effect of intravenous clarithromycin on interdigestive gastroduodenal motility of patients with functional dyspepsia and *Helicobacter pylori* gastritis. Dig Dis Sci 1999;44(12):2439–42.
40. Manabe N, Wong BS, Camilleri M. New-generation 5-HT4 receptor agonists: potential for treatment of gastrointestinal motility disorders. Expert Opin Investig Drugs 2010;19(6):765–75.
41. Shin A, Acosta A, Camilleri M, et al. A randomized trial of 5-Hydroxytryptamine 4-receptor agonist, YKP10811, on colonic transit and bowel function in functional constipation. Clin Gastroenterol Hepatol 2014. [Epub ahead of print].
42. Bouras E, Camilleri M, Burton D, et al. Prucalopride accelerates gastrointestinal and colonic transit in patients with constipation without a rectal evacuation disorder. Gastroenterology 2001;120(2):354–60.
43. Bortolotti M, Cucchiara S, Sarti P, et al. Comparison between the effects of neostigmine and ranitidine on interdigestive gastroduodenal motility of patients with gastroparesis. Digestion 1995;56(2):96–9.
44. Lucey MA, Patil V, Girling K, et al. Does neostigmine increase gastric emptying in the critically ill?–results of a pilot study. Crit Care Resusc 2003;5(1):14–9.

45. Leming S, Broad J, Cozens SJ, et al. GSK962040: a small molecule motilin receptor agonist which increases gastrointestinal motility in conscious dogs. Neurogastroenterol Motil 2011;23(10):958–958.e410.

46. Broad J, Mukherjee S, Samadi M, et al. Regional- and agonist-dependent facilitation of human neurogastrointestinal functions by motilin receptor agonists. Br J Pharmacol 2012;167(4):763–74.

47. Sanger GJ, Westaway SM, Barnes AA, et al. GSK962040: a small molecule, selective motilin receptor agonist, effective as a stimulant of human and rabbit gastrointestinal motility. Neurogastroenterol Motil 2009;21(6):657–64 e30–1.

48. Trudel L, Tomasetto C, Rio MC, et al. Ghrelin/motilin-related peptide is a potent prokinetic to reverse gastric postoperative ileus in rat. Am J Physiol Gastrointest Liver Physiol 2002;282(6):G948–52.

49. Dass NB, Munonyara M, Bassil AK, et al. Growth hormone secretagogue receptors in rat and human gastrointestinal tract and the effects of ghrelin. Neuroscience 2003;120(2):443–53.

50. Tack J, Depoortere I, Bisschops R, et al. Influence of ghrelin on gastric emptying and meal-related symptoms in idiopathic gastroparesis. Aliment Pharmacol Ther 2005;22(9):847–53.

51. Murray CD, Martin NM, Patterson M, et al. Ghrelin enhances gastric emptying in diabetic gastroparesis: a double blind, placebo controlled, crossover study. Gut 2005;54(12):1693–8.

52. Camilleri M, Papathanasopoulos A, Odunsi ST. Actions and therapeutic pathways of ghrelin for gastrointestinal disorders. Nat Rev Gastroenterol Hepatol 2009;6(6): 343–52.

53. Shin A, Camilleri M, Busciglio I, et al. The ghrelin agonist RM-131 accelerates gastric emptying of solids and reduces symptoms in patients with type 1 diabetes mellitus. Clin Gastroenterol Hepatol 2013;11(11):1453–9.

54. Lembo A, Camilleri M, McCallum R, et al. A phase 2, randomized, double-blind, placebo-controlled study to evaluate the safety and efficacy of RM-131 in patients with diabetic gastroparesis. Gastroenterology 2014;146(Suppl 1): S158–9.

55. Ejskjaer N, Wo JM, Esfandyari T, et al. A phase 2a, randomized, double-blind 28-day study of TZP-102 a ghrelin receptor agonist for diabetic gastroparesis. Neurogastroenterol Motil 2013;25(2):e140–50.

56. Longstreth GF, Malagelada JR, Kelly KA. Metoclopramide stimulation of gastric motility and emptying in diabetic gastroparesis. Ann Intern Med 1977;86(2):195–6.

57. Loo FD, Palmer DW, Soergel KH, et al. Gastric emptying in patients with diabetes mellitus. Gastroenterology 1984;86(3):485–94.

58. Watts GF, Armitage M, Sinclair J, et al. Treatment of diabetic gastroparesis with oral domperidone. Diabet Med 1985;2(6):491–2.

59. Soykan I, Sarosiek I, Shifflett J, et al. Effect of chronic oral domperidone therapy on gastrointestinal symptoms and gastric emptying in patients with Parkinson's disease. Mov Disord 1997;12(6):952–7.

60. Kozarek R. Domperidone for symptomatic management of diabetic gastroparesis in metoclopramide treatment failures. Adv Ther 1990;7:61–8.

61. Koch KL, Stern RM, Stewart WR, et al. Gastric emptying and gastric myoelectrical activity in patients with diabetic gastroparesis: effect of long-term domperidone treatment. Am J Gastroenterol 1989;84(9):1069–75.

62. Horowitz M, Harding PE, Chatterton BE, et al. Acute and chronic effects of domperidone on gastric emptying in diabetic autonomic neuropathy. Dig Dis Sci 1985;30(1):1–9.

63. Silvers D, Kipnes M, Broadstone V, et al. Domperidone in the management of symptoms of diabetic gastroparesis: efficacy, tolerability, and quality-of-life outcomes in a multicenter controlled trial. DOM-USA-5 Study Group. Clin Ther 1998;20(3):438–53.
64. Braun AP. Domperidone in the treatment of symptoms of delayed gastric emptying in diabetic patients. Adv Ther 1989;6:51–62.
65. Heer M, Muller-Duysing W, Benes I, et al. Diabetic gastroparesis: treatment with domperidone–a double-blind, placebo-controlled trial. Digestion 1983;27(4): 214–7.
66. Nagler J, Miskovitz P. Clinical evaluation of domperidone in the treatment of chronic postprandial idiopathic upper gastrointestinal distress. Am J Gastroenterol 1981;76(6):495–9.
67. Franzese A, Borrelli O, Corrado G, et al. Domperidone is more effective than cisapride in children with diabetic gastroparesis. Aliment Pharmacol Ther 2002; 16(5):951–7.

Symptomatic Management for Gastroparesis

Antiemetics, Analgesics, and Symptom Modulators

William L. Hasler, MD

KEYWORDS

- Antiemetic medications • Opiates • Tricyclic antidepressants
- Neuropathic pain modulators • Fundus relaxants

KEY POINTS

- A recent series reported reduced nausea and vomiting caused by open-label transdermal granisetron, a 5-hydroxytryptamine-3 (5-HT$_3$) receptor antagonist, in patients with gastroparesis.
- Opiate analgesics are often taken for pain control; however, caution should be exercised because these agents worsen nausea and vomiting and further delay gastric emptying.
- As with antiemetics, support for use of neuromodulatory agents was restricted to individual cases; however, the largely negative findings from a multicenter, randomized, placebo-controlled trial of the tricyclic antidepressant nortriptyline in patients with idiopathic gastroparesis raise doubts about the effectiveness of neuromodulators in this condition.
- Postulated benefits of antiemetic and neuromodulatory therapies must be weighed against adverse outcomes during gastroparesis treatment, which recently have stressed neurologic and cardiac toxicities of these drugs.
- Placebo-controlled trials must be conducted to characterize the usefulness of these drug classes in managing gastroparesis symptoms.

INTRODUCTION

Gastroparesis presents with a range of symptoms referable to the upper gut including nausea, vomiting, early satiety, postprandial fullness, bloating, distention, and upper abdominal pain or discomfort. Although increased gastric retention is mandated for diagnosis, gastroparesis symptom severity correlates poorly with the degree of gastric

Disclosure statement: Dr W.L. Hasler receives research funding from the National Institute of Diabetes and Digestive and Kidney Diseases (grant U01DK073983) as part of the Gastroparesis Clinical Research Consortium. He also receives funding from Given Imaging, Inc (grant MA-501) for a clinical trial validating the WMC recording system as a diagnostic test for delayed gastric emptying. In the past 24 months, Dr W.L. Hasler has been a consultant to Janssen Pharmaceuticals, Inc; Novartis Pharmaceuticals; GSK; and Salix Pharmaceuticals, Inc.
Division of Gastroenterology, University of Michigan Health System, 3912 Taubman Center, SPC 5362, Ann Arbor, MI 48109, USA
E-mail address: whasler@umich.edu

Gastroenterol Clin N Am 44 (2015) 113–126
http://dx.doi.org/10.1016/j.gtc.2014.11.009
0889-8553/15/$ – see front matter © 2015 Elsevier Inc. All rights reserved.

gastro.theclinics.com

emptying delay. In a large gastroparesis cohort comprising both diabetic and idiopathic patients from the multicenter National Institute of Diabetes and Digestive and Kidney Diseases Gastroparesis Consortium, gastric retention measured at 2 and 4 hours showed no relation to overall or individual symptom intensities among 319 patients with delayed emptying and 106 with normal emptying.[1] Likewise in functional dyspepsia, emptying parameters show no correlation or are only weakly associated with fullness but not nausea, pain, or bloating. One investigation calculated that only 10% of the variance in dyspeptic symptoms relates to gastric emptying rates.[2] Other physiologic defects are proposed to contribute to symptom development. In studies in which combined gastric emptying and barostat testing was performed in dyspeptic patients, delayed gastric emptying correlated with nausea, vomiting, and postprandial fullness, whereas impaired gastric fundic accommodation associated with epigastric pain, early satiety, and weight loss.[3] In a different report, the prevalence of hypersensitivity to gastric distention was greatest (44%) among patients who rated abdominal pain as their predominant symptom.[4]

Because of the importance of delayed emptying in diagnosing gastroparesis, the main focus of treating this condition has been on prokinetic agents that promote gastric evacuation. However, in gastroparesis and functional dyspepsia, metoclopramide and domperidone reduce symptoms over the long term even when there is diminution of initial prokinetic effects with time.[5] Many benefits of these agents may therefore stem from antiemetic effects in the central nervous system. Furthermore, agents with only prokinetic treatments without central antiemetic effects (erythromycin, pyloric botulinum toxin) may be less effective than therapies with combined prokinetic and antiemetic action. One systematic review calculated benefits in only 43% of patients with gastroparesis receiving erythromycin.[6]

These investigations raise the possibility that pharmaceuticals with actions unrelated to gastrokinesis may be beneficial for some gastroparesis manifestations. Medications with only antiemetic mechanisms of action would theoretically be effective with prominent vomiting (and nausea). In contrast, central analgesics or drugs targeting other sensorimotor defects, such as enhanced sensitivity or impaired accommodation, might be useful for discomfort or pain.

MANAGEMENT GOALS

Given the disconnect between symptoms and gastric emptying, it is reasonable to propose that the primary goal of treating gastroparesis should focus on symptom reductions rather than stimulation of gastric emptying. Pharmacologic agents in diverse drug classes are available that decrease nausea, vomiting, and abdominal pain by acting as antiemetics, analgesics, or modulators of enteric neuronal function. These medications represent the sole forms of treatment of some individuals or may complement gastric prokinetic drugs in others. Little controlled investigation has been performed to define benefits of these agents in gastroparesis. Thus, use of these medications is based on pathophysiologic plausibility and expert opinion.

PHARMACOLOGIC STRATEGIES

The benefits of antiemetic, analgesic, and neuromodulatory medications in gastroparesis are unproved and may be modest in scope. Because of these limitations, decisions on any gastroparesis therapies rely on defining and assessing the severity of symptoms that represent the target of treatment. Introduction of validated surveys to measure numerical symptom intensity represents an advance in quantifying gastroparesis severity. The Gastroparesis Cardinal Symptom Index (GCSI) comprises

9 questions in 3 domains (nausea/vomiting, fullness/early satiety, bloating/distention) rated from 0 (no symptoms) to 5 (very severe) and shows good test-retest reliability and treatment response.[7] The GCSI–Daily Diary adds a pain/discomfort domain to this survey and is administered daily.[8] In comprehensive evaluations of a large patient cohort from the Gastroparesis Consortium followed for 48 weeks, overall GCSI scores decreased only by an average of 0.3 points while subjects were under the care of clinicians with expertise in managing this condition.[9] Subjects with predominant nausea and/or vomiting more often improved than those with predominant upper abdominal pain. Future controlled investigations of novel therapies will determine whether medications targeting nausea and vomiting are more effective than those that are designed to reduce other gastroparesis symptoms.

Antiemetic Agents

Nausea is the most prevalent gastroparesis symptom, being experienced by 90% to 95% of patients, whereas 55% to 80% report vomiting.[10] Nausea and/or vomiting represent the predominant symptoms, prompting specialist referral of 44% of patients (**Table 1**).[11] In a single-center study, nausea scores averaged 3.4 (on a scale from 0 to 5) over 8 hours daily in patients with both diabetic and idiopathic gastroparesis.[10] Mean daily vomiting frequencies ranged from 3.5 with idiopathic disease to 7.3 for diabetics with gastroparesis. Vomiting with gastroparesis often occurs 30 to 120 minutes after eating. The vomitus may contain partially digested food residue from meals ingested days before.

Because of the prevalence and severity of nausea and vomiting in gastroparesis, antiemetic agents commonly are prescribed. In data on 416 patients from the Gastroparesis Consortium, antiemetics were used similarly with idiopathic disease (61%) and gastroparesis from type 1 (70%) and type 2 (66%) diabetes.[12] However, symptom improvements are not different between gastroparetics who take versus do not take antiemetic drugs over 48 weeks of care.[9] Although not specifically investigated, this suggests that antiemetics provide no more than modest benefits to gastroparetics referred to centers specializing in motility disorders.

Antiemetic drugs acting on several receptor subtypes have been developed for clinical conditions with nausea and vomiting (**Table 2**). Histamine H_1 antagonists (eg, promethazine, meclizine, dimenhydrinate) are useful for vomiting in conditions with activation of the vestibular system (motion sickness, labyrinthitis), uremia, and postoperative settings. Side effects of antihistamines include sedation and mouth dryness. Nonsedating newer antihistamines (astemizole, cetirizine, fexofenadine) are less effective antiemetics. Muscarinic M_1 antagonists given orally or as transdermal patches (scopolamine) also are best characterized in labyrinthine conditions, including motion sickness, and can elicit side effects including sedation, dryness of the eyes and mouth, constipation, urinary retention, and headaches. Dopamine D_2 antagonists in the phenothiazine (eg, prochlorperazine) and butyrophenone (eg, droperidol, haloperidol) classes exert beneficial effects with vomiting from acute gastroenteritis, medication and cancer chemotherapy, radiation therapy, and surgery. Therapy with dopamine antagonists may cause sleep disturbances, mood changes, anxiety, and movement disorders, and gynecomastia, galactorrhea, or menstrual irregularities from drug-induced hyperprolactinemia. Some agents with antidopaminergic activity also evoke antihistaminic and antimuscarinic side effects. Serotonin 5-hydroxytryptamine-3 (5-HT_3) antagonists (eg, ondansetron, granisetron, dolasetron, palonosetron) can be swallowed, dissolved within the mouth, administered intravenously, or applied transdermally. 5-HT_3 antagonists are effective for prophylaxis of emesis and postoperative vomiting induced by chemotherapy and radiotherapy but also have been used

Table 1
Gastroparesis patient-reported symptom predominance

Predominant Symptom Subscale	Predominant Symptom	Individual Symptom (N)	Individual Symptom (%)	Symptom Subscale (N)	Symptom Subscale (%)
Abdominal pain/discomfort	Upper abdominal pain	27	7	81	21
	Abdominal pain location not specified	42	11		
	Lower abdominal pain	6	2		
	Upper abdominal discomfort	2	0.5		
	Abdominal discomfort location not specified	2	0.5		
	Lower abdominal discomfort	2	0.5		
Nausea/vomiting	Nausea	135	34	172	44
	Vomiting	36	9		
	Retching	1	0.3		
Postprandial fullness/early satiety	Stomach fullness	26	7	47	12
	Not able to finish normal-sized meal	8	2		
	Feeling excessively full after meals	8	2		
	Loss of appetite	5	1		
Bloating/distention	Bloating	26	7	27	7
	Stomach or belly visibly larger	1	0.3		
Esophageal symptoms	Heartburn during the day	1	0.3	32	8
	Heartburn, did not specify day vs when lying down	5	1		
	Feeling of discomfort inside chest during day	1	0.3		
	Feeling of discomfort inside chest, did not specify day vs lying down	4	1		
	Regurgitation or reflux during day	4	1		
	Regurgitation or reflux lying down	3	1		
	Regurgitation or reflux, did not specify day vs lying down	12	3		
	Bitter, acid, or sour taste in mouth	2	0.5		
Bowel habit abnormalities	Constipation	18	5	33	8
	Diarrhea	15	4		
Miscellaneous	No symptom specified	1	0.3	1	0.3

From Hasler WL, Wilson LA, Parkman HP, et al. Factors related to abdominal pain in gastroparesis: contrast to patients with predominant nausea and vomiting. Neurogastroenterol Motil 2013;25:433; with permission.

Table 2
Antiemetic medications and gastroparesis

Medication Class	Examples	Published Data in Gastroparesis
Histamine H_1 antagonist	Dimenhydrinate Meclizine Promethazine	None
Muscarinic (cholinergic) M_1 antagonist	Scopolamine	None
Dopamine D_2 antagonist	Prochlorperazine Trimethobenzamide	1 case report (thiethylperazine)
Serotonin 5-HT_3 antagonist	Ondansetron Granisetron Dolasetron	1 case report (intraperitoneal ondansetron) 1 case series (36 patients, granisetron)
Neurokinin NK_1 antagonist	Aprepitant	2 case reports
Cannabinoid CB_1 agonist	Dronabinol	None

Abbreviation: 5-HT, 5-hydroxytryptamine.

for bulimia nervosa, emesis caused by hepatic or renal disease, and nausea with human immunodeficiency virus infection.[13] In contrast, 5-HT_3 antagonists offer only limited benefits to prevent nausea instead of vomiting. 5-HT_3 antagonist use is complicated by constipation, headaches, increased liver chemistries, and cardiac rhythm disturbances secondary to QTc interval prolongation. Neurokinin -1 receptor subtype (NK_1) antagonists show potent antiemetic effects for chemotherapy-induced nausea and vomiting, postoperative nausea and vomiting, and motion sickness given orally (aprepitant) or intravenously (fosaprepitant).[13] Unlike 5-HT_3 antagonists, NK_1 antagonists are effective at reducing nausea as well as vomiting. Side effects of these agents include bowel habit changes, anorexia, and singultus. Cannabinoid-1 receptor subtype (CB1) agonists (eg, dronabinol) are approved for preventing chemotherapy-induced vomiting but side effects include sedation, euphoria, impaired cognition, and rarely syncope and hallucinations in the elderly. A cannabinoid hyperemesis syndrome mimicking cyclic vomiting syndrome occurs with long-standing use of large amounts of cannabis, but this condition has not been reported with prescription agents like dronabinol.[14]

Case reports and series have suggested the utility of selected antiemetic agents for treating gastroparesis. The dopamine D_2 antagonist thiethylperazine produced symptom benefits in 1 diabetic with gastroparesis.[15] In a 32-year-old type 1 diabetic gastroparetic on continuous cycling peritoneal dialysis, long-term intraperitoneal administration of the 5-HT_3 antagonist ondansetron in the dialysate greatly reduced nausea and vomiting without adverse effects.[16] A recent open-label study of a transdermal patch that delivers 3.1 mg per 24 hours of the 5-HT_3 antagonist granisetron for 7 days was performed in 36 patients with gastroparesis and nausea and vomiting unresponsive to standard antiemetics (**Fig. 1**).[17] On therapy, 18 patients reported symptoms that were somewhat better or moderately better, whereas 15 remained the same, 2 worsened, and 1 discontinued therapy because of poor adhesive adherence to the skin. Side effects included constipation (4 cases), rash (3 patients), and headache (2 individuals). Two cases describing antiemetic benefits of the NK_1 antagonist aprepitant in gastroparesis have been published. In the first, a 31-year-old type 1 diabetic with vomiting refractory to cyclizine, haloperidol, metoclopramide, erythromycin, and pyloric botulinum toxin injection experienced 4 months free of nausea

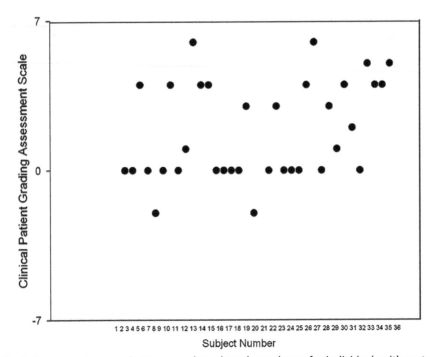

Fig. 1. Responses to a granisetron transdermal patch are shown for individuals with gastroparesis as measured by the Clinical Patient Grading Assessment Scale, ranging from −7 (completely worse) to 0 (no change) to +7 (completely better). Approximately half the patients reported being somewhat to moderately better on therapy. (*From* Simmons K, Parkman HP. Granisetron transdermal system improves refractory nausea and vomiting in gastroparesis. Dig Dis Sci 2014;59:1233; with permission.)

and vomiting on daily aprepitant.[18] In the second case, a 41-year-old woman with idiopathic gastroparesis with vomiting unresponsive to metoclopramide, ondansetron, and promethazine reported significant reductions in symptoms over 2 months on aprepitant before the therapy was withdrawn because of cost.[19] A 4-week placebo-controlled phase 3 trial assessing aprepitant efficacy in patients with chronic nausea and vomiting of presumed gastric origin is being conducted by the Gastroparesis Consortium.

Other prescription pharmaceuticals show antiemetic activity. Corticosteroids and benzodiazepines are frequently included as components of antiemetic programs to prevent delayed chemotherapy-induced emesis or postoperative vomiting. Mechanisms of their antivomiting effects are poorly characterized.

Analgesic and Neuromodulatory Medications

Gastroparesis often presents with symptoms other than nausea and vomiting. Single-center studies report abdominal pain prevalences in gastroparesis ranging from 42% to 89%.[11,20,21] In a report from the Gastroparesis Consortium, upper abdominal pain and discomfort were predominant in 21% of patients (see **Table 1**). Case series have described pain location (epigastric in 36%–43%), timing (postprandial in 24%–80%; nocturnal in 80%), frequency (daily in 43%; weekly in 38%; intermittent in 24%–62%), and characteristics (burning, vague, crampy, sharp, pressure).[20,21] Investigators observe more severe vomiting in diabetics with gastroparesis, whereas pain may be more prominent in idiopathic patients.[10,11] Two-thirds of gastroparetics note

GCSI pain scores of 3 to 5, indicating moderate to very severe intensity, which is associated with impaired quality of life and increased depression and anxiety.[11] The pathophysiology of gastroparesis pain is poorly understood. Most studies, including from the Gastroparesis Consortium, show no relation of pain to gastric emptying.[11,20,21] In diabetics, pain severity does not correlate with neuropathic complications or glycemic control. Twelve percent of gastroparetics report predominant postprandial fullness, early satiety, or anorexia, whereas 7% note bloating or visible distention as their main symptom (see **Table 1**).[11] Extragastric symptoms dominate, with 16% reporting predominance of esophageal symptoms (including heartburn, chest discomfort, regurgitation, or a sour taste in the throat) or bowel habit disturbances.

Because of the prominence of symptoms other than nausea and vomiting, it is reasonable to consider other medication classes that might be beneficial in gastroparesis. Analgesic drugs would be most useful for pain or discomfort. Neuromodulatory agents that act by blunting visceral perception or altering proximal gastric function might also be effective for epigastric pain, but could show utility for fullness, nausea, and vomiting. In data from the Gastroparesis Consortium, 43% of idiopathic patients were taking opiate medications on initial evaluation, compared with 46% of type 1 and 48% of type 2 diabetics with gastroparesis.[12] Higher percentages of patients who reported predominant pain or discomfort expressed opiate use versus those with predominant nausea or vomiting (60% vs 40%).[11] Sixteen percent of idiopathic gastroparetics were on neuropathic pain modulators (duloxetine, gabapentin, pregabalin) versus 27% and 29% of type 1 and 2 diabetics. Use of antidepressants in other classes was reported by 33% to 38%; however, this categorization was not subdivided among agents with versus without analgesic effects.

Prokinetics produce inconsistent reductions in gastroparesis pain, thus agents with analgesic actions often are empirically prescribed.[22] Nonsteroidal antiinflammatory drugs show some beneficial effects on gastric myoelectric function in older studies, but can induce mucosal ulceration or impair renal function. Although often given, opioid agonists retard gastric, small intestinal, and colonic transit and elicit nausea and vomiting.[12,23] In data from the Gastroparesis Consortium, antiemetic agent use was more prevalent among patients with higher abdominal pain scores, perhaps from induction of nausea by the pain or from the opiates prescribed for the pain.[11] Some experts advocate use of weaker opiates like tramadol and tapentadol or longer-acting medications, such as methadone or transdermal fentanyl, to minimize these effects.[23]

Neuromodulatory medications in several classes reduce perception of gastric stimulation or enhance fundic accommodation to meal ingestion (**Table 3**). Many actions relate to modification of serotonergic nerve function in the gut. Tricyclic antidepressants are norepinephrine and serotonin reuptake inhibitors with variable inhibition of dopamine reuptake. In experimental models, tricyclic agents reduce gut sensitivity to mechanical and electrical stimulation.[24] Likewise, prolonged dosing of selective serotonin reuptake inhibitors reduces perception of gut distention, possibly from receptor desensitization to continued serotonin exposure.[25] Other serotonin receptor subtypes represent potential neuromodulatory targets. The 5-HT$_{1A}$ partial agonist buspirone decreases fundic tone, whereas the 5-HT$_{1B/1D/1P}$ agonist sumatriptan augments gastric accommodation and blunts perception of distention in functional dyspepsia.[26]

Because of actions on gastric sensorimotor function, tricyclic medications were thought to have promise in gastroparesis. These drugs showed efficacy in initial uncontrolled reports in related conditions. In a small study in functional dyspepsia, amitriptyline reduced symptoms without altering perception of gastric distention.[27]

Table 3
Neuromodulatory medications and gastroparesis

Medications	Mechanisms of Action	Published Data in Gastroparesis
Tricyclic antidepressants (nortriptyline, amitriptyline, desipramine)	Norepinephrine reuptake inhibition with variable serotonin (and dopamine) reuptake inhibition	Case series in diabetics with nausea and vomiting (29% with delayed emptying) Controlled trial in idiopathic gastroparesis
Mirtazapine	Indirect CNS 5-HT$_{1A}$ agonism, 5-HT$_2$ antagonism, 5-HT$_{2c}$ inverse agonism, 5-HT$_3$ antagonism, alpha-2 antagonism, H$_1$ inverse agonism	Several case reports Preliminary controlled trial in functional dyspepsia
Olanzapine	5-HT$_2$ inverse agonism, 5-HT$_3$ antagonism, M$_1$ antagonism, M$_3$ antagonism, D$_2$ antagonism, H$_1$ inverse agonism	None
Buspirone	5-HT$_1$ partial agonist, presynaptic D$_2$ antagonist, alpha-1 partial agonist	Controlled trial in functional dyspepsia

Abbreviation: CNS, central nervous system.

Tricyclic antidepressants also reduce functional vomiting in retrospective reports.[28] In a follow-up analysis of 24 diabetics with refractory nausea and vomiting, tricyclics at median doses of 50 mg reduced symptoms in 88% and abolished them in nearly one-third.[29] Twenty-nine percent of patients showed delayed gastric emptying. Taken together, these observations suggested potential utility of tricyclics to reduce nausea, vomiting, and pain in gastroparesis.

In the most comprehensive assessment of the utility of neuromodulatory therapy for gastroparesis published to date, investigators from the 7 centers of the Gastroparesis Consortium tested benefits of the tricyclic agent nortriptyline versus placebo in a cohort of patients with idiopathic gastroparesis.[30] One-hundred and thirty patients with symptoms for longer than or equal to 6 months, overall GCSI scores greater than or equal to 21 (mean $\geq$2.33 for 9 symptoms), and delayed emptying (>10% 4-hour retention and/or >60% 2-hour retention) were randomized to nortriptyline or placebo in a 15-week trial. Nortriptyline dosing escalated from 10 mg for 3 weeks, 25 mg for 3 weeks, 50 mg for 3 weeks, and 75 mg at bedtime for 6 weeks if tolerated. Dosage reductions were permitted for medication side effects. The mean baseline GCSI symptom scores were 3.8 for nausea, 3.9 for early satiety, 3.7 for bloating, and 3.4 for upper abdominal pain/discomfort. Sixty-five percent of patients on nortriptyline tolerated the 75 mg dose, 11% reached 50 mg, 11% achieved 25%, and 14% were only able to take 10 mg nightly. A strict primary outcome was set: greater than or equal to 50% reduction in overall GCSI scores on 2 consecutive assessments compared with baseline values. Using this measure, improvements on nortriptyline (23%; 95% confidence interval [CI], 14%–35%) and placebo (21%; 95% CI, 12%–34%) were not different (relative risk of improvement, 1.06; 95% CI, 0.56–2.00; P = .86). On assessing secondary outcomes, GCSI loss of appetite scores improved more on nortriptyline (-1.6; 95% CI, -2.1 to -1.1) versus placebo (-0.9; 95% CI, -1.4 to -0.5; P = .03). Other secondary measures favoring nortriptyline therapy included GCSI inability to finish a meal scores, Gastrointestinal Symptom Rating Scale abdominal pain scores, and overall symptom relief scores on the Clinical Global Patient

Impression survey. Trends to greater increases in body mass index were observed with nortriptyline (0.5 kg/m^2; 95% CI, 0.1–0.8) versus placebo (0.0 kg/m^2; 95% CI, −0.3 to 0.3; $P = .06$). However, other important GCSI symptom subscores, especially nausea and vomiting, showed no differential improvement on nortriptyline (**Fig. 2**). Treatment was stopped more frequently with nortriptyline (29%; 95% CI, 19%–42%) than placebo (9%; 95% CI, 3%–19%; $P = .007$). Five serious adverse events were reported with nortriptyline compared with 1 with placebo. Despite the few positive findings on secondary data analysis, the overall negative trial findings raise doubts about the utility of this neuromodulator class in treating idiopathic gastroparesis.

Another antidepressant, mirtazapine, has been considered as a potential neuromodulatory therapy for gastroparesis. Mirtazapine exerts a complex interaction with several receptors, including indirect central nervous system 5-HT$_{1A}$ agonism, 5-HT$_2$ antagonism, 5-HT$_{2C}$ inverse agonism, 5-HT$_3$ antagonism, alpha-2 antagonism, and H$_1$ inverse agonism.[31] Several case reports have observed gastroparesis symptom reductions with open-label mirtazapine. In an initial report, mirtazapine 15 mg decreased emesis and allowed discontinuation of metoclopramide and lorazepam for 3 months in a 27-year-old diabetic with gastroparesis.[32] Likewise, 3 months of mirtazapine 15 mg nightly reduced nausea and vomiting and promoted adequate oral

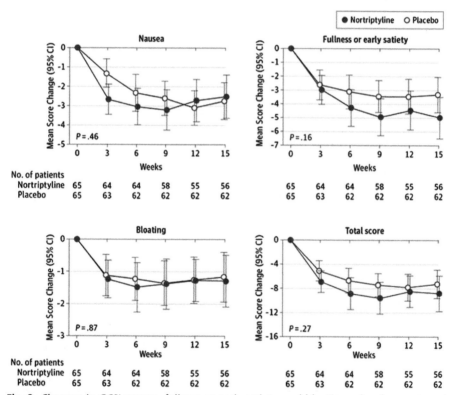

Fig. 2. Changes in GCSI nausea, fullness or early satiety, and bloating subscale scores, and total GCSI scores are shown for nortriptyline versus placebo over 15 weeks. There were no differences in individual or overall symptoms on nortriptyline and placebo (all $P =$ nonsignificant). (*From* Parkman HP, Van Natta ML, Abell TL, et al. Effect of nortriptyline on symptoms of idiopathic gastroparesis: the NORIG randomized clinical trial. JAMA 2013;310:2646; with permission.)

intake in a 52-year-old man with postsurgical gastroparesis.[33] Mirtazapine 30 mg similarly evoked significant antiemetic actions with associated weight gain and improved oral intake in a 34-year-old woman with postinfectious gastroparesis.[34] Mirtazapine has not been investigated in gastroparesis in a controlled fashion, but a preliminary study was reported for functional dyspepsia.[35] Thirty-four functional dyspeptics with greater than or equal to 10% loss of body weight were given mirtazapine 15 mg nightly versus placebo for 8 weeks. Compared with baseline, mirtazapine reduced overall symptoms (on a 24-point scale) from 10.9 ± 0.9 to 7.5 ± 1.1 ($P = .02$), whereas placebo did not produce statistical benefits. Reductions in early satiety and weight increases were better on mirtazapine than placebo. If confirmed, these observations warrant controlled testing in gastroparesis. The mechanisms of mirtazapine on gastric sensorimotor function remain uncertain. Mirtazapine accelerated gastric emptying in healthy dogs and in a canine model of delayed emptying induced by rectal distention.[36] Such prokinetic effects have not been proved in gastroparesis, although mirtazapine reduced gastric residuals during gastrostomy feedings in an 87-year-old diabetic with gastroparesis.[37] Another antidepressant agent with antiemetic effects, olanzapine, acts via $5\text{-}HT_2$ inverse agonism, $5\text{-}HT_3$ antagonism, M_1 antagonism, M_3 antagonism, D_2 antagonism, and H_1 inverse agonism.[38] This agent has efficacy in chemotherapy-induced emesis, but has not been investigated in gastroparesis.

Agents that enhance meal-induced fundic accommodation have been proposed to treat functional dyspepsia and gastroparesis, especially with prominent symptoms related to satiation. Compared with placebo, the $5\text{-}HT_{1A}$ partial agonist buspirone enhances gastric relaxation to nutrient ingestion (229 ± 28 mL vs 141 ± 32 mL) and leads to greater reductions in postprandial fullness, early satiety, and bloating in functional dyspeptics (**Fig. 3**).[39] This agent has no prokinetic action to accelerate solid gastric emptying; buspirone retards emptying of liquids. A placebo-controlled trial of another $5\text{-}HT_{1A}$ agonist, tandospirone, similarly observed decreases in overall symptoms and upper abdominal pain in functional dyspepsia.[40] No controlled investigations have been performed on $5\text{-}HT_{1A}$ agonists in gastroparesis.

Pharmaceuticals in other classes show neuromodulatory effects to reduce pain and discomfort in nongastrointestinal disorders. Medications like gabapentin and pregabalin are prescribed to patients with gastroparesis for symptoms other than nausea and vomiting, but no uncontrolled or controlled trials have assessed their efficacy in this condition.[21,22]

Potential Drug Toxicity

Use of several gastroparesis therapies is limited by side effects and safety concerns in some patients. Many antiemetic, analgesic, and neuromodulatory drugs elicit prominent gastric emptying delays, including M_1 antagonists, some H_1 and D_2 antagonists with overlapping anticholinergic actions, CB_1 agonists, opiates, and tricyclic antidepressants. D_2 antagonists that act centrally may induce a range of movement disorders, including tardive dyskinesia. In 2009, the US Food and Drug Administration issued a black box warning detailing this complication of metoclopramide therapy when given at high doses or for prolonged periods (>18 months), most often in women or individuals more than 70 years old.[41] Because of this concern, metoclopramide prescription rates have decreased from 70% of all gastroparetics before the warning to 24% in 2013.[42] The other prominent safety concern that has been a focus of attention is medication induction of dangerous cardiac rhythm disturbances such as torsades de pointes, most often with electrocardiographic QTc interval prolongation (>450 milliseconds in men, >470 milliseconds in women). This complication has been associated with prokinetics currently in use worldwide (domperidone) or withdrawn except

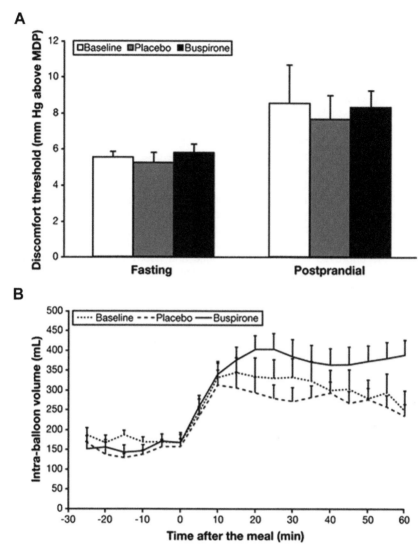

Fig. 3. The effects of the 5-HT$_{1A}$ agonist buspirone are shown on gastric sensitivity to distention (*A*) and gastric accommodation after eating (*B*) in patients with functional dyspepsia. Buspirone had no effect on sensation but enhanced meal-induced gastric relaxation. (*From* Tack J, Janssen P, Masaoka T, et al. Efficacy of buspirone, a fundus-relaxing drug, in patients with functional dyspepsia. Clin Gastroenterol Hepatol 2012;10:1243; with permission.)

in regulated patient-assistance programs (cisapride). QTc prolongation also has been attributed to other antiemetic and neuromodulatory drugs used for gastroparesis, including 5-HT$_3$ receptor antagonists and tricyclic antidepressants.[43] Although increases in sudden cardiac death have been reported, no similar black box warnings have been issued for these medications. Consideration has been advocated for surveillance monitoring of electrolytes and electrocardiographic testing in selected clinical settings during use of some of these drugs.

SUMMARY/DISCUSSION

Antiemetic, analgesic, and neuromodulatory agents commonly are used to manage nausea, vomiting, pain, discomfort, and other symptoms of gastroparesis. Despite their theoretic benefits, evidence for utility of antiemetic drugs has been limited to a few case reports. The recent publication of a case series using short-term transdermal granisetron, a 5-HT$_3$ antagonist, in open-label fashion supports conduct of more controlled trials of antiemetics in gastroparesis. An ongoing placebo-controlled trial of the NK$_1$ antagonist aprepitant in patients with gastroparesis symptoms will provide new information on such benefits. Opiate analgesics are often taken for pain control, but caution should be exercised because this drug class can exacerbate nausea and vomiting and retard gastric emptying. Like antiemetics, support for neuromodulatory agents has been restricted to individual gastroparesis cases. However, negative findings from a meticulously conducted placebo-controlled trial of the tricyclic antidepressant nortriptyline in patients with idiopathic gastroparesis dampen enthusiasm for this type of therapy. Investigations of other neuromodulators are proceeding for treating conditions related to gastroparesis. In addition, the unproved benefits of antiemetic and neuromodulatory gastroparesis treatments must be weighed against potential adverse outcomes that recently have focused on neurologic and cardiac toxicities.

REFERENCES

1. Pasricha PJ, Colvin R, Yates K, et al. Characteristics of patients with chronic un-explained nausea and vomiting and normal gastric emptying. Clin Gastroenterol Hepatol 2011;9:567–76.
2. Delgado-Aros S, Camilleri M, Cremonini F, et al. Contributions of gastric volumes and gastric emptying to meal size and postmeal symptoms in functional dyspepsia. Gastroenterology 2004;127:1685–94.
3. Karamanolis G, Caenepeel P, Arts J, et al. Determinants of symptom pattern in idiopathic severely delayed gastric emptying: gastric emptying rate or proximal stomach dysfunction? Gut 2007;56:29–36.
4. Karamanolis G, Caenepeel P, Arts J, et al. Association of the predominant symptom with clinical characteristics and pathophysiological mechanisms in functional dyspepsia. Gastroenterology 2006;130:296–303.
5. Schade RR, Dugas MC, Lhotsky DM, et al. Effect of metoclopramide on gastric liquid emptying in patients with diabetic gastroparesis. Dig Dis Sci 1985;30:10–5.
6. Maganti K, Onyemere K, Jones MP. Oral erythromycin and symptomatic relief of gastroparesis: a systematic review. Am J Gastroenterol 2003;98:259–63.
7. Revicki DA, Rentz AM, Dubois D, et al. Development and validation of a patient-assessed gastroparesis symptom severity measure: the Gastroparesis Cardinal Symptom Index. Aliment Pharmacol Ther 2003;18:141–50.
8. Revicki DA, Camilleri M, Kuo B, et al. Evaluating symptom outcomes in gastroparesis clinical trials: validity and responsiveness of the Gastroparesis Cardinal Symptom Index—Daily Diary (GCSI-DD). Neurogastroenterol Motil 2012;24:456–63.
9. Pasricha PJ, Nguyen LA, Snape WJ, et al. Changes in quality of life and symptoms in a large cohort of patients with gastroparesis followed prospectively for 48 weeks [abstract]. Gastroenterology 2010;138:1069.
10. Cherian D, Parkman HP. Nausea and vomiting in diabetic and idiopathic gastroparesis. Neurogastroenterol Motil 2012;24:217–22.

11. Hasler WL, Wilson LA, Parkman HP, et al. Factors related to abdominal pain in gastroparesis: contrast to patients with predominant nausea and vomiting. Neurogastroenterol Motil 2013;25:427–38.

12. Parkman HP, Yates K, Hasler WL, et al. Similarities and differences between diabetic and idiopathic gastroparesis. Clin Gastroenterol Hepatol 2011;9:1056–64.

13. Navavi RM. Management of chemotherapy-induced nausea and vomiting: focus on newer agents and new uses for older agents. Drugs 2013;73:249–62.

14. Galli JA, Sawaya RA, Friedenberg FK. Cannabinoid hyperemesis syndrome. Curr Drug Abuse Rev 2011;4:241–9.

15. Lossos IS, Mevorach D, Oren R. Thiethylperazine treatment of gastroparesis diabeticorum. Ann Pharmacother 1992;26:1016.

16. Amin K, Bastani B. Intraperitoneal ondansetron hydrochloride for intractable nausea and vomiting due to diabetic gastroparesis in a patient on peritoneal dialysis. Perit Dial Int 2002;22:539–40.

17. Simmons K, Parkman HP. Granisetron transdermal system improves refractory nausea and vomiting in gastroparesis. Dig Dis Sci 2014;59:1231–4.

18. Chong K, Dharariya K. A case of severe, refractory diabetic gastroparesis managed by prolonged use of aprepitant. Nat Rev Endocrinol 2009;5:285–8.

19. Fahler J, Wall GC, Leman BI. Gastroparesis-associated refractory nausea treated with aprepitant. Ann Pharmacother 2012;46:e38.

20. Cherian D, Sachdeva P, Fisher RS, et al. Abdominal pain is a frequent symptom of gastroparesis. Clin Gastroenterol Hepatol 2010;8:676–81.

21. Bielefeldt K, Raza N, Zickmund SL. Different faces of gastroparesis. World J Gastroenterol 2009;15:6052–60.

22. Anaparthy R, Pehlivanov N, Grady J, et al. Gastroparesis and gastroparesis-like syndrome: response to therapy and its predictors. Dig Dis Sci 2009;54:1003–10.

23. Maurer AH, Krevsky B, Knight LC, et al. Opioid and opioid-like drug effects on whole-gut transit measured by scintigraphy. J Nucl Med 1996;37:818–22.

24. Peghini PL, Katz PO, Castell DO. Imipramine decreases oesophageal pain perception in human male volunteers. Gut 1998;42:807–13.

25. Coates MD, Johnson AC, Greenwood-Van Meerveld B, et al. Effects of serotonin transporter inhibition on gastrointestinal motility and colonic sensitivity in the mouse. Neurogastroenterol Motil 2006;18:464–71.

26. Tack J, Vanden Berghe P, Coulie B, et al. Sumatriptan is an agonist at 5-HT1P receptors on myenteric neurons in the guinea pig gastric antrum. Neurogastroenterol Motil 2007;19:39–46.

27. Mertz H, Fass R, Kodner A, et al. Effect of amitriptyline on symptoms, sleep, and visceral perception in patients with functional dyspepsia. Am J Gastroenterol 1998;93:160–5.

28. Prakash C, Lustman PJ, Freedland KE, et al. Tricyclic antidepressants for functional nausea and vomiting: clinical outcome in 37 patients. Dig Dis Sci 1998; 43:1951–6.

29. Sawhney MS, Prakash C, Lustman PJ, et al. Tricyclic antidepressants for chronic vomiting in diabetic patients. Dig Dis Sci 2007;52:418–24.

30. Parkman HP, Van Natta ML, Abell TL, et al. Effect of nortriptyline on symptoms of idiopathic gastroparesis: the NORIG randomized clinical trial. JAMA 2013;310:2640–9.

31. Fernández J, Alonso JM, Andrés JI, et al. Discovery of new tetracyclic tetrahydrofuran derivatives as potential broad-spectrum psychotropic agents. J Med Chem 2005;48:1709–12.

32. Kim SW, Shin IS, Kim JM, et al. Mirtazapine for severe gastroparesis unresponsive to conventional prokinetic treatment. Psychosomatics 2006;47:440–2.

33. Johnstone M, Buddhdev P, Peter M, et al. Mirtazapine: a solution for postoperative gastroparesis? BMJ Case Rep 2009. http://dx.doi.org/10.1136/bcr.02.2009.1579.

34. Kundu S, Rogal S, Alam A, et al. Rapid improvement in post-infectious gastroparesis symptoms with mirtazapine. World J Gastroenterol 2014;20:6671–4.

35. Ly HG, Carbone F, Holvoet L, et al. Mirtazapine improves early satiation, nutrient intake, weight recovery and quality of life in functional dyspepsia with weight loss: a double-blind, randomized, placebo-controlled pilot study (abstract). Gastroenterology 2013;144:161.

36. Yin J, Song J, Lei Y, et al. Prokinetic effects of mirtazapine on gastrointestinal transit. Am J Physiol Gastrointest Liver Physiol 2014;306:G796–801.

37. Gooden JY, Takahashi PY. Mirtazapine treatment of diabetic gastroparesis as a novel method to reduce tube-feed residual: a case report. J Med Case Rep 2013;7:38.

38. Kaneishi K, Kawabata M, Morita T. Olanzapine for the relief of nausea in patients with advanced cancer and incomplete bowel obstruction. J Pain Symptom Manage 2012;44:604–7.

39. Tack J, Janssen P, Masaoka T, et al. Efficacy of buspirone, a fundus-relaxing drug, in patients with functional dyspepsia. Clin Gastroenterol Hepatol 2012;10:1239–45.

40. Miwa H, Nagahara A, Tominaga K, et al. Efficacy of the 5-HT$_{1A}$ agonist tandospirone citrate in improving symptoms of patients with functional dyspepsia: a randomized controlled trial. Am J Gastroenterol 2009;104:2779–87.

41. Lee A, Kuo B. Metoclopramide in the treatment of diabetic gastroparesis. Expert Rev Endocrinol Metab 2010;5:653–62.

42. Ehrenpreis ED, Deepak P, Sifuentes H, et al. The metoclopramide black box warning for tardive dyskinesia: effect on clinical practice, adverse event reporting, and prescription drug lawsuits. Am J Gastroenterol 2013;108:866–72.

43. Keller GA, Ponte ML, Di Girolamo G. Other drugs acting on nervous system associated with QT-interval prolongation. Curr Drug Saf 2010;5:105–11.

Pyloric Sphincter Therapy

Botulinum Toxin, Stents, and Pyloromyotomy

 CrossMark

John O. Clarke, MD[a], William J. Snape Jr, MD[b],*

KEYWORDS

- Pyloric stent • Botulinum toxin • Pyloroplasty • Pyloromyotomy • Gastroparesis
- Impedance planimetry

KEY POINTS

- A subset of patients with gastroparesis may have pyloric dysfunction.
- Pyloric dysfunction has traditionally been assessed via manometry; however, several promising new technologies, especially wireless capsule motility and impedance planimetry, may make assessment of pyloric function more practical and help better define patients who may respond to targeted intervention.
- Botulinum toxin for gastroparesis has been controversial, and 2 randomized controlled trials do not show benefit; however, both trials were small and the patients studied were not stratified based on pyloric physiology.
- Transpyloric stent placement, endoscopic pyloromyotomy, and surgical pyloroplasty are promising treatment options for select patients; however, more data are needed regarding safety, long-term durability, and applicability.

INTRODUCTION

Gastroparesis is a syndrome characterized by delayed gastric emptying with associated symptoms, including nausea, vomiting, early satiety, bloating, and abdominal pain.[1,2] Although the diagnosis is established by objective measurement of gastric emptying, symptoms can vary significantly among affected individuals and the syndrome itself is heterogeneous. Normal gastric emptying is a complex series of events that requires appropriate function and coordination of multiple interrelated processes, including the smooth muscle of the gut, interstitial cells of Cajal, afferent and efferent neurons, and the sympathetic and parasympathetic nervous systems. Problems with any of these components can lead to impaired emptying and associated symptoms.

[a] Division of Gastroenterology & Hepatology, Johns Hopkins University, 1830 East Monument Street, Room 425, Baltimore, MD 21205, USA; [b] Neurogastroenterology and Motility, California Pacific Medical Center, 2340 Clay Street, Room 210, San Francisco, CA 94115, USA
* Corresponding author.
E-mail address: snapew@sutterhealth.org

Gastroenterol Clin N Am 44 (2015) 127–136
http://dx.doi.org/10.1016/j.gtc.2014.11.010
0889-8553/15/$ – see front matter © 2015 Elsevier Inc. All rights reserved.

Gastroparesis is a functional disorder with a common set of symptoms but likely multiple different pathways by which those symptoms can be achieved.

Multiple mechanisms are thought to be responsible for gastroparesis symptoms in affected individuals. The proposed causes include problems with fundic accommodation, gastric arrhythmia, impaired contractile ability, abnormalities of the small bowel with resultant aberrant gastric feedback, vagal injury/neuropathy, and pyloric dysfunction, with many affected patients potentially having multiple causes.[3] Pyloric dysfunction in particular has received significant attention and may be a significant contributor to symptom pathogenesis in a portion of affected patients with gastroparesis. This dysfunction can consist of pyloric restriction or pylorospasm and may offer the potential for localized therapy for a select subset of patients with gastroparesis.

DIAGNOSTIC EVALUATION

There are multiple modalities by which pyloric function can be assessed but no true gold standard, as the pylorus has multiple properties that can be assessed independently and may be associated with symptom pathogenesis.[4] In routine clinical practice, barium fluoroscopy and endoscopy are the two methods of evaluation most commonly performed. Fluoroscopy can suggest a functional obstruction at the pylorus,[5,6] but interpretation is often subjective and varies across institutions. Likewise, endoscopy may suggest restriction or spasm at the pylorus, but interpretation is subjective and depends on multiple factors, such as the degree of insufflation, that are impossible to standardize in clinical practice. Scintigraphy is currently viewed as the gold standard with regard to gastric emptying but offers scant data with regard to pyloric function.

When objective data are desired to further evaluate pyloric function, the traditional method of evaluation has been antroduodenal or pyloric manometry (ADM). This evaluation involves placement of a manometry catheter, via either endoscopy or fluoroscopy, which traverses the pylorus and enters the proximal small bowel. This study allows measurement of pyloric pressure and coordination. Dooley and colleagues[7] initially evaluated the pyloric pressure in 1985 with a seminal paper, following the next year by Mearin, Camilleri, and Malagelada.[8] Mearin and colleague[8] evaluated 24 patients with diabetes with nausea/vomiting versus 12 healthy controls and found that patients with symptoms were significantly more likely to have prolonged pyloric pressurization and more intense contraction, which they termed *pylorospasm*. Since that publication, manometry has been viewed as the most reliable way to measure pyloric pressures. However, it is not widely available, is limited to tertiary medical centers, is invasive and time consuming, and is associated with frequent catheter migration. The pylorus in particular is challenging to visualize because the length of the sphincter is relatively short (2 cm), migration of the catheter is common, and the sensors are widely spaced apart. Desipio and colleagues[9] from Temple University attempted to eliminate this issue by using a high-resolution ADM catheter. They recruited 12 subjects and were able to place the catheter successfully in 10. Normative data were obtained for pyloric width, basal pressure, and contractile pressure. An abstract published described the squeeze pressure in symptomatic patients, but data with regard to high-resolution ADM data in symptomatic patients are limited.[10] Also, the cost of high-resolution manometry catheters and the high likelihood that sensors could be damaged in the course of endoscopic placement discourage routine clinical usage at this point in time.

Recently, there have been several new developments that have suggested novel methods by which pyloric function could be assessed. The wireless motility capsule (SmartPill, Given Imaging, Israel) is a wireless, ingestible medical device that measures pH, pressure, and temperature throughout the gastrointestinal tract and was approved by the Food and Drug Administration for evaluation of gastric emptying in 2006. As opposed to manometry, this device is mobile and not fixed in space. Most data to date evaluating the wireless motility capsule have used gastric transit time for evaluation of gastric function,[11–14] although limited data also exist with regard to gastric pressure amplitude and contractile frequency.[15] In one intriguing abstract that has not yet been published in manuscript form, Roland and colleagues[16] attempted to measure intrapyloric pressures via the wireless motility capsule and suggested that this measurement seemed to predict scintigraphic meal emptying. At present, the jury is still out as to whether the wireless motility capsule can reliably isolate and measure pyloric pressure; however, if the technique of measuring intrapyloric pressure can be standardized and normative data can be obtained, then it is possible that this device may make measurement of pyloric pressure more practical in clinical practice.

Recently, the Endolumenal Functional Lumen Imaging Probe (EndoFLIP; EndoFlip, Crospon, Ireland) was developed and presents a novel method to assess pyloric function. This device uses impedance planimetry to record cross-sectional area and minimum diameter of any hollow structure. By combining that information with intraballoon pressure and volume measurements, it is possible to measure distensibility and compliance of any sphincter. This device was approved by the Food and Drug Administration in 2010 but has only recently entered routine clinical practice. Most of the data to date using this technology from the gastrointestinal standpoint involve measurement of the esophagogastric junction for patients with achalasia[17,18] or measurement of esophageal distensibility in affected patients with eosinophilic esophagitis.[19–21] However, recently, this technology has also been applied to measurement of pyloric sphincter distensibility. Two abstracts were published on this topic at Digestive Disease Week 2014[22,23] and another at the Federation of Neurogastroenterology and Motility,[24] which suggests that this information may be of clinical utility. Research is rapidly emerging regarding impedance planimetry and gastric distention, and it is hoped that peer-reviewed published information will be available soon to guide decision making.

In summary, although several techniques exist by which pyloric function can be assessed, there are little validated data to reliably guide pyloric evaluation. Endoscopy and barium are usually the first steps in clinical practice but are plagued by subjectivity and lack of clear objective criteria to distinguish abnormality. Antroduodenal/pyloric manometry is considered the reference standard but is limited by invasiveness, space between sensors, catheter migration, and lack of clear normative data. Wireless motility capsule and impedance planimetry are both emerging technologies that seem quite promising; however, most of these data with regard to pyloric function specifically are only available in abstract form, and normative data to guide clinical management have not yet been established.

THERAPY

Despite the difficulty in assessing pyloric function, there has been great interest in therapy aimed at decreasing pylorospasm or disrupting the integrity of the pyloric sphincter. This interest has been largely driven by the limited options available to treat gastroparesis and the significant impairment in quality of life that these patients experience. To date, there has been no evidence that medical or dietary therapy alone makes a difference in pyloric function; therapeutic attempts have been entirely endoscopic or surgical. Currently, there are 4 main approaches that have been explored: endoscopic botulinum toxin injection, transpyloric channel stent placement, surgical pyloromyotomy, and most recently endoscopic pyloromyotomy.

Botulinum Toxin

Botulinum toxin is a neurotoxic protein that binds to presynaptic cholinergic receptors and inhibits acetylcholine release, leading to muscle relaxation.[25] This neurotoxic protein was initially used in the gastrointestinal tract for treatment of achalasia by Pasricha and colleagues[26] approximately 20 years ago. Since that point, it has been used in numerous other gastrointestinal conditions, including esophageal spasm, anal fissures, and constipation. Given the observation that pyloric pressures were sometimes elevated on antroduodenal manometry, a supposition of pyloric spasm, and the relatively safety of botulinum toxin injection in the gastrointestinal system, it was hypothesized that botulinum toxin injection to the pyloric sphincter may potentially relieve pylorospasm, decrease outflow obstruction, and improve gastric emptying in patients with gastroparesis.

Sharma and colleagues[27] presented the first report of intrapyloric botulinum toxin injection for a patient with gastroparesis in 1998 in abstract form at the annual meeting of the American College of Gastroenterology. This initial report was followed in 2002 by 3 manuscripts by other investigators evaluating intrapyloric botulinum toxin injection for patients with delayed gastric emptying. Ezzeddine and colleagues[28] reported on injection of botulinum toxin in 6 patients with refractory symptoms in the context of diabetic gastroparesis. They reported a 55% improvement in symptoms and 52% improvement in gastric emptying after injection and these patients were followed for a total of 6 weeks. Lacy and colleagues[29] reported on injection of botulinum toxin to 3 patients with refractory symptoms in the context of diabetic gastroparesis and objective abnormalities on antroduodenal manometry and scintigraphy. All 3 patients reported clinical improvement, although radiographic improvement was not universal. Finally, Miller and colleagues[30] from Temple University reported on the use of intrapyloric botulinum toxin injection for patients with idiopathic gastroparesis with refractory symptoms and reported improvement in their pilot study in both symptoms and gastric emptying.

Subsequent open-label and retrospective studies followed over the next few years, all of which showed improvement in symptoms and improvement in gastric emptying when measured.[31–33] These data led to 2 randomized, double-blind, placebo-controlled trials. The first was performed by Arts and colleagues[34] from Leuven University in Belgium. They evaluated 23 patients with gastroparesis (19 idiopathic) in crossover fashion. The patients received either 100 units of botulinum toxin or saline on the first endoscopy and then received the second option on a subsequent endoscopy 4 weeks later. Symptom scores and gastric emptying were evaluated at the beginning of the protocol and then 4 weeks after each injection. The patients reported improvement in symptoms and had objective improvement in gastric emptying after receiving both saline injection and botulinum toxin; however, there was no statistically significant difference between saline and botulinum toxin. The second study was performed by Friedenberg and colleagues[35] at Temple University. In their study, 32 patients with gastroparesis were randomized to receive either placebo (saline injection) or botulinum toxin (200 units). At a 1-month follow-up, 37.5% randomized to botulinum toxin achieved improvement as defined by the study, as compared with 56.3% of those patients randomized to placebo. Both groups were also noted to have improvement in objective gastric emptying, without significant difference between the two. These studies did not take into account the possible normal pyloric pressure in approximately 50% of the patients with gastroparesis.[10]

Although the publication of 2 randomized trials showing no benefit for botulinum toxin injection as compared with placebo would seem to be a death blow to the use of botulinum toxin for gastroparesis in clinical practice, other data have been published since that point that suggest that botulinum toxin may improve symptoms in a defined clinical subset. In the largest series published to date and the most intriguing, investigators in Michigan evaluated a retrospective series of 179 patients with gastroparesis who received botulinum toxin injection between 2001 and 2007, with 87 patients of the group receiving 307 follow-up injections. There was a decrease in symptoms 1 to 4 months after injection in 51.4% of patients. When higher doses of botulinum toxin were used, then that percentage increased, with 76.7% of patients reporting improvement after a dose of 200 units. Of those patients who responded to an initial injection and underwent further therapy, 73.4% also responded to a second injection. Other factors that predicted response included female gender, age less than 50 years, and a nondiabetic, nonsurgical cause.[36]

A systematic review published in 2010 evaluated this issue and concluded after review of 15 reports that "there is no evidence to recommend botulinum toxin injection for the treatment of gastroparesis."[37] This finding was highlighted in the recent American College of Gastroenterology's clinical guideline on the management of gastroparesis where they gave a strong recommendation with a high level of evidence that "intrapyloric injection of botulinum toxin is not recommended for patients with gastroparesis based on randomized controlled trials," with the caveat that "there is a need for further study in patients with documented 'pylorospasm'."[2] In practice, however, botulinum toxin injection is still performed at many centers (including the authors' center) for refractory patients with gastroparesis who have not responded to conventional therapy and in whom pyloric dysfunction is suspected; although it is not routine and the data from randomized trials are discouraging, there may be subgroups that benefit, and it is important to recognize that both the published randomized trials had small sample sizes. The authors echo the recommendation of the American College of Gastroenterology's clinical guideline that there is a need for a further study in carefully identified patients with suspected pylorospasm.

Transpyloric Stent Placement

Given the limited data to suggest that distention or disruption of the pylorus can result in symptomatic improvement in patients with refractory symptoms related to gastroparesis, investigators at Johns Hopkins recently hypothesized that transpyloric endoscopic stent placement may improve symptoms in refractory patients with suspected pyloric dysfunction.[38] Three cases were presented wherein a double-layered, full-covered, self-expandable metallic stent was placed through the endoscope and positioned across the pylorus, with improvement in gastric emptying and symptoms in all 3 patients. This presentation was followed by a brief report presented in abstract form only of open-label stent placement in 17 patients with refractory symptoms, with symptom improvement in 14 patients (82%) and radiographic improvement in all patients who underwent follow-up imaging. However, stent migration was a concern and long-term durability was not assessed.[39] The investigators hypothesized that transpyloric stent placement may play a potential role as salvage therapy in patients suspected to have pyloric dysfunction with documented gastroparesis and refractory symptoms; however, further data are required to evaluate efficacy, durability, and safety. A prospective pilot study is planned; but at present, the role of this technique remains unclear until more data are available. Moreover, if benefit is proven in prospective studies, the role of the transpyloric stent will need to be defined as it could potentially serve as both therapy and as a diagnostic test/bridge before pyloromyotomy.

Surgical Pyloroplasty

Surgical pyloroplasty has been used as a gastric drainage procedure after elective vagotomy and in response to mechanical obstruction for the past 4 decades.[40] However, reports of surgical pyloroplasty for gastroparesis are limited. Recently, Hibbard and investigators[41] from the Oregon Clinic presented their retrospective review of 28 patients (21 idiopathic, 7 diabetic) who underwent minimally invasive pyloroplasty alone as the treatment of gastroparesis between 2007 and 2010. The operation was performed entirely laparoscopically (Heineke-Mikulicz pyloroplasty) in 26 patients. In 2 patients, a transoral endoscopic circular stapled pyloroplasty with laparoscopic assistance was used. The investigators reported a significant reduction in prokinetic use, from 89% to 14%. Gastric emptying was assessed via scintigraphy and measured via half-time. This time decreased from 320 minutes to 112 minutes and normalized in 71% of patients. Finally, symptoms improved significantly at 1-month and 3-month intervals. Overall, 83% of patients reported improvement at the 1-month follow-up.[41]

This study was followed by several additional reports suggesting a benefit with surgical intervention directed toward pyloric disruption. Sarosiek and colleagues[42] from Texas Tech University evaluated the addition of surgical pyloroplasty to gastric electrical stimulation for patients with symptomatic gastroparesis undergoing surgical intervention. In their study, 49 patients underwent placement of a gastric electrical stimulator and 26 of those patients also received a surgical pyloroplasty. When the patients who received both a gastric electrical stimulator and pyloroplasty were compared with the control group that received only the gastric electrical stimulator, the gastric emptying time was substantially accelerated (64% improvement vs 7% improvement). Symptoms improved in both groups. Toro and colleagues[43] from Emory University presented their data on laparoscopic surgical pyloroplasty (hand-sewn Heineke-Mikulicz configuration) from 2006 through 2013. Of the 50 patients who underwent surgical intervention, 34 (68%) had prior foregut surgery and 32 (64%) underwent concomitant procedures along with pyloroplasty. Postoperative symptom improvement was reported in 82%. The gastric emptying time was measured by scintigraphy and recorded via half-time. This time decreased from 180 minutes to 60 minutes postoperatively. The readmission rate was 14%, but no patients required conversion to an open procedure or had reported intraoperative complications. Finally, Datta and investigators[44] from the University of Pennsylvania recently reported on their experience with rescue pyloroplasty for the treatment of delayed gastric emptying after esophagectomy. They also performed a Heineke-Mikulicz pyloroplasty and reported on 13 patients who had refractory symptoms despite medical therapy. In addition, before surgery, these patients had undergone 3.4 ± 1.0 endoscopic balloon dilatations and 7 patients (54%) received intrapyloric botulinum toxin injection. After pyloroplasty, nausea, vomiting, bloating, prokinetic use, and parenteral/enteral nutrition dependence decreased. Nine of the 13 patients were identified as pyloroplasty treatment successes.[44]

Putting this information together, there does seem to be decent data to suggest that surgical pyloroplasty can accelerate gastric emptying and improve symptoms in select patients with a suspicion for pyloric dysfunction and refractory symptoms, with the 2 largest studies to date reporting clinical improvement in 82% and 83% of patients, respectively. However, to date, there are no randomized trials evaluating surgical pyloroplasty for delayed gastric emptying; most of the published literature seems to focus on gastroparesis related to an underlying postsurgical cause. Although promising, more data are needed.

Endoscopic Pyloromyotomy

Given recent advancements in submucosal endoscopic dissection techniques, endoscopic myotomy has now become possible. Kawai and colleagues[45] evaluated the feasibility and reported the first animal experiments evaluating endoscopic pyloromyotomy in 8 pigs in 2012. The first human report was from Khashab and colleagues[46] at Johns Hopkins in late 2013. They reported on a single patient with diabetic gastroparesis with multiple hospitalizations related to refractory nausea and vomiting. She underwent placement of a transpyloric stent with resolution of symptoms, but her symptoms recurred several weeks afterward in the context of stent migration. She refused surgical intervention, and after much discussion the decision was made to proceed with endoscopic pyloromyotomy. There were no procedural complications, and the patient was discharged home after 48 hours. At the 12-week follow-up, her symptoms were markedly improved. Postprocedure imaging showed delayed gastric emptying; however, a preprocedure comparison was not available, as she had been vomiting too profusely to tolerate gastric scintigraphy. This initial report was followed by a second report evaluating endoscopic pyloromyotomy in a 38-year-old woman with postsurgical gastroparesis from Chaves and colleagues[47] from Brazil in early 2014 and by a third report in a 54-year-old woman with postesophagectomy gastroparesis from Chung and colleagues[48] in France.

Most recently, Shlomovitz and colleagues[49] from Oregon reported on their experience with 7 patients (4 idiopathic, 2 postsurgical, 1 normal gastric emptying). Technical success was reported in all 7 with no immediate procedural complications, although one patient had a gastrointestinal bleed 2 weeks after the procedure and required endoscopic clipping of a pyloric channel ulcer and one patient developed a hospital-acquired pneumonia. All of the patients also underwent concomitant procedures and, because of this, 6 procedures were performed under laparoscopic guidance (with the seventh procedure being purely endoscopic). Three-month follow-up gastric emptying studies were available for 5 of 7 patients at the time of publication and showed normalization of gastric emptying in 4 of 5 patients (80%) at 4 hours. Six of 7 patients reported significant improvement in symptoms. The lone nonresponder underwent laparoscopic pyloroplasty, which also failed to significantly improve her symptoms.

At present, endoscopic pyloromyotomy seems to be in its infancy; however, given the rapid expansion of per-oral endoscopic myotomy for achalasia and the similar technical skills required, one can assume that this will become more feasible and more widely available in upcoming years. Further data, preferably prospective and controlled, are needed to show efficacy, safety, and durability.

SUMMARY

Gastroparesis is defined by the presence of symptoms in the context of delayed gastric emptying; however, it is clear that multiple mechanisms are likely involved and that there are likely distinct clinical subgroups that may respond more optimally to tailored therapy. Scintigraphy is an imperfect test with loose correlation between gastric emptying, symptoms, and therapeutic response. Pyloric dysfunction may play a role in a subset of patients with gastroparesis. In the past, the diagnosis of pyloric dysfunction was limited because of the technical limitations of pyloric manometry and lack of widespread availability of this technology. However, with the increasing use of high-resolution manometry, the wireless motility capsule, and impedance planimetry, the armamentarium of pyloric evaluation has significantly changed; there may now be the potential to evaluate the pylorus in a manner not previously possible. On the other side of the equation, treatment of pyloric dysfunction has become more robust. Although the use of botulinum toxin is controversial and has not shown a benefit in randomized trials, transpyloric stent placement and pyloroplasty (laparoscopic and endoscopic) are emerging options with good preliminary data.

It is an exciting time for investigators of gastroparesis, and the next steps from the angle of pyloric dysfunction seem clear. Prospective studies need to be done evaluating the diagnostic technologies detailed earlier in well-defined clinical cohorts who are followed prospectively long-term. Therapeutic trials need to be done evaluating the new treatment options for pyloric dysfunction in a prospective randomized controlled fashion. Ideally, the patients entering these trials should also have a thorough pyloric diagnostic evaluation to determine whether any distinct clinical subgroups can be identified who preferentially derive treatment from these modalities. The developments that we have seen in the last few years are very exciting, but they are just a harbinger of what is to come.

REFERENCES

1. Camilleri M. Clinical practice. Diabetic gastroparesis. N Engl J Med 2007;356:820–9.
2. Camilleri M, Parkman HP, Shafi MA, et al. Clinical guideline: management of gastroparesis. Am J Gastroenterol 2013;108:18–37 [quiz: 38].
3. Camilleri M, Bharucha AE, Farrugia G. Epidemiology, mechanisms, and management of diabetic gastroparesis. Clin Gastroenterol Hepatol 2011;9:5–12 [quiz: e7].
4. Ramkumar D, Schulze KS. The pylorus. Neurogastroenterol Motil 2005;17(Suppl 1):22–30.
5. Levin AA, Levine MS, Rubesin SE, et al. An 8-year review of barium studies in the diagnosis of gastroparesis. Clin Radiol 2008;63:407–14.
6. Tougas G, Anvari M, Dent J, et al. Relation of pyloric motility to pyloric opening and closure in healthy subjects. Gut 1992;33:466–71.
7. Dooley CP, Reznick JB, Valenzuela JE. A continuous manometric study of the human pylorus. Gastroenterology 1985;89:821–6.
8. Mearin F, Camilleri M, Malagelada JR. Pyloric dysfunction in diabetics with recurrent nausea and vomiting. Gastroenterology 1986;90:1919–25.
9. Desipio J, Friedenberg FK, Korimilli A, et al. High-resolution solid-state manometry of the antropyloroduodenal region. Neurogastroenterol Motil 2007;19:188–95.
10. Nguyen LB, Parker S, Bunker S, et al. Continuous pyloric manometry determines the effectiveness of botulinum toxin injection in patients with gastroparesis. Gastroenterology 2005;123:A384.
11. Kuo B, McCallum RW, Koch KL, et al. Comparison of gastric emptying of a nondigestible capsule to a radio-labelled meal in healthy and gastroparetic subjects. Aliment Pharmacol Ther 2008;27:186–96.
12. Rao SS, Camilleri M, Hasler WL, et al. Evaluation of gastrointestinal transit in clinical practice: position paper of the American and European Neurogastroenterology and Motility Societies. Neurogastroenterol Motil 2011;23:8–23.
13. Sarosiek I, Selover KH, Katz LA, et al. The assessment of regional gut transit times in healthy controls and patients with gastroparesis using wireless motility technology. Aliment Pharmacol Ther 2010;31:313–22.
14. Stein E, Berger Z, Hutfless S, et al. Wireless motility capsule versus other diagnostic technologies for evaluating gastroparesis and constipation: a comparative effectiveness review. Report No: 13-EHC060-EF; AHRQ Comparative Effectiveness Reviews. Rockville (MD): Agency for Healthcare Research and Quality (US); 2013.
15. Kloetzer L, Chey WD, McCallum RW, et al. Motility of the antroduodenum in healthy and gastroparetics characterized by wireless motility capsule. Neurogastroenterol Motil 2010;22:527–33 e117.

16. Roland BC, Ciarleglio M, Raja S, et al. Intrapyloric pressures are elevated in gastroparesis and reliably predict scintigraphic meal emptying. Gastroenterology 2014;146:S609.
17. Kwiatek MA, Pandolfino JE, Hirano I, et al. Esophagogastric junction distensibility assessed with an endoscopic functional luminal imaging probe (EndoFLIP). Gastrointest Endosc 2010;72:272–8.
18. Lin Z, Nicodeme F, Boris L, et al. Regional variation in distal esophagus distensibility assessed using the functional luminal imaging probe (FLIP). Neurogastroenterol Motil 2013;25:e765–71.
19. Kwiatek MA, Hirano I, Kahrilas PJ, et al. Mechanical properties of the esophagus in eosinophilic esophagitis. Gastroenterology 2011;140:82–90.
20. Lin Z, Kahrilas PJ, Xiao Y, et al. Functional luminal imaging probe topography: an improved method for characterizing esophageal distensibility in eosinophilic esophagitis. Therap Adv Gastroenterol 2013;6:97–107.
21. Nicodeme F, Hirano I, Chen J, et al. Esophageal distensibility as a measure of disease severity in patients with eosinophilic esophagitis. Clin Gastroenterol Hepatol 2013;11:1101–7.e1.
22. Gourcerol G, Tissier F, Touchais O, et al. Measure of fasting pyloric pressure and compliance in gastroparesis. Gastroenterology 2014;146:S261.
23. Malik ZA, Sankineni A, Parkman HP. EndoFlip as a novel method to evaluate the pyloric sphincter in patients with gastroparesis. Gastroenterology 2014;146:S611.
24. Snape WJ, Lin M, Shaw R. The importance of the pylorus in patients with gastroparesis evaluated by concurrent intraluminal pressure and EndoFLIP. Neurogastroenterol Motil 2014;26(Suppl 1):A208.
25. Vittal H, Pasricha PF. Botulinum toxin for gastrointestinal disorders: therapy and mechanisms. Neurotox Res 2006;9:149–59.
26. Pasricha PJ, Ravich WJ, Kalloo AN. Botulinum toxin for achalasia. Lancet 1993; 341:244–5.
27. Sharma VK, Glassman SB, Howden CW, et al. Pyloric intraspincteric botulinum toxin in a patient with diabetic gastroparesis. Am J Gastroenterol 1998;93:456.
28. Ezzeddine D, Jit R, Katz N, et al. Pyloric injection of botulinum toxin for treatment of diabetic gastroparesis. Gastrointest Endosc 2002;55:920–3.
29. Lacy BE, Zayat EN, Crowell MD, et al. Botulinum toxin for the treatment of gastroparesis: a preliminary report. Am J Gastroenterol 2002;97:1548–52.
30. Miller LS, Szych GA, Kantor SB, et al. Treatment of idiopathic gastroparesis with injection of botulinum toxin into the pyloric sphincter muscle. Am J Gastroenterol 2002;97:1653–60.
31. Lacy BE, Crowell MD, Schettler-Duncan A, et al. The treatment of diabetic gastroparesis with botulinum toxin injection of the pylorus. Diabetes Care 2004;27: 2341–7.
32. Bromer MQ, Friedenberg F, Miller LS, et al. Endoscopic pyloric injection of botulinum toxin A for the treatment of refractory gastroparesis. Gastrointest Endosc 2005;61:833–9.
33. Arts J, van Gool S, Caenepeel P, et al. Influence of intrapyloric botulinum toxin injection on gastric emptying and meal-related symptoms in gastroparesis patients. Aliment Pharmacol Ther 2006;24:661–7.
34. Arts J, Holvoet L, Caenepeel P, et al. Clinical trial: a randomized-controlled crossover study of intrapyloric injection of botulinum toxin in gastroparesis. Aliment Pharmacol Ther 2007;26:1251–8.
35. Friedenberg FK, Palit A, Parkman HP, et al. Botulinum toxin A for the treatment of delayed gastric emptying. Am J Gastroenterol 2008;103:416–23.

36. Coleski R, Anderson MA, Hasler WL. Factors associated with symptom response to pyloric injection of botulinum toxin in a large series of gastroparesis patients. Dig Dis Sci 2009;54:2634–42.

37. Bai Y, Xu MJ, Yang X, et al. A systematic review on intrapyloric botulinum toxin injection for gastroparesis. Digestion 2010;81:27–34.

38. Clarke JO, Sharaiha RZ, Kord Valeshabad A, et al. Through-the-scope transpyloric stent placement improves symptoms and gastric emptying in patients with gastroparesis. Endoscopy 2013;45(Suppl 2 UCTN):E189–90.

39. Saxena P, Clarke JO, Penas I, et al. Refractory gastroparesis can be successfully managed with transpyloric stent placement and fixation. Gastroenterology 2014; 146:S771.

40. Binswanger RO, Aeberhard P, Walther M, et al. Effect of pyloroplasty on gastric emptying: long term results as obtained with a labelled test meal 14–43 months after operation. Br J Surg 1978;65:27–9.

41. Hibbard ML, Dunst CM, Swanstrom LL. Laparoscopic and endoscopic pyloroplasty for gastroparesis results in sustained symptom improvement. J Gastrointest Surg 2011;15:1513–9.

42. Sarosiek I, Forster J, Lin Z, et al. The addition of pyloroplasty as a new surgical approach to enhance effectiveness of gastric electrical stimulation therapy in patients with gastroparesis. Neurogastroenterol Motil 2013;25:134–134.e80.

43. Toro JP, Lytle NW, Patel AD, et al. Efficacy of laparoscopic pyloroplasty for the treatment of gastroparesis. J Am Coll Surg 2014;218:652–60.

44. Datta J, Williams NN, Conway RG, et al. Rescue pyloroplasty for refractory delayed gastric emptying following esophagectomy. Surgery 2014;156:290–7.

45. Kawai M, Peretta S, Burckhardt O, et al. Endoscopic pyloromyotomy: a new concept of minimally invasive surgery for pyloric stenosis. Endoscopy 2012;44: 169–73.

46. Khashab MA, Stein E, Clarke JO, et al. Gastric peroral endoscopic myotomy for refractory gastroparesis: first human endoscopic pyloromyotomy (with video). Gastrointest Endosc 2013;78:764–8.

47. Chaves DM, de Moura EG, Mestieri LH, et al. Endoscopic pyloromyotomy via a gastric submucosal tunnel dissection for the treatment of gastroparesis after surgical vagal lesion. Gastrointest Endosc 2014;80:164.

48. Chung H, Dallemagne B, Perretta S, et al. Endoscopic pyloromyotomy for post-esophagectomy gastric outlet obstruction. Endoscopy 2014;46(Suppl 1 UCTN): E345–6.

49. Shlomovitz E, Pescarus R, Cassera MA, et al. Early human experience with peroral endoscopic pyloromyotomy (POP). Surg Endosc 2014. [Epub ahead of print].

Complementary and Alternative Medicine for Gastroparesis

Linda A. Lee, MD[a],*, Jiande Chen, PhD[b], Jieyun Yin, MD[c]

KEYWORDS

- Acupuncture • Gastrointestinal motility • STW 5 • Rikkunshito • Marijuana

KEY POINTS

- Complementary and alternative medicine is used by a significant percentage of individuals with chronic gastrointestinal disorders.
- Acupuncture and electroacupuncture are the modalities that have been most studied with respect to their effect on visceral hypersensitivity, gastric accommodation, and gastric emptying.
- Herbal formulations, such as STW 5 and Rikkunshito, may help improve some symptoms of functional dyspepsia, but more studies are needed to understand their mechanisms of action and clinical efficacy.
- No clinical studies have yet been conducted using marijuana or cannabinoids to treat symptoms of gastroparesis, although endocannibinoids have a wide array of effects on gastrointestinal function.

Complementary and alternative medicine (CAM) is used pervasively throughout the world with a prevalence ranging from 5% to 72%.[1] Despite widespread patient interest, there is a need for health care providers to learn more about the vast array of specific practices, and to better understand why patients express interest in knowing more about them. Studies suggest that it is uncommon for most patients to abandon conventional therapy for alternative practices. For some patients with gastrointestinal (GI) disorders, CAM therapies may help provide a sense of control over their disease.[2] Patients fearing that their questions may not be well received or that their conventional care practitioner is not knowledgeable, sometimes choose not to fully disclose their

[a] Division of Gastroenterology and Hepatology, Johns Hopkins Integrative Medicine & Digestive Center, Johns Hopkins University School of Medicine, 2360 West Joppa Road, Suite 200, Lutherville, MD 20193, USA; [b] Clinical Motility Lab, Division of Gastroenterology and Hepatology, Johns Hopkins University School of Medicine, 4940 Eastern Avenue, A-505, Baltimore, MD 21224, USA; [c] Veterans Research and Education Foundation, VA Medical Center, 921 NE 13th Street, Oklahoma City, OK 73104, USA
* Corresponding author.
E-mail address: llee12@jhmi.edu

Gastroenterol Clin N Am 44 (2015) 137–150
http://dx.doi.org/10.1016/j.gtc.2014.11.011
0889-8553/15/$ – see front matter © 2015 Elsevier Inc. All rights reserved.

interest or their usage. In the United States, this issue resulted in the National Center for Complementary and Alternative Medicine to launch the "Time to Talk" campaign in 2011 to encourage patients and their providers to openly discuss complementary practices. This article is intended to help those involved in the care of those with gastroparesis understand the modalities most commonly used and discussed by patients with gastroparesis.

CAM use by patients with GI disease or symptoms is not uncommon. A multicenter survey of pediatric patients followed in a GI clinic revealed that 40% of parents of pediatric patients with GI disorders use CAM therapies, with the most important predictors being the lack of effectiveness of conventional therapy, school absenteeism, and the adverse effects of allopathic medication.[3] In a UK survey, 26% of patients with GI symptoms sought CAM therapy.[4] A survey at a single UK academic center showed the incidence of CAM use was 49.5% for inflammatory bowel disease, 50.9% for irritable bowel syndrome, 20% for general GI diseases, and 27% for controls.[5]

Studies reporting CAM use by patients with functional bowel disorders have centered primarily on those with irritable bowel syndrome. Relatively few studies exist describing the prevalence of CAM use by those with functional dyspepsia or gastroparesis. In the National Institutes of Health's Clinical Gastroparesis Research Center's registry of more than 600 patients, 22% reported using a CAM therapy at the time of initial enrollment (Lee 2014, unpublished data). Gastroparetic patients who used CAM were more likely to be women, white, college-educated, and nonsmokers. The therapies most commonly used by those in the registry were vitamins, herbal supplements, acupuncture, probiotics, and therapeutic massage (Lee 2014, unpublished data).

Several of these therapies are reviewed here with respect to gastroparesis, their proposed mechanisms of action, and results from clinical trials. Among various methods of CAM, herbal medicine and acupuncture/electroacupuncture (EA) are the only ones that have been applied in animal models of gastroparesis or impaired gastric motility. Compared with herbal medicine, relatively more reports are available in the literature studying the effects and mechanisms of acupuncture/EA on the pathophysiology of gastroparesis. In addition, a discussion of marijuana and cannabinoids also is included because of the general interest expressed by patients and family members and possible relevance to clinical care.

ACUPUNCTURE/ELECTROACUPUNCTURE

Acupuncture/EA affects impaired gastric accommodation, visceral hypersensitivity, and gastric dysmotility (gastric dysrhythmia, antral hypomotility, and delayed gastric emptying).

Electroacupuncture and Gastric Accommodation

When food enters the stomach, the proximal stomach relaxes during eating to accommodate the ingested food without producing a large increase in gastric pressure; this reflex is called gastric accommodation. Impaired gastric accommodation is commonly seen in patients with functional dyspepsia and gastroparesis.[6] Clinically, it is difficult to treat impaired gastric accommodation in patients with gastroparesis or functional dyspepsia due to coexisting condition of antral hypomotility. Treatment of impaired accommodation with muscle relaxants or adrenergic agents would worsen antral hypomotility. On the other hand, treatment of antral hypomotility often worsens impaired gastric accommodation.

In a rodent model of diabetic gastroparesis (1-time injection of streptozotocin), EA at ST36 improved gastric accommodation and the effect was blocked by naloxone.[7] In dogs, the same method of EA restored vagotomy-induced impairment in gastric accommodation but showed no effects on gastric accommodation in normal animals (**Fig. 1**).[8] In a recent clinical study, transcutaneous EA (electrical stimulation performed via electrodes placed on the acupuncture points) increased gastric accommodation in patients with functional dyspepsia, assessed by a nutrient drink test.[9]

Electroacupuncture and Gastric Slow Waves

The gastric slow wave originates in the proximal stomach and propagates distally toward the pylorus. It determines the maximum frequency and propagation direction of gastric contractions. The gastric slow wave has a low frequency of 3 cycles per minute (cpm) in humans, and 5 cpm in dogs and rats. Dysrhythmia in gastric slow waves has been linked to impaired gastric motility, such as antral hypomotility and delayed gastric emptying.[10] The effects of EA on gastric slow waves in patients with gastric motility disorders have been widely studied due to the availability of the noninvasive method of electrogastrography. Both EA and needleless transcutaneous EA have been consistently and robustly shown to improve gastric dysrhythmia.[11]

In diabetic rats, acute EA increased the percentage of normal slow waves from 55% to 69%, and the effect was blocked by naloxone.[7] In dogs, EA at ST36 was reported to reduce gastric dysrhythmia induced by duodenal distention[8] or rectal distention,[12] and the ameliorating effect was mediated via the opioid and vagal pathways. In a rodent study, the effect of EA on gastric slow waves was reported to be site-specific: EA at PC6 showed an inhibitory effect on gastric slow waves, whereas EA at ST36 enhanced gastric slow waves.[13] In rats with thermal injury, EA at ST36 improved gastric slow waves with a concurrent suppression of inflammatory cytokine, interleukin-6.[14]

Electroacupuncture and Gastric Contractions

Coordinated and distally propagated gastric contractions or peristalsis is needed to empty the stomach. Effects and mechanisms of acupuncture/EA on gastric contractions have been investigated in several species, including rats,[15–17] rabbits[18] and dogs.[8,12]

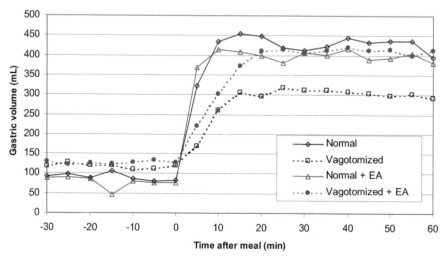

Fig. 1. Effects of EA on gastric accommodation in dogs.

In anesthetized rats, antral contractions were enhanced with acupuncturelike stimulation in the limbs but inhibited with similar stimulation in the abdomen or lower chest region[16]; the excitatory effect was mediated via the vagal pathway, whereas the inhibitory effect was through the activation of sympathetic activity.[19] In an in vitro study with diabetic rats, EA at ST36 at both low and high frequencies increased contractility of muscle strips from the gastric antrum and the effect was noted to involve the stem cell factor/c-kit pathway.[12] In an in vivo study with the measurement of gastric contractions using strain gauge, EA at ST36 was reported to exert dual effects: enhancement of gastric contractions in rats with hypomotility and inhibition of contractions in rats with hypermotility.[17]

In dogs, EA at ST36 improved antral hypomotility induced with rectal distention.[12] Regular antral contractions were measured by a manometric catheter placed in the antrum via a chronically implanted cannula in the middle of the stomach (**Fig. 2**A). Rectal distention substantially inhibited postprandial antral contractions (see **Fig. 2**B) and the effect was reversed by guanethidine (see **Fig. 2**C), suggesting a sympathetic mechanism. EA at ST36 dramatically enhanced antral contractions during rectal distention (see **Fig. 2**D) and the effect was abolished by naloxone (see **Fig. 2**E), suggesting an opioid mechanism.

Electroacupuncture and Gastric Emptying

With appropriate selection of acupoints and stimulation parameters, the prokinetic effect of EA on gastric emptying has been consistent and robust in both humans and animals[8,15,20–22] ST36 is the most commonly used acupoint for improving gastric emptying and other components of gastric motility, such antral contractions and gastric slow waves. The stimulation frequency ranges from 4 Hz to 100 Hz, with the frequencies of 20 to 40 Hz being the most prevalent. The pulse width is typically set at 0.3 to 0.5 ms, although some studies failed to mention this important parameter. The stimulation amplitude is chosen at a level tolerable by the animals, ranging from 1 to 10 mA, depending on preparation.

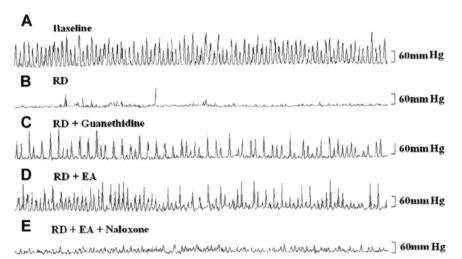

Fig. 2. Effects of EA on antral contractions in the postprandial state. (*A*) No intervention; (*B*) rectal distention (RD) was applied; (*C*) rectal distention in the presence of guanethidine; (*D*) EA at ST36 was applied during RD; (*E*) EA applied in the presence of naloxone.

Gastric emptying was accelerated with EA in normal rats,[20] rats with restrain stress,[15] rats with thermal injury,[14] and diabetic rats with gastroparesis.[7] EA at both PC6 and ST36 or ST36 alone also accelerated gastric emptying in dogs with delayed gastric emptying induced by duodenal distention[8] or rectal distention.[23] A typical example showing the effect and mechanism of EA on rectal distention–induced delay in gastric emptying is presented in **Fig. 3**.

The accelerative effect of EA on gastric emptying may be mediated via the vagal and opioid mechanisms evidenced by the assessment of vagal activity based on the spectral analysis of the heart rate variability and the blockage effect of atropine and naloxone.[8,23] Other mechanisms also have been implicated. In diabetic rats, the accelerative effect of EA at ST36 was shown to involve the rescue of the damaged networks of interstitial cells of Cajal (ICC), such as inhibition of ICC apoptosis and enhancement of ICC proliferation.[24] In rats with thermal injury, the improvement in gastric emptying with EA was noted to involve the inhibition of interleukin-6.[14] Other mechanisms reported in the literature include enhancement of blood flow,[25] activation of A delta and/or C afferent fiber,[26] and involvement of the serotonin pathway.[27]

Electroacupuncture and Visceral Hypersensitivity

The effects and mechanisms of EA on visceral hypersensitivity have been investigated in various animal models without gastroparesis. Acupuncture and EA have been most successfully applied for the treatment of pain. Therefore, in general, they are believed to exert analgesic effects on visceral pain as well.

In rats with neonatal colorectal chemical irritation, EA at ST36 reduced rectal distention–evoked abdominal electromyogram and the expression of 5HT-3 receptors in the colon.[28] In rats with visceral hypersensitivity induced by colorectal distention, EA at ST37 and ST25 improved visceral hypersensitivity assessed by the abdominal withdrawal reflexes and reduced P2X2 and P2X3 receptor expressions in the dorsal root ganglion.[29] The same method of EA also was reported to reduce the number of mucosal mast cells in the colon and the expressions of corticotropin-releasing hormone in the hypothalamus and substance P and substance P receptors in the colon of rats with irritable bowel syndrome.[30] In our own laboratory, in rats with visceral hypersensitivity established by colorectal injection of acetic acid during the neonatal stage, EA at ST36 reduced visceral hyperalgesia and reversed the enhanced excitability of colon dorsal root ganglion neurons.[31]

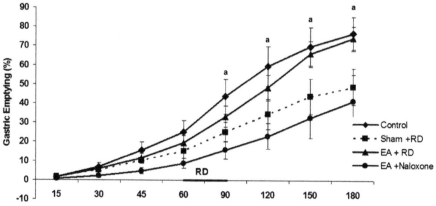

Fig. 3. Effects of EA solid gastric emptying in dogs. [a] P<.03 versus control/sham.

Clinical Studies of Acupuncture for Symptoms of Gastroparesis

Acupuncture has been used for the treatment of gastrointestinal ailments for thousands of years. Most clinical trials have focused on irritable bowel syndrome or the management of nausea and vomiting that arises postoperatively, or as the result of chemotherapy, pregnancy, or motion sickness.[32] The acupuncture point thought to be most responsible for reducing nausea and vomiting is P6 (Pericardium 6), located 3 cm proximal to the wrist between the tendons of the flexor carpi radials muscle and palmaris longus muscle. The mechanisms by which P6 stimulation results in reduced nausea and vomiting have been discussed.[32] Acupuncture also might affect gastric motor activity[8,33] or restore gastric accommodation.[34]

Although there have been several published studies and reviews on the role of acupuncture in postoperative nausea and chemotherapy-induced nausea, comparatively few randomized controlled clinical trials exist examining the effect of acupuncture for the treatment of functional dyspepsia and gastroparesis. The results of some of these trials are summarized here:

- In 15 diabetic individuals with dyspeptic symptoms, cutaneous electrogastrography showed increased percentages of normal frequency, decreased percentages of tachygastria, and increased serum pancreatic polypeptide levels during and after EA.[35] In a randomized controlled study of acupuncture delivered 5 times per week for 4 weeks in 72 patients with functional dyspepsia, significantly greater improvement was seen in the Symptom Index of Dyspepsia (SID) in those who received acupuncture versus sham acupuncture (non–acupuncture points).[36] Quality of life, measured by Nepean Dyspepsia Index (NDI), improved significantly for the acupuncture group only. In that same study, a subset of the patients underwent cerebral positron emission testing after acupuncture. The increase in NDI score was significantly related to the decrease in glycometabolism in the insula, thalamus, brainstem, anterior cingulate cortex, and hypothalamus, suggesting acupuncture has a central effect.[36]
- One of the largest randomized control studies of acupuncture for functional dyspepsia involved 720 patients randomized to 1 of 4 acupuncture treatment arms and 1 sham acupuncture arm. In addition, there was a sixth treatment arm in which patients received itopride, a prokinetic. All 4 active acupuncture arms and itopride resulted in significant improvement in the SID compared with sham acupuncture, particularly with regard to early satiety. In addition, the 4 acupuncture arms resulted in significant improvement in quality of life (NDI) compared with sham acupuncture, but itopride showed no improvement in quality of life.[37]
- Acupuncture was compared with standard promotility drugs in improving gastric emptying in a group of critically ill patients receiving enteral feeding. Delayed gastric emptying was defined as a gastric residual volume greater than 500 mL for 2 days or more. Bilateral prolonged intermittent transcutaneous electrical acupoint stimulation of acupuncture point Neiguan (P6) was delivered daily using a transcutaneous electrical nerve stimulation device for 5 days. There was no statistical difference in the types of drugs delivered to both groups of patients during the study. Acupoint stimulation significantly improved delayed gastric emptying in critically ill patients when compared with standard prokinetics.[38]
- Finally, a small, randomized single-blinded study of EA in diabetic patients with gastroparesis over 2 weeks reduced the dyspeptic symptoms of diabetic gastroparesis and accelerated solid gastric emptying.[21]

Thus, acupuncture continues to be one modality that attracts patients with chronic nausea and vomiting, early satiety, postprandial bloating, and epigastric pain. Its mechanisms of action are not yet fully understood, and it remains uncertain how frequent the acupuncture treatments should be delivered, for how long, and for what duration of each session. Because acupuncture has relatively few side effects, it seems reasonable to recommend this therapy for those individuals strongly interested in using this modality or in those who have exhausted pharmacologic attempts at managing their symptoms.

Herbal Formulations/Supplements (Including Marijuana)

STW 5 (Iberogast)

STW 5 (Iberogast; Steigerwald GmbH, Darmstadt, Germany) is an herbal formulation originating in Germany containing 9 extracts (*Iberis amara planta totalis, Chelidonii herba, Cardui mariae fructus, Melissae folium, Carvi fructus, Liquiritiae radix, Angelicae radix, Matricariae flos, Menthae piperitae folium*). Prescribed primarily to treat the symptoms of functional dyspepsia, its effects may be due to its ability to increase gastric accommodation and perhaps affect anteroduodenal motility, as shown in healthy male volunteers.[39] It does not appear to accelerate gastric emptying of solids, however.[39] STW 5 may have other effects, including modulating intestinal afferent sensitivity as shown in male Wistar rats[40] and some of its components exert antispasmolytic, prosecretory, and anti-inflammatory effects in the small intestine and colon in animal models.[41,42]

A randomized placebo-controlled trial using STW 5 in patients with functional dyspepsia for 8 weeks showed it to have a slightly better improvement in Gastrointestinal Symptom Score (GIS) compared with placebo with no difference in adverse effects.[43] Another randomized placebo double-blind study of patients with functional dyspepsia also documented improvement in the GIS in those randomized to STW 5, but no acceleration in gastric emptying in those with documented gastroparesis.[44] The lack of correlation between symptom improvement and accelerated gastric emptying is not surprising and similar to what has been observed with other therapies, such as electrical gastric stimulation.

Rikkunshito

Rikkunshito (RKT), a Kampo (Japanese herbal) medicine (also known as TJ-43 or Liu-Jun-Zi-Tang, a traditional Chinese herbal medicine), contains extracts of *Atractylodis lanceae rhizoma, Ginseng radix, Pinelliae tuber, Hoelen, Zizyphi fructus, Aurantii nobilis percarpium, Glycyrrhizae radix,* and *Zingiberis rhizoma.* RKT when instilled into the stomachs of dogs has been shown to accelerate gastric emptying and stimulate phasic contractions of the duodenum and jejunum, an effect not blocked by vagotomy.[45] In the isolated guinea pig stomach, Liu-Jun-Zi-Tang enhanced gastric adaptive relaxation induced by luminal distention, which was not seen with metoclopramide, trimebutine, or cisapride.

RKT was compared against domperidone in a randomized controlled trial of 27 patients with functional dyspepsia. After 4 weeks, there was improvement in the symptoms of both groups as measured by their Gastrointestinal Symptom Rating Scale questionnaire scores.[46] However, in a randomized controlled trial of RKT in 247 patients with functional dyspepsia, 2.5 g RKT administered 3 times daily for 8 weeks was associated with reduced symptoms of epigastric pain and postprandial fullness, but the primary end point of reduced global symptom assessment was not met.[47] In a separate randomized controlled trial of patients with proton pump inhibitor refractory gastroesophageal reflux disease (GERD) symptoms, addition of RKT significantly reduced the frequency of GERD symptoms in patients with nonerosive GERD.[48]

How RKT works is not well understood, as a study in healthy volunteers suggested that RKT does not affect esophageal motility, decrease postprandial gastroesophageal acid, nonacid reflux events, or accelerate esophageal clearance time.[49] It was reported to promote gastric adaptive relaxation in patients with functional dyspepsia.[50]

Simotang

Simotang (decoction of 4 powered drugs), one of the most commonly used Chinese herbal formulas, was administrated to chronically stressed mice daily for 7 days for the assessment of its effect on gastrointestinal motility.[51] In comparison with the placebo treatment, Simotang significantly increased gastric emptying and intestinal propulsion, increased serum motilin, and decreased the expressions of cholecystokinin-positive cells and genes in the small intestine, spinal cord, and brain.

Taraxacum officinale

Taraxacum officinale is a traditional herbal medicine commonly used for treating abdominal illness. One special preparation of *Taraxacum officinale* was found to increase gastric emptying in rats with potency comparable to cisapride.[52] In in vitro studies, it increased gastric contractions and decreased pyloric contractions, mediated by the cholinergic mechanism.[52]

Dai-kenchu-to

Dai-kenchu-to is another herbal medicine used to treat gastrointestinal diseases. Its main ingredients include Zanthoxylum fruit, ginseng root, and dried ginger rhizome. In dogs, intraluminal administration of Dai-kenchu-to was reported to induce gastric and intestinal contractions.[53] In another canine study, however, only the main ingredient, dried ginger rhizome, was noted to elicit phase contractions in the stomach and the effect was mediated through cholinergic 5HT-3 receptors.[54]

Modified Xiaoyao San

Modified Xiaoyao San (MXS, or Jiawei xiaoyao san, Jia-Wey Shiau-Yau San, called Kami shoyo san in Japanese) is a Chinese herbal formulation widely prescribed in Asia to treat gastrointestinal symptoms, such as abdominal distention, hiccups, anorexia, and dry or bitter taste in the mouth.[55] MXS is mixture of 14 herbs: *Radix bupleuri, Radix angelicae sinensis, Radix paeoniae alba, Rhizoma atractylodis macrocephalae, Poria, Rhizoma zingiberis recens, Radix glycyrrhizae, Herba menthae, Cortex moutan, Fructus gardeniae, Cortex magnoliae officinalis, Fructus aurantii, Radix puerariae,* and *Fructus jujubae.* Qin and colleagues[55] recently performed a literature review, identified 14 randomized controlled studies in which MXS was used alone or compared with a prokinetic agent, but was unable to draw a conclusion about its efficacy because all studies were of poor quality.

Banxiaxiexin decoction

Banxiaxiexin decoction (BXXD), a traditional Chinese herbal medicine containing 7 commonly used herbs (*Pinellia ternata, Radix scutellariae, Rhizoma zingiberis, Panax ginseng, Radix glycyrrhizae, Coptis chinensis,* and *Fructus jujubae*) has been used for the treatment of diabetic gastroparesis and functional dyspepsia. A recent review of the literature indicated that only small studies have so far been published, from which no definite efficacy or safety conclusions could be made.[56]

Marijuana (Cannibis sativa)

Marijuana is included in this article because of tremendous interest expressed by patients and family members, even though there are no published clinical trials on marijuana and gastroparesis. Legalization of the sales of marijuana in 20 US states, and the perception of increased access and medical endorsement, likely contributes to this interest and may result in greater use by patients with functional GI disorders. *Cannabis* has been used as an herbal remedy in many cultures for the relief of nausea and other GI complaints. *Cannabis* contains several active cannabinoids, such as its major constituent Δ9-tetrahydrocannabinol, and these vary in their pharmacologic effects and. In recent years, the components of the endocannabinoid system have been detailed in several excellent recent reviews to which the reader is directed.[57–60]

Endocannabinoids, such as anandamide and 2-arachidonylglycerol, may affect gastric acid secretion, lower esophageal relaxation, visceral hypersensitivity, intestinal motility, inflammation, and secretion and ion transport.[57] Endocannabinoids exert multiple pharmacologic effects via its primary receptors, CB1 and CB2, but also the Transient Receptor Potential Vanilloid 1 (TRPV1). Effects of cannabinoids on gut motility and visceral sensation are mediated through these receptors, which are expressed on enteric neurons as well as macrophages.[61–64] The highest density of CB1 and CB2 receptors are found in the myenteric and submucosal plexuses. Additionally, activation of TRPV1 receptors in the hippocampus and the periaqueductal gray matter may contribute to the anticonvulsant[65] and anxiolytic effects of cannabinoids,[66] respectively.

In the gut, the endocannabinoid system is modulated by the state of satiety and the presence of intestinal inflammation.[67] Food deprivation increases CB1 receptor expression in vagal afferent neurons and increases anandamide levels.[68] In rodent studies, cannabinoids slow intestinal transit.[61] They also may inhibit production of tumor necrosis factor in the setting of experimentally induced intestinal inflammation.[69]

Perhaps the greatest potential therapeutic effect for patients with gastroparesis may be the effect of cannabinoids on nausea and vomiting. Indirect activation of somatodendritic 5-HT(1A) receptors in the dorsal raphe nucleus may explain its antiemetic effects.[70] Endocannabinoids, such as anandamide, reduce emesis through CB1 or TRPV1 receptors in the brainstem to control vomiting.[71]

Endocannabinoid pathways could theoretically be affected by developing drugs that interfere with production or degradation of endocannabinoids or expression of their receptors. Most clinical trials have focused on using synthetic cannabinoids developed to treat chemotherapy-induced nausea and vomiting. The most clinically relevant studies are those using synthetic cannabinoids as opposed to the whole herb itself. There are 2 cannabinoid derivatives approved by the Food and Drug Administration, dronabinol and nabilone, for chemotherapy-induced nausea and vomiting, but these are no longer considered first-line agents, given the availability of 5HT3 antiemetics that are viewed as safer.[72]

There are no studies of cannabinoids in the treatment of symptoms associated with dyspepsia or gastroparesis. There are still many concerns about the use of cannabinoids for managing symptoms due to functional GI disorders. Furthermore, extrapolating any of the effects observed with synthetic cannabinoids to the whole herb cannot be made. There are safety concerns around marijuana, in that it could be addictive and it may be as harmful as tobacco smoking.[73] Moreover, there are now numerous case reports and series of marijuana hyperemesis syndrome occurring in daily users of marijuana. The symptoms include nausea, vomiting, a need to frequently bathe in hot water, and abdominal pain.[74,75] Cessation of marijuana smoking may improve symptoms.

REFERENCES

1. Frass M, Strassl RP, Friehs H, et al. Use and acceptance of complementary and alternative medicine among the general population and medical personnel: a systematic review. Ochsner J 2012;12(1):45–56.
2. Li FX, Verhoef MJ, Best A, et al. Why patients with inflammatory bowel disease use or do not use complementary and alternative medicine: a Canadian national survey. Can J Gastroenterol 2005;19(9):567–73.
3. Vlieger AM, Blink M, Tromp E, et al. Use of complementary and alternative medicine by pediatric patients with functional and organic gastrointestinal diseases: results from a multicenter survey. Pediatrics 2008;122(2):e446–51.
4. Langmead L, Chitnis M, Rampton DS. Use of complementary therapies by patients with IBD may indicate psychosocial distress. Inflamm Bowel Dis 2002; 8(3):174–9.
5. Kong SC, Hurlstone DP, Pocock CY, et al. The incidence of self-prescribed oral complementary and alternative medicine use by patients with gastrointestinal diseases. J Clin Gastroenterol 2005;39(2):138–41.
6. Tack J, Piessevaux H, Coulie B, et al. Role of impaired gastric accommodation to a meal in functional dyspepsia. Gastroenterology 1998;115(6):1346–52.
7. Yin J, Chen J, Chen JD. Ameliorating effects and mechanisms of electroacupuncture on gastric dysrhythmia, delayed emptying, and impaired accommodation in diabetic rats. Am J Physiol Gastrointest Liver Physiol 2010;298(4):G563–70.
8. Ouyang H, Yin J, Wang Z, et al. Electroacupuncture accelerates gastric emptying in association with changes in vagal activity. Am J Physiol Gastrointest Liver Physiol 2002;282(2):G390–6.
9. Xu F, Tan Y, Huang Z, et al. Ameliorating effect of transcutaneous electroacupuncture on impaired gastric accommodation in patients with postprandial distress syndrome -predominant functional dyspepsia: a pilot study. Evid Based Complement Alternat Med, in press.
10. Chen JD, Pan J, McCallum RW. Clinical significance of gastric myoelectrical dysrhythmias. Dig Dis 1995;13(5):275–90.
11. Yin J, Chen JD. Gastrointestinal motility disorders and acupuncture. Auton Neurosci 2010;157(1–2):31–7.
12. Chen J, Song GQ, Yin J, et al. Electroacupuncture improves impaired gastric motility and slow waves induced by rectal distension in dogs. Am J Physiol Gastrointest Liver Physiol 2008;295(3):G614–20.
13. Shiotani A, Tatewaki M, Hoshino E, et al. Effects of electroacupuncture on gastric myoelectrical activity in healthy humans. Neurogastroenterol Motil 2004;16(3): 293–8.
14. Song J, Yin J, Sallam HS, et al. Electroacupuncture improves burn-induced impairment in gastric motility mediated via the vagal mechanism in rats. Neurogastroenterol Motil 2013;25(10):807-e635.
15. Iwa M, Tateiwa M, Sakita M, et al. Anatomical evidence of regional specific effects of acupuncture on gastric motor function in rats. Auton Neurosci 2007;137(1–2): 67–76.
16. Sato A, Sato Y, Suzuki A, et al. Neural mechanisms of the reflex inhibition and excitation of gastric motility elicited by acupuncture-like stimulation in anesthetized rats. Neurosci Res 1993;18(1):53–62.
17. Tatewaki M, Harris M, Uemura K, et al. Dual effects of acupuncture on gastric motility in conscious rats. Am J Physiol Regul Integr Comp Physiol 2003;285(4): R862–72.

18. Niu WX, He GD, Liu H, et al. Effects and probable mechanisms of electroacupuncture at the Zusanli point on upper gastrointestinal motility in rabbits. J Gastroenterol Hepatol 2007;22(10):1683–9.

19. Imai K, Ariga H, Chen C, et al. Effects of electroacupuncture on gastric motility and heart rate variability in conscious rats. Auton Neurosci 2008;138(1–2):91–8.

20. Tabosa A, Yamamura Y, Forno ER, et al. A comparative study of the effects of electroacupuncture and moxibustion in the gastrointestinal motility of the rat. Dig Dis Sci 2004;49(4):602–10.

21. Wang CP, Kao CH, Chen WK, et al. A single-blinded, randomized pilot study evaluating effects of electroacupuncture in diabetic patients with symptoms suggestive of gastroparesis. J Altern Complement Med 2008;14(7):833–9.

22. Xu S, Hou X, Zha H, et al. Electroacupuncture accelerates solid gastric emptying and improves dyspeptic symptoms in patients with functional dyspepsia. Dig Dis Sci 2006;51(12):2154–9.

23. Yin J, Chen JD. Electroacupuncture improves rectal distension-induced delay in solid gastric emptying in dogs. Am J Physiol Regul Integr Comp Physiol 2011; 301(2):R465–72.

24. Chen Y, Xu JJ, Liu S, et al. Electroacupuncture at ST36 ameliorates gastric emptying and rescues networks of interstitial cells of Cajal in the stomach of diabetic rats. PLoS One 2013;8(12):e83904.

25. Lin YP, Yi SX, Yan J, et al. Effect of acupuncture at Foot-Yangming Meridian on gastric mucosal blood flow, gastric motility and brain-gut peptide. World J Gastroenterol 2007;13(15):2229–33.

26. Li YQ, Zhu B, Rong PJ, et al. Neural mechanism of acupuncture-modulated gastric motility. World J Gastroenterol 2007;13(5):709–16.

27. Sugai GC, Freire Ade O, Tabosa A, et al. Serotonin involvement in the electroacupuncture- and moxibustion-induced gastric emptying in rats. Physiol Behav 2004;82(5):855–61.

28. Chu D, Cheng P, Xiong H, et al. Electroacupuncture at ST-36 relieves visceral hypersensitivity and decreases 5-HT(3) receptor level in the colon in chronic visceral hypersensitivity rats. Int J Colorectal Dis 2011;26(5):569–74.

29. Weng Z, Wu L, Lu Y, et al. Electroacupuncture diminishes P2X2 and P2X3 purinergic receptor expression in dorsal root ganglia of rats with visceral hypersensitivity. Neural Regen Res 2013;8(9):802–8.

30. Ma XP, Tan LY, Yang Y, et al. Effect of electro-acupuncture on substance P, its receptor and corticotropin-releasing hormone in rats with irritable bowel syndrome. World J Gastroenterol 2009;15(41):5211–7.

31. Xu GY, Winston JH, Chen JD. Electroacupuncture attenuates visceral hyperalgesia and inhibits the enhanced excitability of colon specific sensory neurons in a rat model of irritable bowel syndrome. Neurogastroenterol Motil 2009;21(12): 1302-e125.

32. Streitberger K, Ezzo J, Schneider A. Acupuncture for nausea and vomiting: an update of clinical and experimental studies. Auton Neurosci 2006;129(1–2):107–17.

33. Chang CS, Chou JW, Ko CW, et al. Cutaneous electrical stimulation of acupuncture points may enhance gastric myoelectrical regularity. Digestion 2002;66(2): 106–11.

34. Ouyang H, Xing J, Chen J. Electroacupuncture restores impaired gastric accommodation in vagotomized dogs. Dig Dis Sci 2004;49(9):1418–24.

35. Chang CS, Ko CW, Wu CY, et al. Effect of electrical stimulation on acupuncture points in diabetic patients with gastric dysrhythmia: a pilot study. Digestion 2001;64(3):184–90.

36. Zeng F, Qin W, Ma T, et al. Influence of acupuncture treatment on cerebral activity in functional dyspepsia patients and its relationship with efficacy. Am J Gastroenterol 2012;107(8):1236–47.

37. Ma TT, Yu SY, Li Y, et al. Randomised clinical trial: an assessment of acupuncture on specific meridian or specific acupoint vs. sham acupuncture for treating functional dyspepsia. Aliment Pharmacol Ther 2012;35(5):552–61.

38. Pfab F, Winhard M, Nowak-Machen M, et al. Acupuncture in critically ill patients improves delayed gastric emptying: a randomized controlled trial. Anesth Analg 2011;112(1):150–5.

39. Pilichiewicz AN, Horowitz M, Russo A, et al. Effects of Iberogast on proximal gastric volume, antropyloroduodenal motility and gastric emptying in healthy men. Am J Gastroenterol 2007;102(6):1276–83.

40. Liu CY, Muller MH, Glatzle J, et al. The herbal preparation STW 5 (Iberogast) desensitizes intestinal afferents in the rat small intestine. Neurogastroenterol Motil 2004;16(6):759–64.

41. Ammon HP, Kelber O, Okpanyi SN. Spasmolytic and tonic effect of Iberogast (STW 5) in intestinal smooth muscle. Phytomedicine 2006;13(Suppl 5):67–74.

42. Krueger D, Gruber L, Buhner S, et al. The multi-herbal drug STW 5 (Iberogast) has prosecretory action in the human intestine. Neurogastroenterol Motil 2009; 21(11):1203-e110.

43. von Arnim U, Peitz U, Vinson B, et al. STW 5, a phytopharmacon for patients with functional dyspepsia: results of a multicenter, placebo-controlled double-blind study. Am J Gastroenterol 2007;102(6):1268–75.

44. Braden B, Caspary W, Borner N, et al. Clinical effects of STW 5 (Iberogast) are not based on acceleration of gastric emptying in patients with functional dyspepsia and gastroparesis. Neurogastroenterol Motil 2009;21(6):632–8 e25.

45. Yanai M, Mochiki E, Ogawa A, et al. Intragastric administration of rikkunshito stimulates upper gastrointestinal motility and gastric emptying in conscious dogs. J Gastroenterol 2013;48(5):611–9.

46. Arai M, Matsumura T, Tsuchiya N, et al. Rikkunshito improves the symptoms in patients with functional dyspepsia, accompanied by an increase in the level of plasma ghrelin. Hepatogastroenterology 2012;59(113):62–6.

47. Suzuki H, Matsuzaki J, Fukushima Y, et al. Randomized clinical trial: rikkunshito in the treatment of functional dyspepsia–a multicenter, double-blind, randomized, placebo-controlled study. Neurogastroenterol Motil 2014;26(7):950–61.

48. Tominaga K, Iwakiri R, Fujimoto K, et al. Rikkunshito improves symptoms in PPI-refractory GERD patients: a prospective, randomized, multicenter trial in Japan. J Gastroenterol 2012;47(3):284–92.

49. Morita T, Furuta K, Adachi K, et al. Effects of rikkunshito (TJ-43) on esophageal motor function and gastroesophageal reflux. J Neurogastroenterol Motil 2012;18(2):181–6.

50. Hayakawa T, Arakawa T, Kase Y, et al. Liu-Jun-Zi-Tang, a kampo medicine, promotes adaptive relaxation in isolated guinea pig stomachs. Drugs Exp Clin Res 1999;25(5):211–8.

51. Cai GX, Liu BY, Yi J, et al. Simotang enhances gastrointestinal motility, motilin and cholecystokinin expression in chronically stressed mice. World J Gastroenterol 2011;17(12):1594–9.

52. Jin YR, Jin J, Piao XX, et al. The effect of *Taraxacum officinale* on gastric emptying and smooth muscle motility in rodents. Neurogastroenterol Motil 2011;23(8):766-e333.

53. Kawasaki N, Nakada K, Nakayoshi T, et al. Effect of Dai-kenchu-to on gastrointestinal motility based on differences in the site and timing of administration. Dig Dis Sci 2007;52(10):2684–94.

54. Shibata C, Sasaki I, Naito H, et al. The herbal medicine Dai-Kenchu-Tou stimulates upper gut motility through cholinergic and 5-hydroxytryptamine 3 receptors in conscious dogs. Surgery 1999;126(5):918–24.
55. Qin F, Huang X, Zhang HM, et al. Pharmacokinetic comparison of puerarin after oral administration of Jiawei-Xiaoyao-San to healthy volunteers and patients with functional dyspepsia: influence of disease state. J Pharm Pharmacol 2009;61(1): 125–9.
56. Tian J, Li M, Liao J, et al. Chinese herbal medicine banxiaxiexin decoction treating diabetic gastroparesis: a systematic review of randomized controlled trials. Evid Based Complement Alternat Med 2013;2013:749495.
57. Izzo AA, Sharkey KA. Cannabinoids and the gut: new developments and emerging concepts. Pharmacol Ther 2010;126(1):21–38.
58. Vigna SR. Cannabinoids and the gut. Gastroenterology 2003;125(3):973–5.
59. Izzo AA, Camilleri M. Emerging role of cannabinoids in gastrointestinal and liver diseases: basic and clinical aspects. Gut 2008;57(8):1140–55.
60. Coutts AA, Izzo AA. The gastrointestinal pharmacology of cannabinoids: an update. Curr Opin Pharmacol 2004;4(6):572–9.
61. Izzo AA, Fezza F, Capasso R, et al. Cannabinoid CB1-receptor mediated regulation of gastrointestinal motility in mice in a model of intestinal inflammation. Br J Pharmacol 2001;134(3):563–70.
62. Kulkarni-Narla A, Brown DR. Localization of CB1-cannabinoid receptor immunoreactivity in the porcine enteric nervous system. Cell Tissue Res 2000;302(1): 73–80.
63. Croci T, Manara L, Aureggi G, et al. In vitro functional evidence of neuronal cannabinoid CB1 receptors in human ileum. Br J Pharmacol 1998;125(7):1393–5.
64. Burdyga G, Varro A, Dimaline R, et al. Expression of cannabinoid CB1 receptors by vagal afferent neurons: kinetics and role in influencing neurochemical phenotype. Am J Physiol Gastrointest Liver Physiol 2010;299(1):G63–9.
65. Iannotti FA, Hill CL, Leo A, et al. Nonpsychotropic plant cannabinoids, cannabidivarin (CBDV) and cannabidiol (CBD), activate and desensitize transient receptor potential vanilloid 1 (TRPV1) channels in vitro: potential for the treatment of neuronal hyperexcitability. ACS Chem Neurosci 2014;5(11):1131–41.
66. Campos AC, Guimaraes FS. Evidence for a potential role for TRPV1 receptors in the dorsolateral periaqueductal gray in the attenuation of the anxiolytic effects of cannabinoids. Prog Neuropsychopharmacol Biol Psychiatry 2009; 33(8):1517–21.
67. Izzo AA, Coutts AA. Cannabinoids and the digestive tract. Handb Exp Pharmacol 2005;(168):573–98.
68. Burdyga G, Lal S, Varro A, et al. Expression of cannabinoid CB1 receptors by vagal afferent neurons is inhibited by cholecystokinin. J Neurosci 2004;24(11): 2708–15.
69. Croci T, Landi M, Galzin AM, et al. Role of cannabinoid CB1 receptors and tumor necrosis factor-alpha in the gut and systemic anti-inflammatory activity of SR 141716 (rimonabant) in rodents. Br J Pharmacol 2003;140(1):115–22.
70. Parker LA, Rock EM, Limebeer CL. Regulation of nausea and vomiting by cannabinoids. Br J Pharmacol 2011;163(7):1411–22.
71. Sharkey KA, Cristino L, Oland LD, et al. Arvanil, anandamide and N-arachidonoyl-dopamine (NADA) inhibit emesis through cannabinoid CB1 and vanilloid TRPV1 receptors in the ferret. Eur J Neurosci 2007;25(9):2773–82.
72. Todaro B. Cannabinoids in the treatment of chemotherapy-induced nausea and vomiting. J Natl Compr Canc Netw 2012;10(4):487–92.

73. Volkow ND, Baler RD, Compton WM, et al. Adverse health effects of marijuana use. N Engl J Med 2014;370(23):2219–27.
74. Allen JH, de Moore GM, Heddle R, et al. Cannabinoid hyperemesis: cyclical hyperemesis in association with chronic cannabis abuse. Gut 2004;53(11):1566–70.
75. Simonetto DA, Oxentenko AS, Herman ML, et al. Cannabinoid hyperemesis: a case series of 98 patients. Mayo Clin Proc 2012;87(2):114–9.

Surgical Approaches to Treatment of Gastroparesis

Gastric Electrical Stimulation, Pyloroplasty, Total Gastrectomy and Enteral Feeding Tubes

Irene Sarosiek, MD[a], Brian Davis, MD[b], Evelin Eichler, MS, RD, LD[a], Richard W. McCallum, MD[a],*

KEYWORDS

- Gastric electrical stimulation • Gastroparesis • Total gastrectomy pyloroplasty
- Gastrostomy tubes • Jejunostomy tubes • Treatment

KEY POINTS

- Gastric electrical stimulation (GES) is neurostimulation; its mechanism of action is affecting central control of nausea and vomiting and enhancing vagal function.
- GES is a powerful antiemetic available for patients with refractory symptoms of nausea and vomiting from gastroparesis of idiopathic and diabetic causes.
- The need for introducing a feeding tube means that intensive medical therapies are failing, and the implantation of the GES system may be indicated at the time of surgical placement of a feeding tube.
- Because there is no acceleration of gastric emptying with GES neurostimulation by itself, a surgical pyloroplasty should accompany GES surgery to help improve the rate of gastric emptying.
- Total gastrectomy is indicated in that small subset of gastroparetic patients (<5%) when vomiting does not respond to GES in order to prevent hospitalizations and improve quality of life.

INTRODUCTION

This article discusses the surgical approaches to the treatment of gastroparesis (GP). This entails gastric electrical stimulation (GES), pyloroplasty, total gastrectomy, and the placement of gastrojejunal and jejunostomy feeding tubes.

[a] Division of Gastroenterology, Department of Internal Medicine, Paul L. Foster School of Medicine, Texas Tech University Health Sciences Center, 4800 Alberta Avenue, El Paso, TX 79905, USA; [b] Department of Surgery, Paul L. Foster School of Medicine, Texas Tech University Health Sciences Center, 4800 Alberta Avenue, El Paso, TX 79905, USA
* Corresponding author.
E-mail address: richard.mccallum@ttuhsc.edu

Gastroenterol Clin N Am 44 (2015) 151–167
http://dx.doi.org/10.1016/j.gtc.2014.11.012
0889-8553/15/$ – see front matter © 2015 Elsevier Inc. All rights reserved.

HISTORY OF GASTRIC ELECTRICAL STIMULATION

In the clinical world of treatment of severe symptoms of drug-refractory GP, there are not many pharmacologic or surgical options.[1–3] The list of available prokinetic and antiemetic agents has changed very little in the last 30 years. The same medications with their sometimes-severe side effects as well as tachyphylaxis problems provide limited choices for the growing number of gastroparetic patients around the world.[4,5]

There is a need to consider new therapeutic approaches for the 20% to 25% of the gastroparetic population, whose symptoms are not addressed by existing drugs, investigational agents, nutrition support modalities, better diabetic control, as well as lifestyle modifications.

Therefore, the pioneering thinking of surgeon Ayden Bilgutay, MD and his colleagues[6] in the early 1960s provided a new approach. The concept of gastrointestinal pacing by using intraluminal electrical stimulation was first studied in the setting of postoperative ileus. This innovating theory led to more research in a canine model in 1970,[7] laying the foundation to investigate myoelectrical activities, contractility, and finally electrical stimulation of the gastrointestinal tract in humans. The challenge of understanding how gastric peristalsis was regulated by an electrical rhythm led to identifying the pacemaker site located in the corpus along the great curvature 5 to 7 cm from the cardia.[8,9] The interstitial cells of Cajal were also identified as a network controlling the direction, velocity (rate), and frequency of gastric waves and, thus, the frequency and coordination of muscle contractions. This increasing knowledge of gastric electrophysiology inspired, in the late 1990s, a group of scientists and clinicians, such as Qian, Kelly, McCallum, Morison and Familoni, to pursue the potential therapeutic role of gastric pacing and normalization of myoelectrical dysrhythmia.[10–13]

DIFFERENT METHODS OF STIMULATION

The original concept of gastric pacing was based on similar principals to cardiac pacing, namely, strengthening of gastric slow waves and also overcoming electrical dysrhythmias. Two GES parameters have been established: (1) Long-pulse with high energy and a physiologic frequency of stimulation using single or multichannel electrodes. These parameters can entrain slow waves, reverse dysrhythmias, and, hence, accelerate gastric emptying.[10–13] (2) On the other hand, short-pulse low-energy GES at frequencies higher than physiologic is termed neurostimulation, and may alleviate gastroparetic symptoms, specifically nausea and vomiting, without a meaningful improvement in gastric emptying or changing the underlying slow-wave rhythm pattern.[14,15] Hence, the predicted outcome or goals of GES depend on the parameters of the applied stimulation (**Fig. 1**).

Gastric Pacing

Pioneering studies using antegrade stimulation with a long duration or high-energy pulse width of 10 to 600 milliseconds and maximal frequency of 4.3 cpm, thus achieving pacing parameters, have shown a complete entrainment of gastric slow waves, normalization of gastric dysrhythmia, acceleration of gastric emptying, and better control of GP symptoms in initially a dog model and now in humans.[11,16,17]

A clinical trial was reported whereby an external low-frequency and high-energy stimulation device was tested against an implantable high-frequency and low-energy gastric stimulation device.[18] The primary goals were to investigate the effects of 2-channel gastric pacing on gastric myoelectrical activity and energy consumption with the secondary intent to monitor gastric emptying and symptoms in patients with

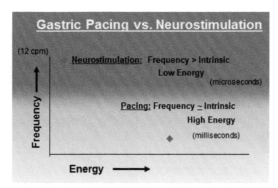

Fig. 1. The 2 GES parameters being used in clinical and animal research.

severe diabetic GP. Four pairs of temporary pacing wires were secured on the serosa of the stomach at the time of laparotomy to place the Enterra System (Medtronic, Inc, Minneapolis, MN) in 19 patients with severe GP who were not responding to standard medical therapies. Two of the pairs were for electrical stimulation and the other two for recording. Five days after surgery, the optimal pacing parameters for the entrainment of gastric slow waves in each patient were identified by serosal recordings. Two-channel gastric pacing was then initiated for 6 weeks using a newly developed external multichannel pulse generator. Key results showed that 2-channel gastric pacing at 1.1 times the intrinsic frequency entrained gastric slow waves and normalized gastric dysrhythmia by decreasing tachygastria in the fasting and postprandial state, significantly reducing GP symptoms and improving mean 4-hour gastric retention in patients with diabetic GP with an excellent safety profile. This observation was also in agreement with the results on multichannel gastric pacing previously published in both healthy and diseased canine models.[18–20]

One of the major drawbacks for single-channel gastric pacing with long pulses is that it needs high stimulation energy to entrain gastric slow waves and normalize dysrhythmias. This is explained by the fact that the stimulating electrode has to be placed in the proximal stomach to avoid reverse pacing.[20] To entrain gastric slow waves, the stimulation energy for the single-channel gastric pacing has to be high enough to ensure the stimulation pulses are propagated a distance of 20 cm or greater from the proximal stomach to the distal antrum. Therefore, multichannel GES was designed to mimic the natural propagation and characteristics of the gastric slow waves. For 2-channel gastric pacing with long pulses used in this study, each stimulation channel was responsible to entrain slow waves at a distance of 8 cm. As a result, the consumption of stimulation energy with 2-channel gastric pacing was much less than that with single-channel gastric pacing and, hence, saving battery life. This concept had already been proposed and studied in a dog model,[21] and research in this area is continuing. Currently, there are no US Food and Drug Administration (FDA)–approved long-pulse–generating implantable devices available on the market (**Fig. 2**).

Neurostimulation

The pulse width in short-pulse stimulation is a few hundred microseconds, and the frequency is 3 to 4 times higher than the physiologic rate of gastric slow waves.[22,23] Reports in dogs had shown strengthening of gastric contractions and acceleration of gastric emptying.[24,25] These findings set the stage for studies GES in humans, although these observations have not been reproducible with subsequent

A   **B**

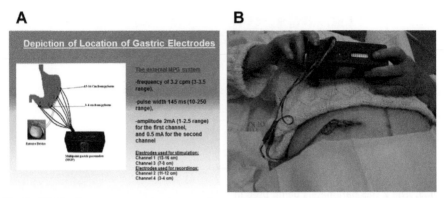

Fig. 2. (A) The Enterra neurostimulator pulse generator as well as an external gastric pacemaker unit connected to 4 pairs of electrodes on the serosa of the stomach; (B) patient with gastric pacemaker connected to external wires. MPG, multichannel pulse generator.

experiments. Investigating gastric stimulation with high-frequency/low-energy parameters, known as Enterra therapy (Medtronic, Inc, Minneapolis, MN), led to many clinical trials. The net result indicates that GES by the Enterra device does produce a significant and sustained improvement in symptoms and nutritional status in the majority of patients with intractable symptomatic GP. These results were initially based on open-label studies[11,12] and in subgroups of patients with diabetic and idiopathic GP (ID-GP).[26] The World Anti-Vomiting Electrical Stimulation Study (WAVESS) was a double-blind crossover study whereby the Enterra system was activated or shammed starting at the time of surgery.[12,14] Based on the positive results of this trial, in March of 2000, this therapy was approved by the US FDA as a humanitarian device exemption (HDE) and it is commercially available as the implantable pulse generator to treat drug-refractory nausea and vomiting secondary to diabetic or ID-GP.[27] As of December 2014, there are more than 8,000 patients implanted worldwide with Enterra therapy.

Because of the paucity of double-blind placebo-controlled data focused on Enterra therapy (GES therapy), in diabetic (DM) and ID-GP, further prospective clinical trials were conducted to evaluate the efficacy and safety of gastric neurostimulation therapy. The primary objectives were to demonstrate an improvement in weekly vomiting frequency (WVF) when the device was turned ON, relative to when the device was turned OFF, during a blinded 3-month crossover phase. The secondary goals were to demonstrate a reduction in symptom scores and to assess changes in quality of life, gastric emptying, number of days in the hospital, and body mass index in the ID-GP cohort when receiving active stimulation for up to 12 months. Unlike the WAVESS design, the double-blind randomization began after 6 weeks of open-labeled Enterra therapy (**Figs. 3** and **4**).

The first message from these trials was that the initiation of GES for 6 weeks caused a rapid and significant reduction of symptoms, which was able to be sustained despite a period of up to 3 months with the device OFF. The second important point was related to the observation that even though the double-blind 3-month crossover period showed a nonsignificant reduction in vomiting in the ON versus OFF period, at 12 months with ON stimulation continuing, there was a significant decrease in vomiting symptoms and days of hospitalizations and improvement of quality of life in patients diagnosed with severe medication-unresponsive GP of DM and ID causes.[28,29]

Since the HDE approval of Enterra therapy for diabetic and ID causes of GP, post-surgical patients with GP were subsequently added to the clinical cohort investigated

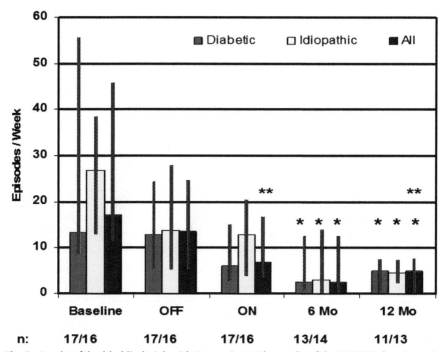

n: 17/16   17/16   17/16   13/14   11/13

Fig. 3. Results of double-blind trials with Enterra in GP. The results of the WAVESS showing a significant improvement when patients are turned ON versus OFF. Also, the reduction in nausea and vomiting was sustained over 12 months. (*From* Abell T, McCallum RW, Hocking M, et al. Gastric electrical stimulation for medically refractory gastroparesis. Gastroenterology 2003;125:421–8; with permission.)

and a trial of gastric stimulation trial was successful. This condition occurs in up to 10% of patients who undergo vagotomy, either intentional or inadvertent, mostly related to Nissen fundoplications. It has also been reported in up to 50% of patients undergoing intentional vagotomy in the setting of Billroth I and II, antral resection, and Roux-en-Y surgeries.[30]

Many investigators made serious attempts to look for any differences in the way diabetic, ID, and postvagotomy patients will respond to the gastric stimulation therapy. The longest and largest single-center report in the world to date reviewed prospectively generated data based on 10 years of experience, whereby 188 patients with GP were followed up for a mean of 56 months.[26] Overall, the clinical outcomes observed by the investigators were consistent with previous shorter-term studies reported from many centers[14,31,32] indicating that there was a >50% symptomatic improvement that can be sustained with GES therapy for as long as 10 years (**Table 1**).

One of the major findings from that study was that patients with DM and post-surgical GP had a superior (>50%) reduction in their symptom scores than patients with ID-GP (60% vs 59% vs 49%, respectively). In the DM group, the better symptom control was also reflected by a reduction in hemoglobin A1c level from 8.5% to 7.8%, which has implications for overall better morbidity and mortality in patients with DM. The improvement in severity of vomiting makes these patients better candidates for renal and/or pancreas transplant because vomiting prevents reliable absorption of immunosuppressant medications. Most of the studied patients (75%) continued to have similar degrees of delayed GE during the follow-up visits.[26] A comparison of

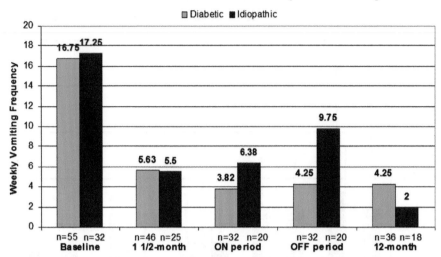

Fig. 4. The results of 2 double-blind crossover studies, one in diabetic patients and one in idiopathic patients with GP. This device was initially ON for 6 weeks. Then the double-blind crossover phase was initiated. No differences seen during 3 months ON or OFF, although a significant reduction in nausea and vomiting continued and was sustained during a further 8 months of neurostimulation. (*From* McCallum RW, Snape W, Brody F, et al. Gastric electrical stimulation with Enterra therapy improves symptoms from diabetic gastroparesis in a prospective study. Clin Gastroenterol Hepatol 2010;8:952; with permission.)

Table 1
The 10-year outcome achieved by the Enterra device on symptoms control and results of gastric emptying in gastroparetic patients. Symptoms were significantly improved in all groups (*P < 0.05) but not gastric emptying

GP Symptoms	Diabetic Gastroparetic Patients (n = 111)	Idiopathic Gastroparetic Patients (n = 41)	Postsurgical GP (n = 30)
Baseline	19.8 ± 5.0	18.6 ± 5.8	19.1 ± 3.4
Follow-up	8.7 ± 6.04*	9.7 ± 6.2*	10.9 ± 7.6*
Improvement (%)	55	47	48
>50% reduction (%)	60	49	59
Follow-up time (mo)	54	57	63
Results of Gastric Emptying			
Gastric Retention (%)	Diabetic Gastroparetic Patients (n = 75)	Idiopathic Gastroparetic Patients (n = 20)	Postsurgical GP (n = 24)
Baseline at 2 h	70.5 (53.0–86.0)!	63.0 (43.0–71.0)	80.5 (68.0–92.0)!
Follow-up at 2 h	68.0 (45.0–84.0)	60.5 (53.5–78.0)	65.0 (35.5–86.0)*
Baseline at 4 h	39.5 (21.0–68.0)!	30.5 (10.0–40.0)	48.0 (33.0–73.0)!
Follow-up at 4 h	30.0 (9.0–57.0)	20.5 (6.2–55.5)	40.0 (4.5–73.0)*

long-term symptom responses among 3 etiologic subgroups (DM, ID, post-vagotomy) showed that the diabetic group responded better than others; hence, the expectation of a therapeutic response based on cause is important for selecting patients to receive GES. One explanation for the limited improvement in patients with ID-GP might be the fact that the ID group consists of a relatively heterogeneous mix of patients and often with more concomitant abdominal pain complaints than seen in other subgroups with GP.[27,33,34] It is well known that abdominal pain is the least likely complaint to be improved by GES.[15,35,36]

SURGICAL IMPLANTATION OF GASTRIC ELECTRICAL STIMULATION AND ITS PARAMETERS

The *implantation technique* of GES is included in all published manuscripts where patients receive the Enterra therapy system (Model 7425G or Model 3116; Medtronic, Inc Minneapolis, MN) via the surgical, laparotomy, or laparoscopy approach. Two intramuscular leads (Model 4351; Medtronic, Inc) are inserted into the muscularis propria of the stomach using either laparoscopy or laparotomy as previously described.[11,15] The 2 electrodes are sutured 9 and 10 cm from the pylorus on the greater curvature of the stomach and connected by leads of 35 cm in length to the pulse generator placed subcutaneously in the abdominal wall, usually in the right upper quadrant. The device is programmed to standardized parameters (5 mA, 14 Hz, 330 µs, cycle on 0.1 second, cycle off 5 seconds) using a programmer (Model 7432 or Model 8840, Medtronic, Inc) (**Fig. 5**).

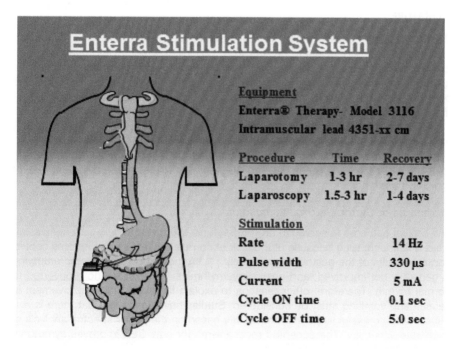

Fig. 5. The specific location of the gastric electrodes, the pulse generator for the surgical placement of the Enterra gastric neurostimulation system, as well as the programming parameters for the pulse generator.

The programming parameters are usually set as the default at surgery and are reevaluated approximately 3 months after surgery. Also, it is suggested by the manufacturer that the voltage should be adjusted during interrogation of the system, based on impedance (resistance between 2 electrodes) to maintain a 5-mA current. Some investigators proposed specially designed algorhythms[37,38]; but because of the lack of any controlled trials, these are presented as suggestions only for clinically nonresponding patients. Over time and specifically during a 10-year observation,[26] the current is increased approximately 20% to 30% during intermittent interrogations based on a perception by the clinician that symptoms are not optimally controlled and more voltage might help. This practice is not based on any supportive evidence.

Adverse Events

Based on the experiences of many investigators, there is a consensus on what adverse events may occur: (1) dislodgement of GES electrodes (trauma, tingling/braiding of the leads), (2) penetration of electrodes through the gastric mucosa, (3) lead insulation damage, (4) lead or neurostimulator erosion or migration, and (5) bowel obstruction. The main complication is the 6% risk of infection at the pulse generator site. This complication is a little more likely to occur in the immediate postoperative setting but can also occur at any time, particularly in patients with diabetes, or secondary to trauma, injuries and falls, or it could be related to systemic infections. The major concern is related to comorbidities, especially in the diabetic group of patients.

SURGERY- OR THERAPY-RELATED SERIOUS ADVERSE EVENTS REPORTED IN LITERATURE

Reasons for the removal of the pulse generator of the GES system include (1) infection of the pulse generator or electrode sites (6%); (2) lack of symptom improvement (2%); (3) lead dislodgement, small bowel obstruction, peptic ulcer, and penetration of the electrode into the lumen of the stomach (total of 3%); (4) total gastrectomy because of treatment failure (4%); (5) repositioning of GES system related to the lead dislodgement secondary to trauma or twisted wires (2%); and (6) migration of the device (1%).

Therefore, overall up to 16% of the patients initially implanted with GES underwent another surgery of some type over the course of time.

In addition, depleted batteries are replaced without changing electrodes. The life expectancy of these batteries is up to 10 years, but it depends on the settings of the GES parameters.

Mechanism of Gastric Electrical Stimulation

The clinical outcome observed in drug-refractory GES gastroparetic patients was always a little confusing because of the lack of correlation between symptoms control and the results of the gastric emptying test.[6–8] We now know that gastric emptying is generally not improved, and gastric dysrhythmias are definitely not converted to normal rhythm. Therefore, other reasons to explain the substantial improvement in nausea and vomiting must be considered. Studies have confirmed that there is evidence GES increases vagal efferent activity based on the power spectral analysis of heart rate variability. The accepted mechanisms for how GES improves symptoms of GP are the following (**Fig. 6**)[39–41]:

1. Activation of the thalami reflects stimulation of the visceral afferent component of the vagal nerve fibers transmitting impulses to the nucleus tractus solitaries

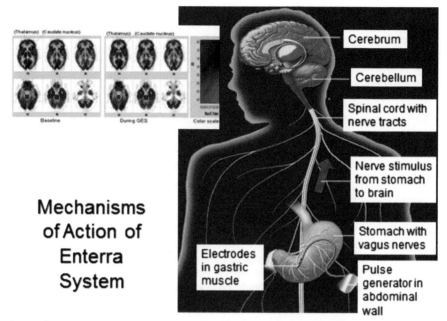

Mechanisms of Action of Enterra System

Cerebrum

Cerebellum

Spinal cord with nerve tracts

Nerve stimulus from stomach to brain

Stomach with vagus nerves

Electrodes in gastric muscle

Pulse generator in abdominal wall

Fig. 6. The Enterra stimulator in place and summary of the mechanisms of how it leads to decreased symptoms in GP: (1) increased vagal nerve activation, (2) fundic relaxation, and (3) effect on centers for nausea and vomiting based on changes in thalamic and caudate nuclei imaging.

(NTS), which then project to the thalami via the reticular formation and in turn exert an inhibitory influence on nausea and vomiting control mechanisms.

2. There is enhanced vagal autonomic function causing increased gastric accommodation and enhancing better food intake.
3. There is enhanced vagal autonomic function which leads to better postprandial adaptation and decreased gastric sensitivity to volume distention.

Advances in Gastric Electrical Stimulation

Pyloroplasty

The lack of acceleration of the delayed gastric emptying by GES begs the question as to how much better the outcome would be if gastric emptying could be accelerated. This is the rationale for the addition of a surgical pyloroplasty (PP) performed at the time when GES is implanted. This approach can be supported by the following data in the literature:

1. Injection of Botox into the pylorus causes a transient but substantial decrease in symptoms and gastric retention rate. This effect was most pronounced in the post-vagotomy subset.[42]
2. Surgical papers[43,44] suggested that PP alone could have a role in patients with GP.
3. Pylorospasm is hypothesized to be present in diabetes.[1]
4. A subset of ID-GP was suspected of having pyloric dysfunction based on pyloric motility findings.[5,6]

However, the question could be asked whether PP alone without Enterra therapy could generate similar results. In the most recent publication addressing this question,[45] the investigators present a retrospective review of prospectively collected data and a very short-term follow-up to assess laparoscopic Heineke-Mikulicz PP. Improvement in GP symptoms and the mean half-life of gastric emptying time was evident during 3 months of follow-up but a number of patients then required Enterra placement.[42,43]

Only one clinical investigation has tested whether PP combined with GES could enhance the outcomes of GES.[46] This study showed the following:

1. Gastric emptying improved in all subgroups, especially in postsurgical patients with GP; more than 50% of patients normalized their gastric emptying test.
2. No adverse events related to the additional surgery were observed.
3. Oral intake and nutritional status were improved by PP, along with a continued reduction in nausea and vomiting achieved through GES.

A double-blind and randomized study should be performed in the future to follow up on these excellent results.

In summary, it can be concluded that the addition of a Heineke-Mikulicz PP to the standard GES procedure markedly improves and often normalizes delayed gastric emptying, especially in postvagotomy gastroparetic patients, thus, enhancing long-term symptom control and augmenting the central mechanism of nausea and vomiting by GES.[47] It is recommended to be routinely added to the standard GES method. A controlled and randomized study should be done in the future to follow up on these excellent results.

Temporary stimulation with endoscopic placement of electrodes

A very interesting approach is the research on endoscopically placed, temporary GES as a predictor of permanent GES outcome introduced in 2005 by Abell's group.[48] This technique delivers electrical stimulation through a cardiac pacing lead placed endoscopically at the junction of the antrum and the body of the stomach. The lead is brought out through the mouth and attached to an external pacemaker for the duration of the study (8 days), which was a randomized, placebo-controlled crossover trial. The investigators concluded that this technique did have some role in predicting the patients' response to permanent GES in the future, although the outcome of the trial was equivocal, often because the electrodes became detached. Pretesting in this manner is not required to make the decision to proceed to permanent GES therapy for GP.

FACTORS INFLUENCING OUTCOME

- In the last 14 years of Enterra therapy, some studies have focused on what preoperative parameters correlate best with a good post- Enterra outcome. Most of the investigators agree that the diabetic cause of GP, representing a relatively homogeneous group of patients in respect to pathophysiology, provides the best indication to benefit from GES.[26,33] The efficacy in the ID group is not as predictable because they have multifactorial causes, have more abdominal pain and narcotic use, often have many past surgeries, and may have accompanying psychiatric disorders. Also patients who have additional narcotic dependency from back pain or peripheral neuropathy have a less-favorable response to stimulation. It cannot be re-emphasized enough that the most important predictor of success is to make the right diagnosis. GES does not help vomiting explained by rumination syndrome, cyclic vomiting syndrome, dumping syndrome, and bulimic/anorexia-related vomiting.
- Other identified negative factors which impair the outcome are concomitant migraine headaches, menstrual cycle–driven vomiting and endometriosis-induced abdominal pain.

- Abdominal pain overall is not an appropriate symptom to improve. If vomiting is prevented, then this could lead to less pain. However, the goal of GES is not to control abdominal pain.

Dysrhythmias (tachygastria) are markers for loss of interstitial cells of Cajal and correlate with less-than-optimal nausea control. It is suggested to perform electrogastrogram testing on all patients before implantation of GES. A dysrhythmic slow-wave pattern may forecast a less-optimal clinical outcome with continued impaired gastric emptying thus reemphasizing the need for additional PP.

AUTHORS' SUMMARY

GES is effective therapy, but technology is still evolving. Progress in nonsurgical (endoscopic) methods of insertion of electrodes, smaller size of hard drive, longer life of batteries, and remotely conducted interrogation of the devices with the possibility to tailor stimulation parameters based on the patients' preference and tolerance are developing. Some investigators are creating high-resolution gastric maps for modeling of electrical events to understand how the GES electrode current affects the underlying gastric dysrhythmias. In the future, combinations of true gastric pacing methodology during and after the meals to empty the stomach, combined with electrical neurostimulation to reduce nausea between meals could deliver the best long-lasting therapy with acceptable battery life duration for patients with GP.

JEJUNOSTOMY FOR GASTROPARESIS

Feeding jejunostomy is a critical adjunct to the treatment of GP as a means to maintain hydration, nutrition, and glycemic control. These tubes can be placed surgically through a mini-laparotomy, laparoscopically or endoscopically. The largest series of GP (26 patients) followed with jejunostomy was studied by Fontana and Barnett[47] (1996) who demonstrated subjective perception of improved health with improved nutrition in 57% and decreased hospitalizations in 52%. Notably, this series had 23 major complications requiring hospitalization and surgery. Complications included intestinal obstruction, tube dislodgement, wound abscesses, and cellulitis.[47]

Jejunostomy can be performed by a variety of techniques with indications and complications. Techniques for laparotomy are usually used with concomitant gastric surgery for GP. The 3 common techniques are a longitudinal Witzel tunnel, the Roux-en Y technique, and the needle catheter technique. The Witzel technique involves creating a longitudinal tunnel in the small bowel that covers a length of tube so that inadvertent tube removal causes collapse and seal of the enterostomy.[49] Gerndt and Orringer[50] (1994) demonstrated that routine use of the Witzel tunnel resulted in complications in only 2.1% of 523 patients to include intestinal obstruction, intraperitoneal leak, and local and intra-abdominal abscess.[50] The Roux-en-Y jejunostomy has few indications and is mostly used for pediatric patients with severe neurologic malformations and injury. Britnall and colleagues[51] reported a high rate of complications, with 15% stoma prolapse and 6% leakage rates with the Roux-en-Y technique.[51]

The needle catheter technique involves the use of the Seldinger technique whereby a needle is tunneled through the serosa and submucosal space for a distance of 5 cm until entering the enteric lumen. A wire is passed through the needle followed by a narrow lumen catheter. Needle catheter jejunostomies are often used for feedings after oncologic procedures and are plagued by complications, including tube blockage, tube dislodgement, and pneumatosis. Meyers and colleagues[52] (1995) reported on the findings of 2022 patients with needle catheter jejunostomies with complications in only 1.5% of patients, including bowel obstruction, fistula, pneumatosis intestinalis, bowel necrosis, and abdominal wall infection.[52] The laparoscopic approach uses the needle catheter technique for jejunostomy placement resulting in small incisions and early return of bowel function with similar complications.

Per-endoscopic gastrostomies with jejunal extensions (PEGJ) are technically less demanding to perform but plagued with the difficulties of tube migration into the stomach. One of the major negatives with per-endoscopic jejunostomies is that it is generally positioned in the distal duodenum or very proximal jejunum and the force of active vomiting often leads to displacement or coiling of the tubing back into the proximal duodenum or the stomach, resulting in the enteral fluid being vomited. It also partially compromises the size of the pylorus. This specific aspect is relevant because, as oral intake is introduced and PEJ feedings are being tapered off, the usually 14- to 16-French tube is still located in the pylorus interfering with the gastric emptying process and the mechanism of the pylorus. The skin site is often also more difficult to manage because of the larger tube diameter with seeping or discharge of very acidic fluids onto the skin. The tube is large and needs to be taped to the skin and is very cosmetically obtrusive.

The theory that there is a need for a gastric tube placement to provide venting in patients with GP to alleviate symptoms has not been proven to be beneficial. The bloating that patients with GP experience has now been determined to be secondary to small bowel bacterial overgrowth. Venting also causes electrolyte imbalance, particularly potassium, imbalances that are a major health risk. Patients claim they have the ability to eat a meal, but removing or draining it by suction or venting is a very misleading indication of the patients' progress. This sets up a very dangerous cycle when patients will use venting in the name of relieving all pressure and nausea, and this becomes an addictive habit. The stomach itself is also not being adequately re-educated to begin to work again and regain some motor function.

Percutaneous endoscopic jejunostomies (PEJs) are technically more difficult to place but provide a more direct route for enteral alimentation without the need for laparotomy. Fan and colleagues[53] (2002) reported the outcomes of PEGJ versus PEJ with findings for reintervention rates of 39.5% versus 9.0%, respectively. Toussaint and colleagues[54] (2012) reported on the use of PEJ for GP with a success rate of 78.6% and a complication rate of 36.4%, including jejunal volvulus and jejuno-colic fistula. In summary, jejunostomies are a critical adjunct to the management of GP but need knowledgeable medical support to minimize long-term complications.

TOTAL AND SUBTOTAL GASTRECTOMY FOR GASTROPARESIS

Gastrectomy has traditionally been reserved for patients that have experienced refractory postsurgical GP.[45,55,56] Common operations resulting in postsurgical GP include Nissen fundoplication, vagotomy for ulcer disease, and Billroth I and II gastric reconstructions for ulcer disease and gastric cancer. Extensive subtotal or completion gastrectomy provides symptomatic improvement in 67% of these patients but not always a beneficial effect in terms of weight gain according to the largest series (62 patients) by Forstner-Barthell and colleagues[57] (1999). The combination of nausea, need for total parenteral nutrition, and retained food at endoscopy were negative prognostic factors. Complications occurred in 25 patients (40%) and included the following: narcotic withdrawal syndrome (18%), ileus (10%), wound infection (5%), intestinal obstruction (2%), and anastomotic leak (5%). Symptoms were relieved in 43% (Visick grade I or II), but 57% of the patients remained in Visick grade III or IV. Nausea, vomiting, and postprandial pain were reduced from 93% to 50%, 79% to 30%, and 58% to 30%, respectively (P<.05); but chronic pain, diarrhea, and dumping syndrome were not significantly affected.[57]

Subtotal gastrectomy involves resection of 70% of the stomach including the antrum and pylorus with closure of the duodenum and restoration of continuity with a Roux-en-Y jejunal loop. Watkins and colleagues[58] (2003) reported the largest longitudinal experience with subtotal gastrectomy in diabetic GP. This study demonstrated that 6 out of 7 patients had immediate resolution of vomiting symptoms with improvement in quality of life persistent up to 6 years postoperatively.[58] Zehetner (2013) compared 2 groups treated with both gastric electrical stimulation (GES) and laparoscopic subtotal gastrectomy (103 patients). Thirty-one received laparoscopic subtotal gastrectomy compared with 72 that received GES. Comparison demonstrated that 30-day morbidity was significantly greater in the gastrectomy group than GES (23% vs 8%), but this difference decreased over time. Two-thirds (63%) of the GES group achieved symptom improvement, whereas 87% of those in the gastrectomy group reported significant improvement in nausea, vomiting, and epigastric pain. In the GES group, 19 (26%) had to have the device removed because of device malfunction, infection, or failure to respond; these patients received laparoscopic subtotal gastrectomies, and 100% reported symptom improvement. The success with laparoscopic gastrectomy has prompted Lipham to propose this approach as first-line therapy for the surgical treatment of GP.[59]

Recent observations of increased gastric emptying in bariatric surgical patients have prompted several case series and case reports that describe the use of longitudinal sleeve gastrectomy for the treatment of patients with GP. Sleeve gastrectomy involves removal of the body and fundus of the stomach and stapling along the lesser curvature to create a tubular stomach. Bagloo and colleagues[60] (2010) reported an initial case series of sleeve gastrectomy in 4 patients with diabetes with GP. Three of the authors' 4 patients had resolution of their symptoms after a minimum follow-up of 6 months. This series was followed by another one by Meyer and colleagues[61] (2012) that demonstrated resolution of GP symptoms and improved gastric emptying studies in 9 morbidly obese patients with diabetes that received laparoscopic longitudinal sleeve gastrectomy. The advent of laparoscopic gastric resection with reconstruction allows for decreased morbidity in populations with complex diabetic histories prone to complications and morbidity secondary to chronic malnutrition.

McCallum and colleagues[62] reported their experience on 8 patients with GP who underwent completion gastrectomy after failing to respond to both available and experimental medical therapies with prokinetic agents.[50] They concluded that completion gastrectomy, although a radical approach, provides successful therapy for relief of symptoms in a select group of patients with chronic refractory GP following partial gastric resection for gastric outlet obstruction secondary to peptic ulcer disease. Subsequently these authors reported on their own experience at a gastrointestinal motility referral center. They had 9 of 200 patients (4.5%) who received GES for GP and then underwent a total gastrectomy with placement of a jejunostomy tube as a last resort to control their symptoms.[63] All patients had a significant reduction in the number of emergency room visits and hospitalizations. Their nausea and vomiting improved by an average of 55%; all became nutritionally stable, and the jejunostomy tube could be removed. The quality of life was such that they all would recommend the procedure.

In conclusion, when all treatments, including GES, have failed to provide a quality of life outside the hospital, a total gastrectomy may be indicated, although some nausea may continue, and backup jejunostomy tube feeding is initially recommended.

REFERENCES

1. McCallum RW, Soffer E, Pasricha J, et al. Treatment of gastroparesis: a multidisciplinary clinical review. Neurogastroenterol Motil 2006;18:263–83.
2. Bortolotti M. Gastric electrical stimulation for gastroparesis: a goal greatly pursued, but not yet attained. World J Gastroenterol 2011;17(3):273–82.
3. Jayanthi NV, Dexter SP, Sarela AI. Gastric electrical stimulation for treatment of clinically severe gastroparesis. J Minim Access Surg 2013;9(4):163–7.
4. Parkman HP, Hasler WL, Fisher RS. American gastroenterological association medical position statement: diagnosis and treatment of gastroparesis. Gastroenterology 2004;127:2589–91.
5. Hasler WL. Gastroparesis: symptoms, evaluation, and treatment. Gastroenterol Clin North Am 2007;36:619–47.
6. Bilgutay AM, Wingrove R, Griffen WO, et al. Gastrointestinal pacing: a new concept in the treatment of ileus. Ann Surg 1963;158(3):338–48.
7. Quast DC, Beall AC, DeBakey ME. Clinical evaluation of the gastrointestinal pacer. Surg Gynecol Obstet 1965;120:35–7.
8. Hocking MP, Vogel SB, Sninski CA. Human gastric myoelectric activity and gastric emptying following gastric surgery and with pacing. Gastroenterology 1992;103:1811–6.
9. Kelly KA. Pacing the gut. Gastroenterology 1992;103:1967–9.
10. Familoni BO, Abell TL, Nemoto D, et al. Electrical stimulation at a frequency higher than basal rate in human stomach. Dig Dis Sci 1997;42:885–91.
11. McCallum RW, Chen JD, Lin Z, et al. Gastric pacing improves emptying and symptoms in patients with gastroparesis. Gastroenterology 1998;114:456–61.
12. Abell T, McCallum RW, Hocking M, et al. Gastric electrical stimulation for medically refractory gastroparesis. Gastroenterology 2003;125(2):421–8.
13. Soffer EE. Gastric electrical stimulation for gastroparesis. J Neurogastroenterol Motil 2012;18(2):131–7.
14. Abell TL, Van Cutsem E, Abrahamsson H, et al. Gastric electrical stimulation in intractable symptomatic gastroparesis. Digestion 2002;66:204–12.
15. Soffer E, Abell T, Lin Z, et al. Review article: gastric electrical stimulation for gastroparesis – physiological foundations, technical aspects and clinical implications. Aliment Pharmacol Ther 2009;30(7):681–94.
16. Lin ZY, McCallum RW, Shirmer BD, et al. Effects of pacing parameters in the entrainment of gastric slow waves in patients with gastroparesis. Am J Physiol 1998;274:G186–91.
17. Miedema BW, Sarr MG, Kelly KA. Pacing the human stomach. Surgery 1992;111: 143–50.
18. Lin Z, Sarosiek I, Forster J, et al. Two-channel gastric pacing in patients with diabetic gastroparesis. Neurogastroenterol Motil 2011;23:912.
19. Xu J, Ross RA, McCallum RW, et al. Two-channel gastric pacing with a novel implantable gastric pacemaker accelerates glucagons induced delayed gastric emptying in dogs. Am J Surg 2008;195:122–9.
20. Song GQ, Hou X, Yang B, et al. A novel method of 2-channel dual-pulse gastric electrical stimulation improves solid gastric emptying in dogs. Surgery 2008;143:72.
21. Chen JD, Xu X, Zhang J, et al. Efficiency and efficacy of multi-channel gastric electrical stimulation. Neurogastroenterol Motil 2005;17:878.
22. Yau SK, Ke MY, Wang ZE, et al. Visceral sensitivity to gastric stimulation and its correlation with alterations in gastric emptying and accommodation in humans. Obes Surg 2005;15:247–53.

23. Sun Y, Chen JD. Gastric electrical stimulation reduces gastric tone energy dependently. Scand J Gastroenterol 2005;40:154–9.

24. Zhu HB, Sallam H, Chen JD. Synchronized gastric electrical stimulation enhances gastric motility in dogs. Neurogastroenterol Motil 2005;17:628.

25. Lin XM, Peters L, Zhang M, et al. Entrainment of small intestinal slow waves with electrical stimulation in dogs. Dig Dis Sci 2000;45:652–6.

26. McCallum RW, Lin Z, Forster J, et al. Gastric electrical stimulation improves outcomes of patients with gastroparesis for up to 10 years. Clin Gastroenterol Hepatol 2011;9:314.

27. Hejazi RA, McCallum RW. Does grading the severity of gastroparesis by gastric emptying predict outcome of gastroparesis treatment. Dig Dis Sci 2011;56:1147–56.

28. McCallum RW, Snape W, Brody F, et al. Gastric electrical stimulation with Enterra therapy improves symptoms from diabetic gastroparesis in a prospective study. Clin Gastroenterol Hepatol 2010;8:947–54.

29. McCallum RW, Sarosiek I, Parkman HP, et al. Gastric electrical stimulation with Enterra therapy improves symptoms of idiopathic gastroparesis. Neurogastroenterol Motil 2013;25:815.

30. McCallum RW, Lin Z, Wetzel P, et al. Clinical response to gastric electrical stimulation in patients with postsurgical gastroparesis. Clin Gastroenterol Hepatol 2005;3:49–54.

31. Lin ZY, Forster J, Sarosiek I, et al. Treatment of diabetic gastroparesis by high-frequency gastric electrical stimulation. Diabetes Care 2004;27:1071–6.

32. Anand C, Al-Juburi A, Familoni B, et al. Gastric electrical stimulation is safe and effective: a long-term study in patients with drug-refractory gastroparesis in three regional centers. Digestion 2007;75:83–9.

33. Maranki JL, Lytes V, Meilahn JE, et al. Predictive factors for clinical improvement with Enterra gastric electric stimulation treatment for refractory gastroparesis. Dig Dis Sci 2008;53:2072–8.

34. Bityutskiy L, Soykan I, McCallum RW. Viral gastroparesis: a subgroup of idiopathic gastroparesis, clinical characteristics and long-term outcome. Am J Gastroenterol 1997;92:1501–4.

35. Hoogerwerf WA, Pasricha PJ, Kalloo AN, et al. Pain: the overlooked symptom in gastroparesis. Am J Gastroenterol 1999;94:1029–33.

36. Lahr CJ, Griffith J, Subramony C, et al. Gastric electrical stimulation for abdominal pain in patients with symptoms of gastroparesis. Am Surg 2013;79:457–64.

37. Schnelldorfer T, Abell TL, Limehouse VM, et al. Gastric electrical stimulation for gastroparesis: experience with higher setting [abstract]. Neurogastroenterol Motil 2006;18:481.

38. Abidi N, Starkebaum WL, Abell TL. An energy algorithm improves symptoms in some patients with gastroparesis and treated with gastric electrical stimulation. Neurogastroenterol Motil 2006;18:334–8.

39. Xing JH, Brody F, Brodsky J, et al. Gastric electrical stimulation at proximal stomach induces gastric relaxation in dogs. Neurogastroenterol Motil 2003;15:15.

40. McCallum RW, Dusing RW, Sarosiek I, et al. Mechanisms symptom improvement after high-frequency electrical stimulation of the stomach in gastroparetic patients. Neurogastroenterol Motil 2010;227:161–9.

41. Qin C, Chen JD, Zhang J, et al. Modulatory effects and afferent pathways of gastric electrical stimulation on rat thoracic spinal neurons receiving input from the stomach. Neurosci Res 2007;57:29.

42. Reddymasu S, Shailender S, Sankula R, et al. Endoscopic pyloric injection of botulinum toxin A for the treatment of post vagotomy gastroparesis. Am J Med Sci 2009;337(3):161–4.

43. Hibbard ML, Dunst CM, Swanstrom LL. Laparoscopic and endoscopic pyloroplasty for gastroparesis results in sustained symptoms improvement. J Gastrointest Surg 2011;15:1513–9.

44. Toro JP, Lytle NW, Patel AD, et al. Efficacy of laparoscopic pyloroplasty for the treatment of gastroparesis. J Am Coll Surg 2014;218:652–62.

45. Borrazzo EC. Surgical management of gastroparesis: gastrostomy/jejunostomy tubes, gastrectomy, pyloroplasty, gastric electrical stimulation. J Gastrointest Surg 2013;17:1559–61.

46. Sarosiek I, Forster J, Lin Z, et al. The addition of pyloroplasty is a new surgical approach to enhance effectiveness of gastric electrical stimulation therapy in patients with gastroparesis. Neurogastroenterol Motil 2013;25:134–134.e80.

47. Fontana RJ, Barnett JL. Jejunostomy tube placement in refractory diabetic gastroparesis: a retrospective review. Am J Gastroenterol 1996;91:2174–8.

48. Abell TL, Johnson WD, Kedar A, et al. A double-masked, randomized, placebo-controlled trial of temporary endoscopic mucosal gastric electrical stimulation for gastroparesis. Gastrointest Endosc 2011;74:496.

49. Tapia J, Marguia R, Garcia G, et al. Jejunostomy: techniques, indications and complications. World J Surg 1999;23(6):596–602.

50. Gerndt SJ, Orringer MB. Tube jejunostomy as an adjunct to esophagectomy. Surgery 1994;115(4):164–9.

51. Britnall ES, Daum K, Womack NA. Maydl jejunostomy; technical and metabolic considerations. AMA Arch Surg 1952;65:367.

52. Myers JG, Page CP, Stewart RM, et al. Complications of needle catheter jejunostomy in 2,022 consecutive applications. Am J Surg 1995;170(6):547–50.

53. Fan AC, Baron TH, Rumalia A, et al. Comparison of direct percutaneous endoscopic jejunostomy and PEG with jejunal extension. Gastrointest Endosc 2002; 56(6):890–4.

54. Toussaint E, Van Gossum A, Ballarin A, et al. Percutaneous endoscopic jejunostomy in patients with gastroparesis following lung transplantation: feasibility and clinical outcome. Endoscopy 2012;44(8):772–5.

55. Camilleri M, Parkman HP, Shafi MA, et al. Clinical guideline: management of gastroparesis. Am J Gastroenterol 2013;108(1):18–37.

56. Hejazi RA, McCallum RW. Treatment of refractory gastroparesis: gastric and jejunal tubes, Botox, gastric electrical stimulation, and surgery. Gastrointest Endosc Clin N Am 2009;19(1):73–82.

57. Forstner-Barthell AW, Murr MM, Nitecki S, et al. Near total completion gastrectomy for severe postvagotomy gastric stasis: analysis of early and long-term results in 62 patients. J Gastrointest Surg 1999;3(1):15–21.

58. Watkins PJ, Bruxton-Thomas MS, Howard ER. Long-term outcome after gastrectomy for intractable diabetic gastroparesis. Diabet Med 2003;20(1):58–63.

59. Zehetner J, Ravari F, Ayazi S, et al. Minimally invasive surgical approach for the treatment of gastroparesis. Surg Endosc 2013;27(1):61–6.

60. Bagloo M, Besseler M, Ude A. Sleeve gastrectomy for the treatment of diabetic gastroparesis. Proceedings 12th World Congress of Endoscopic Surgery April 14 – 17, 2010 Landover (MD). p. 521.

61. Meyer A, Pallati P, Shaligram A, et al. Partial longitudinal gastrectomy: a novel curative approach for gastroparesis. Proceedings of the 2012 Annual Meeting of the Society of American Gastrointestinal Endoscopic Surgeons, San Diego (CA). p. 249.

62. McCallum RW, Polepalle SC, Schirmer B. Completion gastrectomy for refractory gastroparesis following surgery for peptic ulcer disease. Long-term follow-up with subjective and objective parameters. Dig Dis Sci 1991;36(11):155.
63. Pawan S, Hejazi R, Sarosiek I, et al. Is total gastrectomy a good option for refractory gastroparesis? One site experience. Am J Gastro 2008; abstract #135.

Gastric Arrhythmias in Gastroparesis

Low- and High-Resolution Mapping of Gastric Electrical Activity

Gregory O'Grady, MBChB, PhD, FRACS[a], Thomas L. Abell, MD[b],*

KEYWORDS

- Electrogastrography • Interstitial cells of Cajal • Tachygastria • Slow wave

KEY POINTS

- The discovery that interstitial cells of Cajal are depleted in gastroparesis provides mechanistic insights into arrhythmogenesis, and reinvigorates clinical interest in gastric electrical testing.
- Gastric arrhythmias may play a role in the pathophysiology and symptom generation in gastroparesis, particularly chronic nausea.
- Electrogastrography (EGG) has been the dominant clinical method, demonstrating an association between arrhythmias and gastroparesis; however, EGG is summative and has incomplete sensitivity.
- The advent of high-resolution (HR; multi-electrode) mapping has been a key advance, and is enabling new insights and classifications.
- HR mapping is invasive; low-resolution recordings are being assessed as a bridging method until endoscopic HR recording systems become available for clinical use.

INTRODUCTION

Gastroparesis remains a complex clinical and research challenge, with few effective therapies.[1,2] Among several underlying factors, considerable interest over recent decades has focused on a putative role for gastric electrical arrhythmia.[3] Although the nature and significance of gastric arrhythmia has been a source of considerable

Disclosures: T.L. Abell is a licensor, consultant, and investigator for Medtronic, Inc.
Funding: This work was principally supported by the NIH (R01 DK64775) and the New Zealand Health Research Council.
[a] Department of Surgery, University of Auckland, Private Bag 92019, Auckland 1142, New Zealand;
[b] Division of Gastroenterology, GI Motility Clinic, University of Louisville, 220 Abraham Flexner Way, Suite 300, Louisville, KY 40202, USA
* Corresponding author.
E-mail address: thomas.abell@louisville.edu

controversy, an enhanced understanding is now emerging that could contribute diagnostic and therapeutic value to the problem of gastroparesis.

This review discusses current knowledge of gastric arrhythmia in the context of gastroparesis, and evaluates potential clinical implications in diagnostic testing. Future diagnostic and therapeutic directions for this rapidly evolving field are also considered.

THE HUMAN "GASTRIC CONDUCTION SYSTEM"

Recent advances in normal human gastric electrophysiology have been significant, such that most textbooks are outdated and a brief overview here is warranted. Although several details await clarification, current progress represents a useful foundation for performing and interpreting tests of gastric electrical function.

Gastric contractions are coordinated by bioelectrical slow waves, which are generated and propagated by networks of interstitial cells of Cajal (ICC). Slow waves are transmitted from ICC to the electrically coupled smooth muscle cells, which generate secondary responses that are integrated with other modulatory factors to effect contractions.[4] In humans, ICC anastomose throughout abundant networks within the gastric myenteric plexus (ICC-MP), as well as running parallel to smooth muscle fibers in the longitudinal and circular muscular layers (intramuscular ICC; ICC-IM).[5] Propagation within these layers is also facilitated by a further "septal" subclass of ICC that encase and connect muscle bundles. Animal studies have shown that a break in ICC continuity occurs at the pylorus, serving as an isolating electrical barrier from the distinct slow wave patterns of the duodenum.[6]

In health, gastric slow waves arise in a defined pacemaker region that is located at the mid to upper corpus of the greater curvature (**Fig. 1**).[7] Antegrade propagation

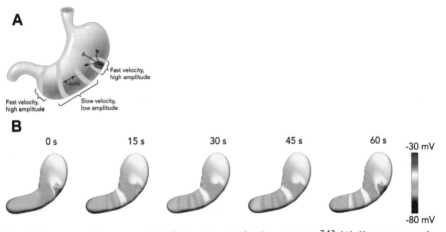

Fig. 1. The normal human gastric slow wave conduction pattern.[7,13] (A) Slow waves arise from a pacemaker region in the corpus at the greater curvature. Slow waves initially propagate in all directions, and rapidly in the circumferential axis, forming complete ring wavefronts in the mid corpus. Multiple wavefronts accrue, spaced approximately 6 cm apart, before a transition to rapid activation within the antrum. Higher amplitude signals are observed whenever conduction velocity is rapid.[13] (B) Simulations demonstrating this activation pattern over time.[13,30] Multiple wavefronts propagate as successive rings around the lumen, with each cycle taking 1 minute to reach the pylorus. (*From* Cheng LK, Du P, O'Grady G. Mapping and modeling gastrointestinal bioelectricity: from engineering bench to bedside. Physiology (Bethesda) 2013;28:312; with permission.)

from this site is facilitated by an underlying frequency gradient within ICC, with cells in the pacemaker region dominating because they have the highest intrinsic frequency.[8] Slow waves propagate toward the pylorus at intervals of around 20 seconds (ie, 3 cycles per minute [cpm]), and at a constant speed of approximately 3 mm/s, such that successive wavefronts become evenly spaced at intervals of around 6 cm. Within the antrum, there is an acceleration in velocity and the wave spacing then becomes greater (see **Fig. 1B**).[7] Slow waves do not normally excite the fundus in vivo.

Considerable discussion has focused on what slow wave frequency ranges should be considered normal in humans, with a commonly cited reference range being 2.5 and 3.6 cpm, such that "bradygastric" or "tachygastric" frequencies are defined outside this range.[9] Although these classifications remain useful, particularly for electrogastrography (EGG) interpretation, their importance in humans may have been overstated in the past, because it now seems that much abnormal activity in humans occurs within this normal range.[10]

An important, recent finding for arrhythmia analysis has been to clarify the role of velocity anisotropy in normal human gastric conduction. Studies in several species initially documented the presence of rapid conduction in the vicinity of the normal pacemaker, compared with the surrounding corpus (see **Fig. 1**),[7,11,12] and it is now known that this occurs because conduction is approximately 2.5 times more rapid in the transverse direction of the human stomach than in the longitudinal (organoaxial) direction.[10] Wavefronts spread out rapidly and circumferentially from the pacemaker; however, by the mid corpus, complete rings of activation have formed such that the rapid circumferential conduction ceases, and the rings thereafter move slowly and longitudinally down the stomach (see **Fig. 1B**).[11,13] Importantly, during gastric arrhythmias, rapid circumferential propagation reemerges to become a major determinant of conduction patterns, as a consequence of either ectopic pacemaking or disruption to the normal ring wavefronts by conduction blocks (**Fig. 2**).[10,13]

It is probable that two complimentary gastric conduction pathways are active to explain these anisotropic velocity properties. For example, ICC-MP and ICC-IM might form a bidirectionally coupled network, such that the leading network switches between ICC-MP (dominant during longitudinal conduction) and circular ICC-IM (dominant during circumferential conduction), depending on the presence or absence of complete gastric ring wavefronts.[13] However, this hypothesis awaits experimental validation, and the role of other ICC populations must be clarified.

THE PATHOLOGIC BASIS FOR ARRHYTHMIAS IN GASTROPARESIS

Research by the US Gastroparesis Clinical Research Consortium has recently clarified the cellular pathologies underlying idiopathic and diabetic gastroparesis. A reduced density of ICC was found to be the most prominent cellular abnormality in both etiologies, with remaining ICC also showing injury.[14,15] Other abnormalities were also routinely documented, including a decreased density of nerve fibers, inflammatory infiltrate, and a marked stromal fibrosis.[14,15] However, the ICC loss may be of particular functional significance to gastroparesis because it has been correlated with delayed gastric emptying in humans,[16] as well as in experimental models.[17]

Given the central role played by ICC in generating and propagating slow waves, these pathologic abnormalities now provide a rational basis for the genesis of arrhythmias in gastroparesis. This concept is also supported by a study showing that the severity of ICC loss correlates with the presence of arrhythmias when assessed by EGG.[18] Although the exact chain of events responsible for these relationships requires

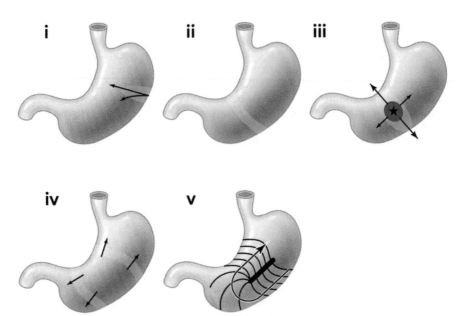

Fig. 2. Velocity anisotropy during normal and arrhythmic gastric conduction.[10,13] In human stomach, conduction is 2.5 times more rapid in the circumferential gastric axis. (*i*) At the normal pacemaker site, conduction occurs rapidly in the circumferential axis. (*ii*) Complete ring wavefronts rapidly form by the mid corpus, such that circumferential conduction ceases and slow longitudinal conduction dominates. (*iii*) Rapid circumferential propagation accompanies ectopic pacemaking, inducing elliptical wavefront patterns. (*iv*) Organized ring wavefronts may arise from ectopic sources that propagate in both antegrade and retrograde directions. (*v*) In conduction blocks, rapid circumferential propagation occurs beneath the site of block. (*From* Cheng LK, Du P, O'Grady G. Mapping and modeling gastrointestinal bioelectricity: from engineering bench to bedside. Physiology (Bethesda) 2013;28:313; with permission.)

further investigation, recent work discussed herein indicates several plausible mechanisms may be contributing.

One helpful classification for understanding gastric arrhythmias, adapted from cardiac rhythm analysis, is to consider them as either "disorders of initiation" or "disorders of conduction" (**Fig. 3**).[10,19] Under this schema, it can be surmised that disorders of slow wave initiation result from abnormalities to intrinsic ICC frequencies, whereas disorders of conduction result from disruption to slow wave entrainment through ICC networks.[20]

In view of these histopathologic findings recently elucidated in gastroparesis, distinct mechanisms may be proposed to contribute to ICC initiation and conduction abnormalities. In terms of initiation disorders, it is known that nonlethal stressors can promote aberrant frequency responses within ICC, including in humans, adversely affecting intrinsic frequency gradients.[21,22] Cholinergic regulation is also known to modulate ICC-IM frequencies, potentially inducing arrhythmias,[23] and a role for autonomic neuropathy in aberrant slow wave initiation therefore deserves further investigation. In terms of conduction abnormalities, biophysically based modeling studies have shown that slowed haphazard conduction occurs in states of ICC loss,[24] potentially promoting arrhythmias. In addition, conduction blocks must result when ICC loss falls

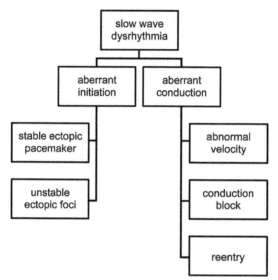

Fig. 3. Arrhythmia classification system based on spatial analyses of abnormal patterns.

below a critical threshold.[10] The presence of fibrosis might also be significant; in cardiac electrophysiology, fibrosis is well-known to slow electrical conduction and to play an important role in arrhythmogenesis.[25]

Of clinical interest, another patient group where ICC pathologies may be relevant are those with chronic unexplained nausea and vomiting. It was recently shown that this poorly characterized disease state, in which gastric emptying is normal, shows substantial clinical overlap with gastroparesis, being equivalent in terms of demographics, symptoms, disease duration, health care utilization, and quality of life.[26] Emerging work now further suggests that chronic unexplained nausea and vomiting might even be considered within the same disease category as gastroparesis, because these patients also seem to display reduced ICC and electrical arrhythmias that are similar to those described in gastroparesis.[27] Accumulating evidence points to a threshold of ICC loss at which failure of gastric emptying becomes likely, at around approximately 3 cell bodies per high-powered field within circular muscle, which may be reached in gastroparesis but not in chronic unexplained nausea and vomiting.[27,28]

These preliminary findings currently await formal publication.

CLINICAL METHODS FOR GASTRIC ELECTRICAL TESTING
Electrogastrography

EGG has long been the most widely researched and practiced technique for assessing gastric electrical activity and arrhythmias, involving the placement of cutaneous electrodes over the surface of the epigastrium.[29] A detailed explanation of how to conduct and interpret EGG is available elsewhere.[9,29]

EGG is clinically attractive owing to its low invasiveness; however, this lack of invasiveness also underlies its several limitations. Because cutaneous signals are recorded at a distance from their gastric sources, they offer only a fundamentally limited and highly summative representation of gastric activation, and it is currently difficult to relate the meaning of these highly integrated signals back to the underlying slow wave events.[30] This problem is further compounded by the fact that 3 wavefronts may be simultaneously active in the human stomach at any 1 time, and possibly more during arrhythmia, which are then summated within a single EGG waveform (**Fig. 4**).[7]

Despite these considerable limitations, EGG can reliably reflect the underlying dominant slow wave frequency[31] and, for this reason, the primary focus of EGG analyses to date have been in the frequency domain, include analyzing the stability of frequency.[9,29] Although such data are useful, the recent evidence that human gastric arrhythmias routinely occur at normal frequencies means that frequency-focused approaches may generally underestimate arrhythmia occurrence.[10] Nevertheless, a

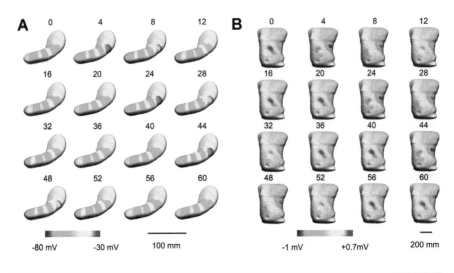

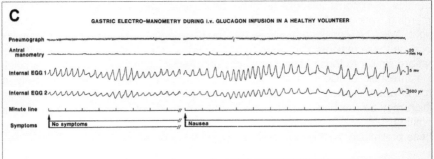

Fig. 4. (*A, B*) The relationship between slow waves and electrogastrography (EGG) analyzed by a virtual model. Multiple slow waves propagate in the human stomach at any 1 time; however, EGG achieves only a summative view. (*A*). Gastric pattern over 60 seconds of propagation. Red represents depolarized activity, blue the resting membrane potentials. (*B*) Simulated resultant body surface EGG potentials of this same activity. Red represents positive potentials and the blue negative potentials in the torso field. The contour lines represent 0.1-mV increments. (*C*) Example slow wave traces showing arrhythmic frequencies associated with nausea after glucagon infusion in a healthy volunteer. Although reflective of frequency, the summative detail achieved by current EGG methods is in contrast to the rich spatial detail achieved in high-resolution mapping (see **Figs. 5–7**). ([*A,B*] *From* Du P, O'Grady G, Cheng LK, et al. A multi-scale model of the electrophysiological basis of the human electrogastrogram. Biophys J 2010;99:2788; with permission.)

large number of successful EGG studies have accrued in the literature in recent decades that do consistently demonstrate clear associations between arrhythmic EGG parameters and gastroparesis (eg, Koch and colleagues[32] and Chen and colleagues[33]).

Despite its diagnostic promise, clinical adoption of EGG has remained weak, with practice limited to a small number of specialist referral and research centers. In addition to the limitations discussed, other factors have contributed to this lack of general clinical interest. The signals are of low amplitude and susceptible to artifacts, such that analyses can be difficult in nonspecialist hands.[34] The test is also perceived as having an incomplete sensitivity and specificity, inconsistent associations with symptoms, and validated protocols defining the role of EGG in clinical algorithms are lacking.[9] The positive predictive value of EGG for normal gastric emptying ranges from 65% to 100% in published studies, versus 50% to 80% for predicting abnormal gastric emptying,[9] although it should be noted that EGG and gastric emptying measure different aspects of motility physiology.

Nevertheless, EGG retains an active and useful role, particularly in research studies, as well as clinically in the screening and diagnosis for motility disorders.[9,29] The promise and limitations of EGG also continue to motivate the development of improved foundations and clinical methods of conducting the test, for example, by introducing multichannel approaches.[30,35] However, more accurate and invasive tests of gastric electrical function are much needed to further progress this field.

Extracellular Recordings

Extracellular recordings taken directly from the gastric surface provide the most useful method of analyzing gastric electrical activity in clinical practice. Extracellular recordings may be undertaken at the mucosal or serosal surfaces, classically by using a small number of electrodes placed at sparse intervals[3,36] or, more recently, by applying dense arrays of electrodes to achieve multi-electrode (high-resolution [HR]) mapping.

The biophysical basis of extracellular recordings was recently addressed, demonstrating robust knowledge of how this technique relates to the underlying electrical activation.[37] Extracellular recordings reflect the localized conduction of slow waves through a defined area of tissue beneath and around the electrode. The potentials approximate the second derivative of the intracellular slow wave time-course, typically adopting a biphasic or triphasic morphology, with the steep negative descent in these signals corresponding with the time of arrival of a wavefront beneath the electrode.[37]

As with EGG, several studies using sparse electrodes have clearly linked arrhythmia with gastroparesis.[36,38] However, the limitations of such studies must again be appreciated. Single point or linear reconstructions from sparse electrodes give no spatial detail about gastric slow wave patterns, meaning that these analyses have again been largely limited to frequency and rhythm domains, which are not always reliable predictors of arrhythmic onset.[10] Spatial aliasing of sparse data can also lead to misinterpretations.[7,13]

Mucosal Recordings and "Low-Resolution Mapping"

Clinically relevant extracellular techniques have evolved over the last several decades, particularly approaches to measuring mucosal electrical activity. Different systems to secure mucosal electrodes have been studied, including 1 early system utilizing external rare earth magnets that enabled a comparison of internal (mucosal) and external (cutaneous) recordings simultaneously, providing validity for these approaches.[39]

Some mucosal recording techniques have utilized more than 1 electrode, thus allowing low-resolution reconstructions of propagation to be estimated. More recently, with the advent of temporary gastric electrical stimulation, mucosal recordings, both single point and multiple sites, have been obtained at the time of surgery as part of routine clinical practice.[40,41] In addition, the same low-resolution approaches can be used serosally, often at the time of gastric stimulator insertion, and with the delivery of energy through proximal to distal electrodes.

High-Resolution Electrical Mapping

In recent years, the limitations with the sparse electrode techniques led Lammers and colleagues[42] to introduce multi-electrode (HR) mapping of slow wave activity. HR mapping involves the placement of dense arrays of many electrodes to track the propagation of slow wave propagation patterns with fine spatiotemporal accuracy.[43] These techniques are well-established in the clinical management of modern cardiac arrhythmias, and are now showing similar potential in the gastroenterology.[44]

Progress in gastrointestinal HR mapping is currently accelerating owing to engineering achievements. These advances include mass producing HR arrays suitable for human applications,[43] and automated methods for analyzing and visualizing the vast volumes of retrieved data.[45] The steps involved in HR mapping analyses are summarized in **Fig. 5**.

The outputs of HR mapping are proving a critical advance in this field, initiating a new era in understanding the events underlying arrhythmic initiation and maintenance.[44] A surprising complexity to gastric arrhythmias is being revealed, necessitating new terms and classification schemes adapted from cardiology, including focal events and reentry as mechanisms of tachygastria and conduction block and retrograde escape rhythms as mechanisms of bradygastria.[19,46] It has also been possible to assess the dynamic evolution of arrhythmic patterns through time, including defining wavefront interactions and collisions.

Despite its clear advantages, the major limitation of HR mapping is its invasiveness. All studies to date have been performed in fasted, anesthetized subjects subjected to surgery. To achieve clinical translation, major technical advances are still required to enable effective endoscopic approaches that can be routinely employed in clinical practice for accurate arrhythmia analysis.

HIGH-RESOLUTION MAPPING IN GASTROPARESIS

Recently, clinical translation of HR mapping was achieved in patients with gastroparesis who were mapped at the time of gastric stimulator implantation.[10] This work enabled several novel, clinically relevant insights into the nature and mechanisms of arrhythmias, some of which have been discussed previously, and which can be summarized as follows:

- Gastric arrhythmias may be usefully classified as disorders of initiation and disorders of conduction (see **Fig. 3**). Both of these classes seem to be prevalent in gastroparesis; however, most past EGG and sparse electrode analyses had focused disproportionately on disorders of initiation.
- In humans, gastric arrhythmias routinely occur at normal slow wave frequencies. Therefore, many arrhythmic events may be missed by techniques focused mainly on frequency-based analyses, including EGG and sparse electrode studies. This issue party explains inconsistencies seen in past arrhythmia investigations.

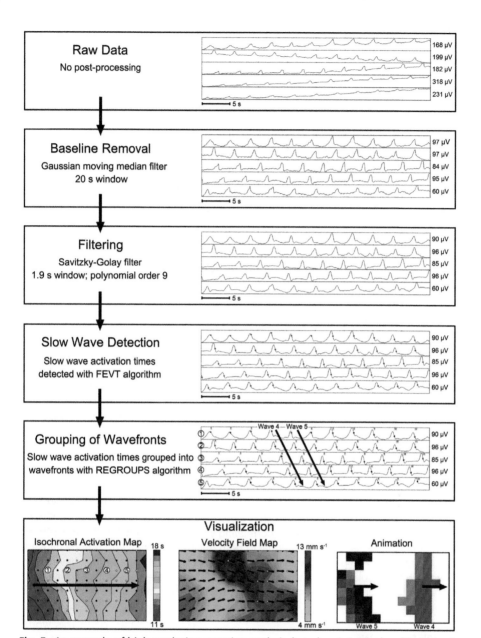

Fig. 5. An example of high-resolution mapping analysis, based on intestinal multi-electrode recordings. First, raw data are filtered to remove baseline wander and extraneous noise.[57] Slow-wave "activation times" are then marked at the point of steepest negative descent (*red dots*), before "grouping" of individual events into their propagation cycles. Algorithms and software are now available to automate these time-intensive tasks,[58,59] but careful manual review and correction are required currently for accurate results in humans. Three forms of visualization are illustrated. Isochronal activation maps (*bottom left*), which quantify propagation patterns in spatiotemporal detail. Each dot represents an electrode, and each color band shows the "isochronal interval" (area propagated per unit time; here 0.5 second).[59] Velocity field maps (*bottom center*) display speed using a color gradient and propagation direction using arrows at each electrode.[60] Propagation patterns may also be animated (*bottom right*),[45] with multiple waves passing through this mapped area concurrently. (*From* Angeli TR, O'Grady G, Du P, et al. Circumferential and functional re-entry of in vivo slow-wave activity in the porcine small intestine. Neurogastroenterol Motil 2013;306; with permission.)

- Rapid circumferential conduction of slow wave activity (ie 2.5 times the velocity of longitudinal conduction) is a determining feature of arrhythmic activation patterns, always emerging at sites of ectopic pacemaking or when normal gastric ring wavefronts are disrupted (**Fig. 6**).
- This rapid circumferential conduction may serve to quickly restore normal antegrade propagation during arrhythmia, but may also lead to organized retrograde propagations that interfere with proximal wavefronts (see **Fig. 6**C). In addition, rapid circumferential conduction is always accompanied by a large increase in the amplitude of the extracellular potentials during arrhythmia (see **Fig. 6**C).[13]
- In general, however, the amplitude of extracellular slow wave recordings seems to be reduced in gastroparesis compared with healthy controls, possibly reflecting a reduced bulk of excited cells, consistent with the underlying pathology of the disease.

Representative examples of tachygastric patterns mapped in gastroparesis using HR methods are shown in **Figs. 6** and **7**.

DO GASTRIC ARRHYTHMIAS CAUSE GASTROPARESIS SYMPTOMS?

One of the areas of controversy regarding gastric arrhythmias has been concerning their role in symptom generation. Previous studies have demonstrated somewhat inconsistent associations with symptoms, possibly reflecting the limitations of past research techniques, and leading some to consider arrhythmias a mere epiphenomenon.

The strongest links between arrhythmias and symptoms are concerning nausea.[47] In general, arrhythmias are measurable whenever nausea occurs, including in chronic disease states such as gastroparesis, as well as in more acute states such as motion sickness, after chemotherapy, and nausea of pregnancy.[20,48] Arrhythmias are therefore a useful objective biomarker for nausea, and can be considered an important potential therapeutic target for antinausea therapies.[47]

Supporting a true role for arrhythmias in nausea genesis is the observation that during motion sickness simulations, rhythm disturbances clearly arise and peak before symptoms occur, with their severity correlating with nausea intensity.[49,50] In addition, gastric pacing seems to have potential to both revert arrhythmia and reduce nausea, and in patients with gastroparesis, improvements in EGG parameters have been linked with the resolution of nausea and vomiting.[32,51] Further research is still needed to confirm these findings, and correlations between arrhythmias and symptoms other than nausea are less certain.

FUTURE DIRECTIONS

Knowledge of gastric arrhythmias is now evolving rapidly, underpinned by the recent technical advances describe herein. The crucial challenge now is to translate this knowledge into improved clinical methods of testing gastric electrical activity.

The essential step must include the development of an endoscopic approach to HR mapping. This goal constitutes a major engineering challenge, owing to the difficulties of safely instrumenting a complex device via the esophagus, and the problem of resolving satisfactory signals at the high-impedance mucosal interface. Nevertheless, published approaches have shown proof of principle, suggesting that it is feasible.[52]

In the meantime, low-resolution methods may serve as an effective bridging technique, such as by using serial placements of sparse electrodes, with the analyses

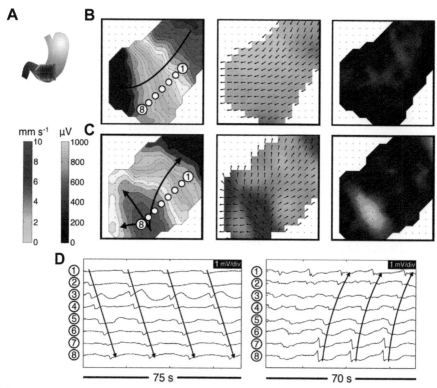

Fig. 6. An example of regular tachygastria mapping at high resolution in a patient with diabetic gastroparesis. Isochronal intervals = 1 second. (*A*) Array position. (*B*) Normal activity was initially mapped for 280 seconds (3.3 cpm); isochronal, velocity, and amplitude maps are shown. (*C*) Regular tachygastria followed owing to an ectopic pacemaker (4.0 cpm). Isochronal maps show organized retrograde propagation, with velocity and amplitude maps demonstrating the emergence of rapid circumferential propagation and associated high-amplitude potentials near the ectopic focus. (*D*) Representative electrograms from these normal (*left*) and arrhythmic activities (*right*). (*From* O'Grady G, Angeli T, Du P, et al. Abnormal initiation and conduction of slow wave activity in gastroparesis, defined by high-resolution electrical mapping. Gastroenterology 2012;143:593; with permission.)

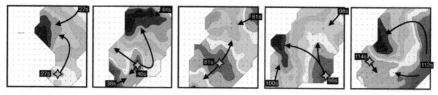

Fig. 7. An example of an irregular tachygastria defined by high-resolution mapping, owing to unstable ectopic events arising at multiple locations (duration >200 seconds). The activity was mapped from the same patient and in the same location as that shown in **Fig. 6**. Isochronal maps of 5 representative cycles (isochronal intervals = 1 s) showing chaotic tissue activation and wave collisions, resulting in a range or frequencies across the mapped field (1.4–5.7 cpm). (*From* O'Grady G, Angeli T, Du P, et al. Abnormal initiation and conduction of slow wave activity in gastroparesis, defined by high-resolution electrical mapping. Gastroenterology 2012;143:593; with permission.)

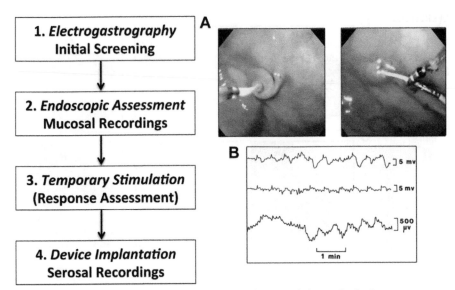

Fig. 8. A preliminary clinical protocol being implemented for arrhythmia management. There is a current need to advance methods for each of these components (*1–4*), including applying mapping-based strategies. (*A*) Examples of mucosal slow wave recording (*left*) and temporary stimulator placement (*right*). (*B*) Example electrograms from mucosal recordings (*top 2 rows*) and simultaneous electrogastrography trace (*bottom row*). (*From* Ayinala S, Batista O, Goyal A, et al. Temporary gastric electrical stimulation with orally or PEG-placed electrodes in patients with drug refractory gastroparesis. Gastrointest Endosc 2005;61(3):457; with permission.)

guided by current HR mapping methods. For example, the knowledge that slow wave amplitudes increase nearly 2.5 times near arrhythmic foci, as a consequence of resultant rapid circumferential conduction, could become a useful biomarker of arrhythmic onset in sparse electrodes.[10,13] A number of strategies, such as laparoscopic and wireless telemetry mapping systems, are now being developed to exploit such information in clinical trials within coming years.[53,54]

Future work must also address therapies; at present, few studies have been designed to reverse arrhythmias and/or their symptoms. Both gastric pacing and high-frequency (low-energy) electrical stimulation approaches have been attempted, but require further investigation using HR techniques before their potential can be fully established.[55,56] There are also few trials of pharmacologic agents to treat arrhythmias, although target pathways of potential therapeutic value have been identified.[20]

Much work is needed before these advances translate to improved care. However, a preliminary clinical protocol has been proposed and implemented for arrhythmia management, serving as a potential template for future advances (**Fig. 8**).

SUMMARY

There has been substantial recent progress in gastric arrhythmia owing to complementary pathologic, engineering, physiologic, and clinical advances. As a result, the opportunity now exists to definitively define the role and value of new electrical diagnostic tests in clinical practice. However, it remains to be seen whether arrhythmias can be meaningfully treated in a way that improves organ function and quality of life in patients.

REFERENCES

1. Hasler WL. Gastroparesis: pathogenesis, diagnosis and management. Nat Rev Gastroenterol Hepatol 2011;8:438–53.
2. Camilleri M, Parkman HP, Shafi MA, et al. Clinical guideline: management of gastroparesis. Am J Gastroenterol 2013;108:18–37 [quiz: 38].
3. You CH, Lee KY, Chey WY, et al. Electrogastrographic study of patients with unexplained nausea, bloating, and vomiting. Gastroenterology 1980;79: 311–4.
4. Huizinga JD, Lammers WJ. Gut peristalsis is coordinated by a multitude of cooperating mechanisms. Am J Physiol Gastrointest Liver Physiol 2009;296:1–8.
5. Torihashi S, Horisawa M, Watanabe Y. c-Kit immunoreactive interstitial cells in the human gastrointestinal tract. J Auton Nerv Syst 1999;75:38–50.
6. Wang XY, Lammers WJ, Bercik P, et al. Lack of pyloric interstitial cells of Cajal explains distinct peristaltic motor patterns in stomach and small intestine. Am J Physiol Gastrointest Liver Physiol 2005;289:G539–49.
7. O'Grady G, Du P, Cheng LK, et al. The origin and propagation of human gastric slow wave activity defined by high-resolution mapping. Am J Physiol Gastrointest Liver Physiol 2010;299:585–92.
8. Hinder RA, Kelly KA. Human gastric pacesetter potential. Site of origin, spread, and response to gastric transection and proximal gastric vagotomy. Am J Surg 1977;133:29–33.
9. Parkman HP, Hasler WL, Barnett JL, et al. Electrogastrography: a document prepared by the gastric section of the American Motility Society Clinical GI Motility Testing Task Force. Neurogastroenterol Motil 2003;15:89–102.
10. O'Grady G, Angeli T, Du P, et al. Abnormal initiation and conduction of slow wave activity in gastroparesis, defined by high-resolution electrical mapping. Gastroenterology 2012;143:589–98.
11. Lammers WJ, Ver Donck L, Stephen B, et al. Origin and propagation of the slow wave in the canine stomach: the outlines of a gastric conduction system. Am J Physiol Gastrointest Liver Physiol 2009;296:1200–10.
12. Egbuji JU, O'Grady G, Du P, et al. Origin, propagation and regional characteristics of porcine gastric slow wave activity determined by high-resolution mapping. Neurogastroenterol Motil 2010;22:e292–300.
13. O'Grady G, Du P, Paskaranandavadivel N, et al. Rapid high-amplitude circumferential slow wave conduction during normal gastric pacemaking and dysrhythmia. Neurogastroenterol Motil 2012;24:e299–312.
14. Grover M, Farrugia G, Lurken MS, et al. Cellular changes in diabetic and idiopathic gastroparesis. Gastroenterology 2011;140:1575–85.e8.
15. Faussone-Pellegrini MS, Grover M, Pasricha PJ, et al. Ultrastructural differences between diabetic and idiopathic gastroparesis. J Cell Mol Med 2012;16: 1573–81.
16. Grover M, Bernard CE, Pasricha PJ, et al. Clinical-histological associations in gastroparesis: results from the Gastroparesis Clinical Research Consortium. Neurogastroenterol Motil 2012;24:531–9.e249.
17. Choi KM, Gibbons SJ, Nguyen TV, et al. Heme oxygenase-1 protects interstitial cells of Cajal from oxidative stress and reverses diabetic gastroparesis. Gastroenterology 2008;135:2055–64, 2064.e1.
18. Lin Z, Sarosiek I, Forster J, et al. Association of the status of interstitial cells of Cajal and electrogastrogram parameters, gastric emptying and symptoms in patients with gastroparesis. Neurogastroenterol Motil 2010;22:56–61.e10.

19. O'Grady G, Egbuji JU, Du P, et al. High-resolution spatial analysis of slow wave initiation and conduction in porcine gastric dysrhythmia. Neurogastroenterol Motil 2011;23:e345–55.

20. O'Grady G, Wang TH, Du P, et al. Recent progress in gastric dysrhythmia: pathophysiology, clinical significance and future horizons. Clin Exp Pharmacol Physiol 2014;41(10):854–62.

21. Xue S, Valdez DT, Tremblay L, et al. Electrical slow wave activity of the cat stomach: its frequency gradient and the effect of indomethacin. Neurogastroenterol Motil 1995;7:157–67.

22. O'Grady G, Pullan AJ, Cheng LK. The analysis of human gastric pacemaker activity. J Physiol 2012;590:1299–300.

23. Forrest AS, Ordog T, Sanders KM. Neural regulation of slow-wave frequency in the murine gastric antrum. Am J Physiol Gastrointest Liver Physiol 2006;290:G486–95.

24. Du P, O'Grady G, Gibbons SJ, et al. Tissue-specific mathematical models of slow wave entrainment in wild-type and 5-HT2B knockout mice with altered interstitial cell of Cajal networks. Biophys J 2010;98:1772–81.

25. Munoz V, Zlochiver S, Jalife J. Fibrosis and fibroblast infiltration: an active structural substrate for altered propagation and spontaneous tachyarrhythmias. In: Zipes DP, Jalife J, editors. Cardiac electrophysiology, from cell to bedside. Philadelphia: Saunders Elsevier; 2009. p. 215–21.

26. Pasricha PJ, Colvin R, Yates K, et al. Characteristics of patients with chronic unexplained nausea and vomiting and normal gastric emptying. Clin Gastroenterol Hepatol 2011;9:567–76.

27. Angeli TR, Cheng LK, Du P, et al. High-resolution mapping reveals gastric slow wave dysrhythmias in chronic nausea and vomiting. Neurogastroenterol Motil 2014;25(S1):12.

28. Gomez-Pinilla PJ, Gibbons SJ, Sarr MG, et al. Changes in interstitial cells of Cajal with age in the human stomach and colon. Neurogastroenterol Motil 2011;23:36–44.

29. Chen JD, Lin Z, Yin Y. Electrogastrography. In: Parkman HP, McCallum RW, Rao SC, editors. GI motility testing: a laboratory and office handbook. Thorofare (NJ): SLACK Incorporated; 2011. p. 81–92.

30. Du P, O'Grady G, Cheng LK, et al. A multi-scale model of the electrophysiological basis of the human electrogastrogram. Biophys J 2010;99:2784–92.

31. Smout AJ, Van der schee EJ, Grashuis JL. What is measured in electrogastrography? Dig Dis Sci 1980;25:179–87.

32. Koch KL, Stern RM, Stewart WR, et al. Gastric emptying and gastric myoelectrical activity in patients with diabetic gastroparesis: effect of long-term domperidone treatment. Am J Gastroenterol 1989;84:1069–75.

33. Chen JD, Lin Z, Pan J, et al. Abnormal gastric myoelectrical activity and delayed gastric emptying in patients with symptoms suggestive of gastroparesis. Dig Dis Sci 1996;41:1538–45.

34. Verhagen MA, van Schelven LJ, Samsom M, et al. Pitfalls in the analysis of electrogastrographic recordings. Gastroenterology 1999;177:453–60.

35. Simonian HP, Panganamamula K, Chen JZ, et al. Multichannel electrogastrography (EGG) in symptomatic patients: a single center study. Am J Gastroenterol 2004;99:478–85.

36. Bortolotti M, Sarti P, Barara L, et al. Gastric myoelectrical activity in patients with chronic idiopathic gastroparesis. Neurogastroenterol Motil 1990;2:104–8.

37. Angeli TR, Du P, Paskaranandavadivel N, et al. The bioelectrical basis and validity of gastrointestinal extracellular slow wave recordings. J Physiol 2013;591: 4567–79.

38. Lin ZY, McCallum RW, Schirmer BD, et al. Effects of pacing parameters on entrainment of gastric slow waves in patients with gastroparesis. Am J Physiol 1998;274:G186–91.

39. Abell TL, Malagelada JR. Glucagon-evoked gastric dysrhythmias in humans shown by an improved electrogastrographic technique. Gastroenterology 1985; 88:1932–40.

40. Daram SR, Tang SJ, Abell TL. Video: temporary gastric electrical stimulation for gastroparesis: endoscopic placement of electrodes (ENDOstim). Surg Endosc 2011;25:3444–5.

41. Abell TL, Johnson WD, Kedar A, et al. A double-masked, randomized, placebo-controlled trial of temporary endoscopic mucosal gastric electrical stimulation for gastroparesis. Gastrointest Endosc 2011;74:496–503.e3.

42. Lammers WJ, al-Kais A, Singh S, et al. Multielectrode mapping of slow-wave activity in the isolated rabbit duodenum. J Appl Physiol (1985) 1993;74: 1454–61.

43. Du P, O'Grady G, Egbuji JU, et al. High-resolution mapping of in vivo gastrointestinal slow wave activity using flexible printed circuit board electrodes: methodology and validation. Ann Biomed Eng 2009;37:839–46.

44. Lammers WJ. Arrhythmias in the gut. Neurogastroenterol Motil 2013;25:353–7.

45. Yassi R, O'Grady G, Paskaranandavadivel N, et al. The Gastrointestinal Electrical Mapping Suite (GEMS): software for analysing and visualising gastrointestinal multi-electrode recordings. BMC Gastroenterol 2012;12:60.

46. Lammers WJ, Ver Donck L, Stephen B, et al. Focal activities and re-entrant propagations as mechanisms of gastric tachyarrhythmias. Gastroenterology 2008; 135:1601–11.

47. Koch KL. Gastric dysrhythmias: a potential objective measure of nausea. Exp Brain Res 2014;232(8):2553–61.

48. Koch KL, Stern RM. Handbook of electrogastrography. Oxford (United Kingdom): Oxford University Press; 2004.

49. Owyang C, Hasler WL. Physiology and pathophysiology of the interstitial cells of Cajal: from bench to bedside. VI. Pathogenesis and therapeutic approaches to human gastric dysrhythmias. Am J Physiol Gastrointest Liver Physiol 2002;283: G8–15.

50. Hasler WL, Kim MS, Chey WD, et al. Central cholinergic and alpha-adrenergic mediation of gastric slow wave dysrhythmias evoked during motion sickness. Am J Physiol 1995;268:G539–47.

51. McCallum RW, Chen JD, Lin Z, et al. Gastric pacing improves emptying and symptoms in patients with gastroparesis. Gastroenterology 1998;114:456–61.

52. Coleski R, Hasler WL. Coupling and propagation of normal and dysrhythmic gastric slow waves during acute hyperglycaemia in healthy humans. Neurogastroenterol Motil 2009;21:492–9.e1.

53. O'Grady G, Du P, Egbuji JU, et al. A novel laparoscopic device for measuring gastrointestinal slow-wave activity. Surg Endosc 2009;23:2842–8.

54. Farajidavar A, O'Grady G, Rao SM, et al. A miniature bidirectional telemetry system for in vivo gastric slow wave recordings. Physiol Meas 2012;33:N29–37.

55. O'Grady G, Du P, Lammers WJ, et al. High-resolution entrainment mapping for gastric pacing: a new analytic tool. Am J Physiol Gastrointest Liver Physiol 2010;298:314–21.

56. Cheng LK, Du P, O'Grady G. Mapping and modeling gastrointestinal bioelectricity: from engineering bench to bedside. Physiology (Bethesda) 2013; 28:310–7.

57. Paskaranandavadivel N, O'Grady G, Du P, et al. Comparison of filtering methods for extracellular gastric slow wave recordings. Neurogastroenterol Motil 2013;25: 79–83.
58. Erickson JC, O'Grady G, Du P, et al. Falling-edge, variable threshold (FEVT) method for the automated detection of gastric slow wave events in serosal high-resolution electrical recordings. Ann Biomed Eng 2010;38:1511–29.
59. Erickson JC, O'Grady G, Du P, et al. Automated cycle partitioning and visualization of high-resolution activation time maps of gastric slow wave recordings: the Region Growing Using Polynomial Surface-estimate stabilization (REGROUPS) Algorithm. Ann Biomed Eng 2011;39:469–83.
60. Paskaranandavadivel N, O'Grady G, Du P, et al. An improved method for the estimation and visualization of velocity fields from gastric high-resolution electrical mapping. IEEE Trans Biomed Eng 2012;59:882–9.

Future Directions in the Treatment of Gastroparesis

Pankaj Jay Pasricha, MD

KEYWORDS

- Gastroparesis • Gastric emptying • Prokinetics • Future treatment
- Functional dyspepsia

KEY POINTS

- The pathophysiology of gastroparesis is complex and requires more sophisticated approaches than current being used.
- Treatments aimed at symptomatic relief have to go beyond simply improving gastric emptying.
- Disease modifying therapies that address the root cause of inflammation and ICC loss are needed.

INTRODUCTION

Effective and rational drug therapy is based on the identification of key molecules or processes involved in the pathogenesis of the disorder being treated. This basis clearly does not apply in gastroparesis, in which neither the biological basis of the condition nor the pathophysiologic basis of its cardinal symptoms where is fully understood. At this point it is therefore important to acknowledge that all current therapy for gastroparesis is palliative as well as empirical. Many of these treatments have been covered elsewhere in this edition. Nevertheless, it is a useful exercise to briefly review the knowledge of existing targets before considering what the future might hold (**Box 1**). These targets can be classified into the following categories, recognizing that they are not mutually exclusive and pathophysiologic contributions from both may exist in different proportions in individual patients.

APPROACHES TO IMPROVE MOTILITY

The intramural structures responsible for motility that are potentially affected in gastroparesis are diverse and in close proximity to each other, representing an environment

Dr P.J. Pasricha is supported by a grant from the NIH (NIDDK 073983).
Department of Medicine, Johns Hopkins Center for Neurogastroenterology, Johns Hopkins School of Medicine, 720 Rutland Street, Ross 958, Baltimore, MD 21205, USA
E-mail address: ppasric1@jhmi.edu

Gastroenterol Clin N Am 44 (2015) 185–189
http://dx.doi.org/10.1016/j.gtc.2014.11.014
0889-8553/15/$ – see front matter

Box 1
Potential therapeutic targets: pathophysiologic changes in patients with gastroparesis

- Impaired relaxation
- Fundic hypocontractility
- Antral hypomotility
- Pylorospasm
- Antropyloroduodenal incoordination
- Gastric arrhythmia
- Autonomic neuropathy
  - Vagal motor
  - Vagal sensory
  - Sympathetic
- Spinal sensory neuropathy

---

that is unlike any other in the body in its complexity. These structures include the enteric nervous system (neurons, glia, and interstitial cells of Cajal [ICC]), associated extrinsic nerves (vagal and spinal), and smooth muscle. The state of knowledge does not yet permit clinicians to identify which of these elements, if any, represents the primary or predominant site of disease. However, much of the current evidence points to a pivotal role for the ICC, which seem to be most consistently affected in both animal models and humans with gastroparesis.[1] Further, diabetic gastroparesis is associated with hypofunctional variations in anoctamin-1, a chloride channel that contributes to slow wave generation and proliferation of ICC.[2] In addition, loss of ICC correlates with delay in gastric emptying.[3] Thus, specific drugs that address ICC loss, dysfunction, or channelopathies/arrhythmias could potentially be useful in treating gastroparesis. In this context, perhaps gastroenterologists can learn from cardiologists about antiarrhythmics. In contrast with ICC, little attention has been paid to smooth muscle dysfunction in gastroparesis as a therapeutic target. Restoring impaired contractility and responsiveness to neurotransmitters in gastroparesis remains a desirable but unexplored objective.[4]

On the neural side, much attention has been paid to the role of loss of nitric oxide in the pathogenesis of gastroparesis, as reviewed by Farrugia elsewhere in this issue. Although pathologic studies in humans have revealed mixed evidence of loss of nitrinergic neurons,[1] loss of nitric oxide can occur even without loss of protein expression.[5] The enzyme neuronal nitric oxide synthase is a complex molecule and requires other cofactors, such as tetrahydrobiopterin (BH4), to maintain a functional dimeric state. BH4 deficiency, seen in diabetes, can therefore result in loss of nitric oxide production; conversely, BH4 supplementation in animal models can reverse gastroparesis.[6,7] In this regard, a pilot study of BH4 treatment in a small group of patients with diabetic gastroparesis has shown promising results.[8]

Similar concepts can be extended to augmenting cholinergic neural activity. Inhibition of acetylcholinesterase can be achieved by classic agents such as pyridostigmine as well as by several other drugs, such as the H2-receptor antagonist, nizatidine, and the dopaminergic antagonist, itopride. The efficacy of these drugs in gastroparesis remains unproved. Acotiamide is a newer acetylcholinesterase inhibitor that can accelerate gastric emptying and has been shown to be of benefit in patients with functional dyspepsia. Other drugs that can enhance cholinergic activity or act via other mechanisms include prucalopride and various motilides in development. These drugs are reviewed elsewhere in this issue and by other investigators.[9]

THE FUTURE OF PROKINETICS: REGIONAL AND RATIONAL NEUROMUSCULAR TARGETING

In the past, physicians focused almost exclusively on delayed gastric emptying as the primary pathophysiologic abnormality in gastroparesis. However, it is becoming increasingly clear that this perspective is simplistic at best and perhaps even misleading, and has led to crude attempts to accelerate gastric emptying such as pyloric stenting or pyloromyotomy, which may be helpful in a subset of patients but can result in significant new or additional morbidity. This topic is discussed elsewhere in this issue. However, just because gastric emptying does not correlate with symptoms does not mean that abnormal motility is not relevant for their pathogenesis. Dysmotility is not synonymous with delayed emptying. The stomach is a complex organ in terms of motor function, with distinct regionally and temporally activated programs (fundic accommodation, fundoantral transfer, antral grinding, pyloric sieving, and so forth) and disturbances in any one of them can potentially be symptomatic without necessarily delaying overall emptying. These programs may have distinct neuropharmacologic profiles, and it is hoped that future prokinetics will be tailored accordingly. As an example, contractility in the gastric fundus is more responsive to serotonin and 5-hydroxytryptamine type 4 receptor agonism than that in the antrum (in mice at least).[10] These differences may be further compounded in the presence of diabetes and, by implication, in idiopathic gastroparesis as well.[11] As another example, sildenafil, a phosphodiesterase inhibitor that augments the effects of nitric oxide by stabilizing cyclic GMP levels, may not change gastric emptying but can potentially accelerate fundoantral transfer of food.[12]

APPROACHES FOR SENSORY MODULATION

A prominent but neglected pathophysiologic concept in gastroparesis is visceral hypersensitivity. This concept applies to spinal as well as vagal afferents and can help explain the pain and nausea that can be so debilitating in these patients. In response to gastric distention with an experimental balloon, diabetic patients experience nausea, pain, and bloating at volumes that produce little or no symptoms in controls.[13] However, the molecular basis of this sensitization remains unknown, particularly on the vagal side. The recently published NORIG (Nortryptiline for Idiopathic Gastroparesis) trial conducted by the Gastroparesis Consortium failed to show the efficacy of low-dose nortriptyline, an antidepressant and neuromodulator.[14] Many other neuromodulators have been used, as reviewed by Hasler elsewhere in this issue. Some of these, such as mirtazapine, have the potential to address multiple symptoms (pain, nausea, poor appetite) and may even improve gastric emptying.[15,16] Dronabinol (a mixed cannabinoid receptor agonist) acts via both central and peripheral (vagal) mechanisms to attenuate nausea but may retard gastric emptying.[15] Aprepitant, an neurokinin-1 receptor antagonist, in contrast may attenuate nausea without significant effect on gastrointestinal transit.[17] A rational approach to the use of these agents may emerge from ongoing clinical trials, such as the GPCRC (Gastroparesis Clinical Research Consortium) conducted APRON (Aprepitant for the Relief of Nausea; ClinicalTrials.gov Identifier:NCT01149369), but true advances will require a deeper understanding of the molecular basis of pain and nausea in these patients, using functional brain imaging and other techniques. At present, this area remains a so-called black box with little or no ongoing research, in part because of the inordinate focus on gastric emptying. The only class of agents that has been shown to be clinically useful is the D2 receptor antagonists; future developments should lead to modifications that eliminate the neurologic and cardiovascular adverse effects that have limited their use.

Nonpharmacologic means of modulating vagal and spinal afferent function may also have promise, particularly using neuromodulatory approaches such as electrical stimulation. However, current devices have failed to allow progress because of a lack of scientific clarity in terms of technological parameters and clinical outcomes, and an absence of any meaningful innovation since their introduction. Novel and more rational devices that can also be placed endoscopically are eagerly awaited. An alternative to electrical modulation is sensory ablation using vanilloid agents (capsaicin or resiniferatoxin) that target spinal and vagal nerve terminals expressing TRPV1 (transient receptor potential cation channel subfamily V member 1). This agent has been tested in humans for painful bladder conditions[18] and experimental evidence suggests that intragastric resiniferatoxin may be helpful for reducing emesis.[19]

TOWARD DISEASE-MODIFYING THERAPY

Almost all of the previous discussion has focused on approaches that are palliative in nature. Although a cure for gastroparesis is still elusive, recent advances in understanding of the pathology of gastroparesis have for the first time raised hopes for rational, disease-modifying therapy. In particular, as described by Farrugia elsewhere in this issue, experimental studies suggest a role for macrophage polarization and activation, and highlight the importance of the enzyme heme oxygenase 1 (HO1) in protecting ICC and other cells against oxidative stress induced by diabetes. The prominent presence of macrophages in stomachs from patients with gastroparesis suggests that similar mechanisms may apply to humans, opening up new pharmacologic targets. These targets could include suppression of subsets of macrophages and upregulation of HO1 by agents such as hemin or carbon monoxide, and clinical trials are eagerly awaited.[20]

SUMMARY

A new era in the study of gastroparesis is beginning. Advances in understanding of the pathogenesis of the disease and pathophysiology of symptoms have opened up the possibility of new, more effective ways to control symptoms as well as, for the first time, improving the prospects of attenuating the underlying disease process.

REFERENCES

1. Grover M, Farrugia G, Lurken MS, et al. Cellular changes in diabetic and idiopathic gastroparesis. Gastroenterology 2011;140:1575–85.e8.
2. Mazzone A, Bernard CE, Strege PR, et al. Altered expression of Ano1 variants in human diabetic gastroparesis. J Biol Chem 2011;286:13393–403.
3. Grover M, Bernard CE, Pasricha PJ, et al. Clinical-histological associations in gastroparesis: results from the Gastroparesis Clinical Research Consortium. Neurogastroenterol Motil 2012;24:531–9 e249.
4. Horvath VJ, Vittal H, Lorincz A, et al. Reduced stem cell factor links smooth myopathy and loss of interstitial cells of Cajal in murine diabetic gastroparesis. Gastroenterology 2006;130:759–70.
5. Gangula PR, Maner WL, Micci MA, et al. Diabetes induces sex-dependent changes in neuronal nitric oxide synthase dimerization and function in the rat gastric antrum. Am J Physiol Gastrointest Liver Physiol 2007;292:G725–33.

6. Gangula PR, Mukhopadhyay S, Ravella K, et al. Tetrahydrobiopterin (BH4), a cofactor for nNOS, restores gastric emptying and nNOS expression in female diabetic rats. Am J Physiol Gastrointest Liver Physiol 2010;298:G692–9.
7. Gangula PR, Mukhopadhyay S, Pasricha PJ, et al. Sepiapterin reverses the changes in gastric nNOS dimerization and function in diabetic gastroparesis. Neurogastroenterol Motil 2010;22:1325–31 e351–2.
8. Nguyen L, Pasricha PJ. Sapropterin improves gastric accommodation and symptoms in women with diabetic gastroparesis. Neurogastroenterol Motil 2013;25:36.
9. Stevens JE, Jones KL, Rayner CK, et al. Pathophysiology and pharmacotherapy of gastroparesis: current and future perspectives. Expert Opin Pharmacother 2013;14:1171–86.
10. James AN, Ryan JP, Crowell MD, et al. Regional gastric contractility alterations in a diabetic gastroparesis mouse model: effects of cholinergic and serotoninergic stimulation. Am J Physiol Gastrointest Liver Physiol 2004;287:G612–9.
11. Cellini J, DiNovo K, Harlow J, et al. Regional differences in neostigmine-induced contraction and relaxation of stomach from diabetic guinea pig. Auton Neurosci 2011;160:69–81.
12. Cho SH, Park H, Kim JH, et al. Effect of sildenafil on gastric emptying in healthy adults. J Gastroenterol Hepatol 2006;21:222–6.
13. Samsom M, Salet GA, Roelofs JM, et al. Compliance of the proximal stomach and dyspeptic symptoms in patients with type I diabetes mellitus. Dig Dis Sci 1995; 40:2037–42.
14. Parkman HP, Van Natta ML, Abell TL, et al. Effect of nortriptyline on symptoms of idiopathic gastroparesis: the NORIG randomized clinical trial. JAMA 2013;310: 2640–9.
15. Wong BS, Camilleri M, Eckert D, et al. Randomized pharmacodynamic and pharmacogenetic trial of dronabinol effects on colon transit in irritable bowel syndrome-diarrhea. Neurogastroenterol Motil 2012;24:358–e169.
16. Yin J, Song J, Lei Y, et al. Prokinetic effects of mirtazapine on gastrointestinal transit. Am J Physiol Gastrointest Liver Physiol 2014;306:G796–801.
17. Rojas C, Raje M, Tsukamoto T, et al. Molecular mechanisms of 5-HT(3) and NK(1) receptor antagonists in prevention of emesis. Eur J Pharmacol 2014;722:26–37.
18. Kuo HC, Liu HT, Yang WC. Therapeutic effect of multiple resiniferatoxin intravesical instillations in patients with refractory detrusor overactivity: a randomized, double-blind, placebo controlled study. J Urol 2006;176:641–5.
19. Hawari R, Yin J, Sallam H, et al. Topical intragastric application of the TRPV1 agonist, resiniferatoxin (RTX), attenuates experimental nausea and vomiting. Gastroenterology 2007;132:A-688.
20. Neshatian L, Gibbons SJ, Farrugia G. Macrophages in diabetic gastroparesis - the missing link? Neurogastroenterol Motil 2014. [Epub ahead of print].

Index

Note: Page numbers of article titles are in **boldface** type.

Gastroenterol Clin N Am 44 (2015) 191–201
http://dx.doi.org/10.1016/S0889-8553(15)00009-6
0889-8553/15/$ – see front matter © 2015 Elsevier Inc. All rights reserved.

Moving?

Make sure your subscription moves with you!

To notify us of your new address, find your **Clinics Account Number** (located on your mailing label above your name), and contact customer service at:

Email: journalscustomerservice-usa@elsevier.com

800-654-2452 (subscribers in the U.S. & Canada)
314-447-8871 (subscribers outside of the U.S. & Canada)

Fax number: 314-447-8029

Elsevier Health Sciences Division
Subscription Customer Service
3251 Riverport Lane
Maryland Heights, MO 63043

Printed and bound by CPI Group (UK) Ltd, Croydon, CR0 4YY

03/10/2024

01040497-0001